2,50

C0-AVE-889

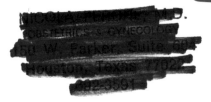

NICOLA PUCKET, M.D.
OBSTETRICS & GYNECOLOGY
150 W. Parker, Suite 604
Houston, Texas 77022
692-3591

OFFICE GYNECOLOGY

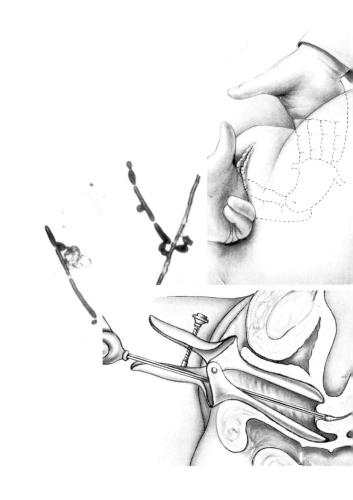

OFFICE GYNECOLOGY

J. P. GREENHILL

B.S., M.D., F.A.C.S., F.I.C.S. (HON.), F.A.C.O.G.

Senior Attending Obstetrician and Gynecologist, Michael Reese Hospital; Professor of Gynecology, Cook County Graduate School of Medicine; Consulting Gynecologist, Cook County Hospital; Editor of the Year Book of Obstetrics and Gynecology; *Author of* Surgical Gynecology *(4th ed.) and* Obstetrics *(13th ed.)*

NINTH EDITION, REVISED AND ENLARGED

YEAR BOOK MEDICAL PUBLISHERS · INC.

35 EAST WACKER DRIVE · CHICAGO

Copyright © 1939, 1945, 1948, 1954, 1959, 1965 and 1971 by Year Book Medical Publishers, Inc. All rights reserved. No part of this publication may be reproduced, stored in a retrieval system, or transmitted, in any form or by any means, electronic, mechanical, photocopying, recording, or otherwise, without prior written permission from the publisher. Printed in the United States of America.

SECOND EDITION, JANUARY, 1940

THIRD, REVISED EDITION, OCTOBER, 1940

REVISED AND REPRINTED, AUGUST, 1943

FOURTH, REVISED EDITION, SEPTEMBER, 1945

REPRINTED, NOVEMBER, 1946

FIFTH, REVISED EDITION, SEPTEMBER, 1948

SIXTH, REVISED EDITION, JULY, 1954

SEVENTH, REVISED EDITION, 1959

EIGHTH, REVISED EDITION, 1965

NINTH, REVISED EDITION, 1971

REPRINTED, APRIL, 1974

Library of Congress Catalog Card Number: 77-138937

International Standard Book Number: 0-8151-3951-9

Preface to Ninth Edition

IT IS MOST GRATIFYING to be asked to prepare a ninth edition of this book. As in all previous editions, every page has been scrutinized and innumerable corrections, deletions, and additions have been made. Several chapters have been deleted, some chapters have been rewritten, and a chapter on Haemophilus Vaginalis Vaginitis has been added. Several illustrations have been removed and new ones added. All surgery that does not apply to everyday practice has been removed.

I am greatly indebted to Robert A. Greenblatt, who rewrote his chapters on Gynecologic and Obstetric Endocrinology and Intersexuality, and to Arnold H. Kegel, who thoroughly revised his chapter on Exercise in the Treatment of Genital Relaxation, Urinary Stress Incontinence, and Sexual Dysfunction. I want also to thank the following specialists who read and corrected a few of the chapters: Sam W. Banks (Backache), Jan Behrman (Immunologic Infertility), William Caro (Diseases of the Skin, Pruritus Vulvae, and Leukoplakia), Melvin A. Cohen (Sterility), William A. Kroger (Psychosomatic Gynecology), John MacLeod (Semen Evaluation), and Peter Segal (Contraception).

It is with the greatest pleasure that I again thank the Year Book Medical Publishers for their invaluable assistance and cooperation in the preparation of this book.

J. P. GREENHILL

Table of Contents

1

Office Equipment Necessary for Gynecologic Practice

EACH YEAR a few thousand young physicians begin the private practice of medicine. The majority have completed an internship of 1 or more years, and many have had a residency in obstetrics and gynecology. A large proportion of these young physicians rent office space in an already established physician's office and use the equipment available in that office. However, many young physicians open new offices for themselves, whether they go into general practice or into the special practice of obstetrics and gynecology. It is not a simple matter to know what to purchase in order to have a well-equipped office from the beginning. Most physicians learn what they need only over a variable period of time and after a few embarrassments. To help young physicians equip their offices, whether they are specialists in gynecology or general practitioners who care for gynecologic patients, I recommend the following office equipment.

1. Examination table with footrests and drop leaf. The table may or may not have compartments for towels, drapes, medicines, gloves, and instruments. A pad, preferably of sponge rubber, should be placed on top of the table and covered with a zippered slip cover; on top of this, a bath towel or disposable covering should be placed.
2. Footstool, to help the patient onto the table.
3. Stool or chair, preferably of metal, for the physician.
4. Metal waste container with top controlled by foot action.
5. Electric light bulb on a gooseneck stand or a head mirror for inspection of the cervix and vagina.
6. Small side table with shelf halfway down. On the top of this table is placed a white towel, or disposable sheet, then on it an electric cautery box with nasal tips, a basin with balls of cotton and tampons, a container with long applicator sticks, a metal box of disposable gloves and bottles of medications, such as silver nitrate, gentian violet, and a mild antiseptic. On the shelf there should be a white towel or disposable sheet on which are placed a number of sterilized 7-in. Miller speculums and long Bozeman curved forceps. There should be at least one small (5-in. Miller) and a virgin-sized speculum. All of these instruments should be covered with another towel or disposable sheet.

7. A washbowl, above which should be a shelf for a tube of lubricant and small bottle or pitcher of liquid green soap or pHisoHex. There should also be a rack for cloth towels and, alongside the washbowl, a container of paper towels.
8. A mirror above the washbowl for the patient's convenience.
9. A rack with hooks and coat hangers for the patient's clothing. These should be placed on a wall or the back of the door leading into the room.
10. A surgical cabinet for instruments and drugs. This may be part of the examination table or a separate piece of equipment, preferably built into one wall or occupying a corner of the room. In this cabinet are stored the speculums, long forceps, which are placed on the small side table during office hours, and other instruments and paraphernalia. These instruments include:

    A stethoscope, preferably a head stethoscope
    Outlet pelvimeter
    One or more scalpels
    Two pairs of tissue forceps, one with and one without teeth
    Several clamps of different sizes
    A needle holder
    Needles of different sizes
    Tubes of surgical gut and silk or silkworm gut
    Two or three of the smallest Hegar dilators
    Uterine probe
    Two tenaculums
    Metal catheter
    Rubber catheter
    Ampules of procaine (Novocain) hydrochloride
    Punch instrument for cervical biopsies
    Randall or Novak suction curet for endometrial biopsies
    Two cannulas with metal or rubber acorn tips for the Rubin test (or the Colvin cannula)
    Asepto syringe
    Platinum loop for obtaining urethral or vaginal secretions
    Scissors, flat and curved, large and small
    Urethroscope (not essential)
    Lugol's solution for Schiller stain
    Lumbar puncture needle for intraspinal alcohol injection (not essential)
11. Laboratory equipment
    Microscope with low-power, high-power, and oil-immersion lenses
    Lens paper
    Slides, both ordinary and hollow ground
    Cover slips
    Rack with test tubes and test-tube holder

Reagents or tablets for testing urine for albumin and sugar
Centrifuge with extra tubes
Oil for oil immersion
Stains such as Gram, methylene blue, and special stains
Hematimeter, pipets, and solutions for counting blood corpuscles and spermatozoa
Bunsen burner
Tripod or metal stand with wire top
Short and long pipets
Paraphernalia for rapid pregnancy tests
Ethyl chloride spray
Sterilizer, 18 in.; also a container with long forceps immersed in mild antiseptic for handling sterile syringes and instruments
Bicarbonate of soda and cleansing fluid for sterilizer
Distilled water for use in sterilizer
Green soap for cleansing purposes
Basins of different sizes
Biopsy bottles containing fixative solution
Disposable syringes (2.5, 5 and 10 ml. with attached disposable needles, 20 and 21 gauge, $1\frac{1}{2}$ and 2 in. long)
Rubber tourniquet (sphygmomanometer cuff may be used for this)
Tubes for blood for Wassermann, Kahn test, blood type, and Rh determination
Bottle of saline solution and KOH for diluting hanging drops of vaginal secretion
Scale for weighing patients
Sphygmomanometer
Paraphernalia for making Papanicolaou smears (see p. 306)
12. Cabinets, to contain:
Sheets (linen or disposable) for draping patients
Bath towels or disposable drapes to be placed under patients
Cloth and paper towels
Facial tissue for patients to dry vulva after examination.
Large piece of rubber or plastic sheeting to be placed under patients who are bleeding or have a profuse vaginal discharge
Disposable gloves
Vulvar pads or vaginal plugs
Sterile dressings
Band-Aids or similar adhesive dressings
Tampons
Absorbent cotton
Adhesive rolls
Box of vaginal pessaries, including Smith, Hodge, Findley, Gynefold,

bee cell, and round pessaries of different sizes. Special pessaries such as the Gellhorn or stem pessary may be purchased as needed.

Tongue depressors

Rubin or other apparatus for determining tubal patency

Electric nasal tip cautery

Instruments for pediatric gynecology (see p. 56 ff.)

Deodorant spray for use after examination of patients with bad odor

Medication

Hormones

Silver nitrate in liquid and on applicators

Gentian violet

Liquid or powder for local treatment of trichomonas vaginitis

Narcotics such as codeine, morphine, and dilaudid (small amounts of each)

Analgesics such as acetylsalicylic acid

Contraceptive devices, including diaphragms, sizes 65–85, inserters, tubes of jelly, and a model of the pelvic organs for demonstration purposes

Stationery, including letterheads, statements, envelopes, and stamps

Record cards or sheets for patients' histories, preferably kept in a metal cabinet

Several textbooks of obstetrics and gynecology and a large medical dictionary

Desk pad and pen and pencil holders

Desk clock

Scratch pads

Pens

Pencils

Correspondence file

Books for accounts

Space for storing roentgenograms, electrocardiograms, and other reports of patients

Space for reprints

Ante- and postpartum books for obstetric patients

Waking-temperature charts

13. Hamper for dirty linen
14. Clothes closet for physician, nurse, and assistant
    White or gray coats—short or long
15. Magazine rack in reception room and current magazines
    Ample ash trays for careless smokers, in both reception and consultation rooms
    Rug outside the door for wiping shoes on rainy or muddy days
    Umbrella rack in reception room

2

Taking a History

IT IS ASSUMED that every physician keeps a permanent record of each patient he sees. The only excuse for a chapter on history taking is that a gynecologic patient frequently has intimate and embarrassing (to her) complaints or confessions to make. It is most important for a practitioner to realize this, and, therefore, he should attempt to obtain a history in a manner different from his approach to men. For this purpose, tact is often of paramount importance. Unless the physician can gain the confidence and respect of his female patients, he may fail utterly in his attempt to help them. Naturally, the approach to all women is not the same. At the time of first contact with the patient, the physician will have to take into consideration many factors, such as age, marital status, the nature of the complaint, the patient's past experience with physicians, her temperament, social status, and so on. Whenever possible, it is best to talk to the patient alone when securing a history, even though she is accompanied by her mother, husband, or someone else. On the other hand, a physician should always have a female attendant or assistant present during the examination of a female patient who is a stranger to him. In this way he will avoid any possible attempts at blackmail.

When the patient is asked to discuss the complaint that made her seek medical aid, she should be permitted to describe it in her own way. However, if she brings into the story many unessential details, it is not difficult for the physician to guide her tactfully back to essential facts. If, however, the patient has enough confidence in the physician to talk about her domestic troubles, including sex difficulties, financial problems, trouble with relatives, or other intimate affairs, the physician should listen patiently and make only a few notes concerning these things. It is best not to write these facts on the record until the patient is out of the room in order to avoid giving her the impression that the secretary or someone else may read about her private affairs. Ordinarily, however, all the facts about a patient's history and physical examination should be written down as soon as they are obtained and not at the end of office hours. Otherwise, many important data may be omitted from the records.

The physician who assumes the capacity of a gynecologist must realize that frequently he is called on to act not as a physician, but as a minister, a parent, a lawyer, a psychiatrist, and an all-around adviser.

A routine should be followed in eliciting all the necessary information. There is no need to emphasize that, in many cases, to make an accurate diagnosis and to prescribe proper therapy, it is important to obtain much more information than the patient gives in the recital of the illness that led her to consult a physician. Hence, in every case a detailed history should be obtained. This requires only a few minutes, and, aside from its medical importance, it may save the physician from making embarrassing statements. All information should be written down and kept permanently. It is immaterial whether one uses cards or sheets for this purpose, but as long as a physician is in the practice of medicine, he should never destroy these records. If the files become too bulky, every year or two the records of patients who have not visited the physician for that length of time should be removed from the active file and stored away. Patients not infrequently return to a physician after a lapse of many years, and it is important (and a sign of efficiency to the patient) to have the old records. Furthermore, a physician may be called on by a court of law to give certain facts about a patient, and written records are important for this.

I use the following routine in taking a history. (In most instances a secretary can obtain most of the information, except that concerning the present illness, which the physician himself should elicit from the patient.)

1. Date of first visit and by whom referred.

2. Last name of patient, first name, and, if the patient is married, the first name of her husband.

3. Address and telephone number.

4. Age, single or married, years married, widow or divorcee, and how long without a husband.

5. Family history, especially concerning cancer, diabetes, etc.

6. Past illnesses and operations.

7. Menstrual history: age of onset; frequency of menses; regularity; duration of flow; amount of flow; any pain and, if so, whether before or during the flow, for how long and the character of the pain; date of beginning of last menses and of previous menstrual period; any associated symptoms, such as nausea, headache, and so on.

8. Obstetric history: brief account of each pregnancy, abortion or labor, with dates, information about the types of deliveries, complications during pregnancy, labor or the puerperium, Rh status (and of the husband if the wife is Rh-negative) and blood type (if known), weight and condition of the babies, breast feeding, the number of spontaneous and induced abortions, and complications, if any.

9. Present illness. This record is first written down in the patient's own words. To it is added information obtained by questions from the physician. Specific questions should be asked about pain, abnormal uterine bleeding, vaginal discharges and sterility in nulliparous women because these are the

four most frequent complaints of women. If the patient has pain, the physician must find out its location, character, duration, relation to menstruation or other occurrence, associated symptoms, and how relief is obtained. If abnormal bleeding is present, it is essential to determine whether or not it occurs between the menses or only at the time of the flow, its duration, the number of pads or vaginal tampons used daily, the color of the blood, the presence of clots and their size, associated symptoms (such as pain), and signs and symptoms of secondary anemia. If leukorrhea is annoying, it is important to find out how long it has been present, its character, the color, its relation to menstruation and associated symptoms such as pruritus vulvae, excoriation of the skin, and foul odor.

The subject of sterility is covered in Chapter 16.

In eliciting information about the illness that caused the patient to seek aid, inquiry should be made about the regularity of bowel movements, any rectal or urinary disturbances, abnormal loss or gain of weight, and, if the physician believes it is essential, information concerning the patient's sex life.

One important matter that may prevent embarrassment is to find out if the patient has visited other physicians for the same ailment. If she has, it is worth while to ask the patient what the opinions of these other physicians were and also what treatment these other physicians gave or advocated.

Before concluding this chapter, I should like to emphasize that occasionally a woman will lie deliberately about her history if she believes she has something to gain by it. For example, a woman who wants to have an early pregnancy terminated may deny having missed any periods. She may even go further and maintain that she has had profuse hemorrhages, because she believes that excessive bleeding may lead a physician to perform a curettement or even a hysterectomy. Nowadays, unmarried girls who are pregnant usually admit that they have had intercourse, although there was a time when most single girls stoutly denied such contact. Much more reliance should generally be placed on the findings of a physical examination than on what the patient has told the physician. When the results of a bimanual examination conflict with the patient's history (or story), the patient should be told frankly of the findings. Nearly all women who have lied will then admit the truth.

A physician must be extremely careful of the way he speaks to a patient about a pregnancy that she appears to be concealing. Nearly always, early pregnancy can be detected by bimanual examination. However, once in a while a uterus may be enlarged and slightly softened and still the patient may not be pregnant. Therefore, one must be careful about telling a woman that she is pregnant when she has denied this possibility. In every such instance, the physician should have a rapid immunologic or other pregnancy test performed and ask the patient to return in a week for another examination. If the woman rebels at this, one may be fairly certain that she has lied and wants to have some operative procedure performed without delay. In such a case, if the patient refuses to wait at least for the result of the pregnancy test, it is best to tell her to seek medical care elsewhere. Otherwise, she may cause the physician grief.

If a woman stoutly denies the possibility of a pregnancy despite the physician's contrary belief from his bimanual examination, the physician should not commit himself definitely until he has obtained a positive response to a pregnancy test. If the result is negative and the physician still believes he is right, the test should be repeated. Also, another bimanual examination should be made. If the uterus is the same size and the result of the second test is negative, the patient is almost certainly not pregnant.

3

The Gynecologic Examination

JUST AS IN taking a history, a definite plan should be followed in examining a patient. Regardless of the patient's complaint, it is highly desirable to spend the necessary time to make a proper physical examination. As previously mentioned, a female patient not known to the physician should be examined in the presence of a nurse, secretary, or other woman. Not infrequently, doctors are blackmailed by women who pose as patients and who, when disrobed and alone with them, threaten to yell and "expose" them immediately. Other women attempt to make trouble for physicians a few days after their visits. Young physicians should be especially careful to avoid such pitfalls.

The results of the examination should be written down in detail. There should first be a statement concerning the patient's general appearance and constitutional type, such as decidedly feminine, masculine, asthenic, obese, unusually tall, very short, dark skinned, and so on. If abnormalities of gait or posture are observed, they should be noted. The pulse, blood pressure, weight, and temperature should be taken as routine, and if the patient did not bring a specimen of urine and there are no facilities for obtaining it in the office, a specimen should be sent or brought in later.

An important detail is that the physician wash his hands before every examination. It is to his benefit to have the patient see him do this before he examines her. Before the patient is placed on the table for examination, she should be asked to empty her bladder. This should be done immediately before the bimanual examination. A cloth or disposable sheet should always be placed over the abdomen and legs.

The head should first be examined, including the mucous membranes of the eyes (for anemia and jaundice) and the skin (for excess hair, acne, and discoloration). The thyroid gland should be palpated, and then the chest is examined. The heart and lungs should be examined by percussion and auscultation if this was not done recently by an internist. A note should be made concerning scars from breast abscesses, biopsies, or mastectomy. The breasts and axillas should be carefully, systematically, and gently palpated. (See Chapter 4.)

The abdomen is inspected and examined by palpation and percussion. On inspection, it is important to determine irregularities in contour, bulging areas, lineae albicantes, the linea nigra, other discolorations, and skin eruptions.

Special attention should be paid to postoperative scars, and they should be examined for evidence of previous drainage and for possible hernias. While examining the abdomen, it is best to have the thighs and knees flexed partly, and the patient should be asked to breathe slowly through her mouth. The physician should be gentle and, in cold weather, should first wash his hands in hot water. Palpation must be gentle not only to avoid hurting the patient but also to secure her co-operation. Both hands should be used at the same time and only the flat of the hand and the palmar surfaces of the fingers, never the finger-tips, should be used. The patient's face should be watched constantly to observe any expression of pain. If it is known that one area is tender, this should be palpated last. Generally it is best to proceed from the left lower quadrant to the left upper quadrant, the epigastrium, the right upper quadrant, the right lower quadrant, the suprapubic area, the inguinal regions, the umbilical region, and the costovertebral angles last (Fig. 1). By this plan the entire abdomen is gone over; if this is done as routine, it will become a habit and require little time. If a tumor is felt abdominally, it should be described minutely on the record so that from time to time comparisons may be made with accuracy and not from memory. A small sketch should be made of all masses in the breasts and abdomen, showing their size and relation to anatomic landmarks such as the nipples, the umbilicus, and the iliac crests. Particular

FIG. 1.—Method of systematic examination of abdomen. Begin at **(1)** left lower quadrant, then proceed to **(2)** left upper quadrant, **(3)** epigastrium, **(4)** right upper quadrant, **(5)** right lower quadrant, **(6)** suprapubic region, **(7)** inguinal regions, **(8)** umbilical region and **(9)** costovertebral angles.

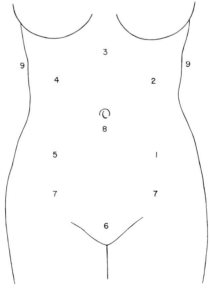

attention should be paid to the inguinal regions in women, especially for inguinal and femoral hernias and for enlargement of nodes. If large nodes are found, they may indicate gonorrhea, syphilis, malignancy of the vulva, vagina or urethra, or granuloma inguinale. In gonorrhea there are usually only one or two large, painful, often suppurating, nodes. In syphilis, the nodes are multiple, small, hard, not tender, and they do not suppurate as a rule.

A bimanual pelvic examination is made last. If a woman is having a regular menstrual flow, this examination may or may not be made. If a woman is bleeding and this flow is not a regular menses, an examination should certainly be made because in most instances intermenstrual bleeding is an indication of some pathologic condition. Even if the patient is menstruating, there is no harm in making a bimanual vaginal examination.

For a bimanual pelvic examination, the patient is placed in the lithotomy or dorsal position with the head slightly elevated and the buttocks over the edge of the table. The patient should be as comfortable as possible, the bladder should be empty, and also the rectum. Good light is essential. The external genitals should be inspected without touching them (Fig. 2). One should note the character of hair distribution and the size of the clitoris and look for congenital abnormalities, lacerations, discoloration, varicose veins, inflammation, edema, excoriations, leukorrheal discharges, blood, chronic vulvar dystrophy commonly called kraurosis vulvae, and leukoplakia, evidence of scratching, neoplasms, and Bartholin's duct abscesses or cysts. Then the labia should be separated gently with gloved fingers. Gloves are essential for the protection of both the patient and the doctor.

Disposable gloves should be used because they are cheaper than rubber gloves, they do not require time and trouble for sterilization, and psychologically they make a favorable impression on the patient. In fact, as much office equipment as possible should be disposable; this is especially applicable to syringes and needles and the paraphernalia used to obtain blood because of the danger of subsequent hepatitis. If nondisposable linens are used for a patient who has gonorrhea they should not be used again until they have been properly laundered. It is better to use disposable drapes and towels for all patients. Whenever possible, "clean" patients should be examined before infected ones.

Every woman should have Papanicolaou smears made at least once a year, but more often when indicated for abnormal bleeding from the vagina. Smears should always be made before the fingers are inserted into the vagina. When patients make an appointment, they should be told not to take a douche the day before or the day of the visit. A warmed speculum should be inserted into the vagina without any lubricant on it. Plain warm water will usually moisten the speculum sufficiently so that it can be inserted without difficulty and without discomfort if gentleness is used and if the speculum of proper

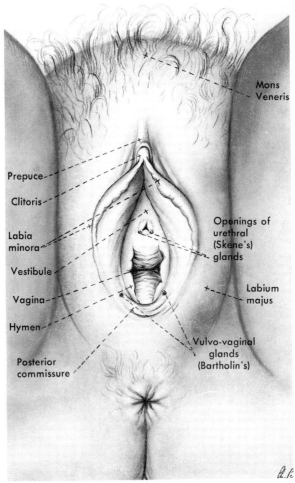

Mons
Veneris

Prepuce

Clitoris

Labia
minora

Vestibule

Vagina

Hymen

Posterior
commissure

Openings of
urethral
(Skene's)
glands

Labium
majus

Vulvo-vaginal
glands
(Bartholin's)

FIG. 2.—External genitals of a multiparous woman with a cystocele and rectocele.

size is inserted vertically and then rotated horizontally after it is all the way in the vagina. (For details on obtaining Papanicolaou smears, see Chapter 36.) The speculum is removed and a vaginal examination is now made as follows:

The labia are separated, revealing the hymen or its remains and the urethral orifice. Then one well-lubricated finger, after warming under hot water, is inserted into the vagina. An excellent lubricant is diluted tincture of green soap, which is cheap, not messy, stainless, and easily removed. The external urinary meatus is gently wiped dry with the hand outside the vagina, and, with the finger in the vagina, gentle but firm pressure is exerted on the under

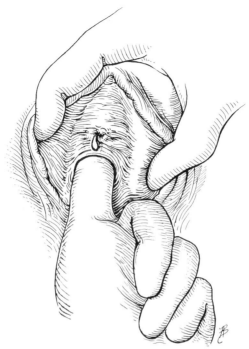

FIG. 3.—Method of squeezing pus out of urethra. External urinary meatus is gently wiped dry before finger in vagina presses on under surface of urethra.

surface of the urethra toward the orifice to squeeze out any pus that may be present (Fig. 3). If pus escapes, smears are made and stained for gonococci, or, if a large amount of pus is present, some of it is used for culture. After this is done, the index and middle fingers (well lubricated) are placed in the vagina in such a way that one finger is above the other. It is best to insert the two fingers thus because the entrance into the vagina is longer in the vertical diameter. After the fingers are in the vagina, they are turned transversely because the large diameter of the inside of the vagina is transverse. With the two fingers in the vagina and the thumb on the outside, first one Bartholin's gland and then the other is palpated to determine whether any cystic enlargement or abscess is present. Then the perineum and pelvic floor are palpated, and the condition of the anterior and posterior vagina walls is determined. A cystocele, urethrocele, rectocele, enterocele, or prolapse can be detected. The patient is asked to bear down hard. Sometimes if urinary incontinence is present, it may be revealed on straining by leakage or flow of urine.

When a patient complains of incontinence on coughing, sneezing, laughing, or straining, it is important to determine if an operation is necessary. With the bladder full and the patient in the lithotomy position, the labia are separated and the patient is asked to cough hard or bear down hard. With stress incontinence, urine will escape as a jet or as a dribble. Then the physician should place an index finger in the vagina and press up on the urethra. The patient is again asked to cough or strain. If no urine escapes, an operation will usually cure the incontinence. The vaginal examination should be repeated with the patient standing up, with one foot on the floor and the other on a stool or chair. This will reveal not only incontinence but also prolapse of the cervix and uterus (Fig. 4), cystocele, rectocele, and varicose veins on the labia and the mons veneris.

Continuing with the bimanual examination, the fingers with palmar surfaces up are gently extended up in the hollow of the sacrum toward the cervix and vault of the vagina (Fig. 5). The cervix is palpated all around to determine its position, size, shape, consistency, lacerations, movability, tenderness or pain on motion, and the presence of polyps. The culdesac and uterosacral ligaments are palpated to determine if they are tender or if there is any bulging of the culdesac from a tumor or fluid. The body of the uterus and the adnexa are then outlined, but for this purpose the other hand is necessary. The hand outside should be placed on the abdomen above the pubis and the pelvic organs pushed down within reach of the fingers in the vagina. The function of the fingers in the vagina should be that of palpation and not of pushing; hence, to make satisfactory bimanual examinations, it does not matter much whether one's fingers are long or short. Of great assistance, especially for individuals with short fingers, is the knowledge that much less force is necessary, and the patient experiences much less discomfort if, during the examination, the patient's perineal body is pushed inward by the flexed third and fourth fingers, which rest against the perineal body. A simple way to accomplish this without interfering with the tactile sense of the two fingers in the vagina is to force the elbow of this hand inward by means of the corresponding hip. Another way is to raise the corresponding foot on a stool or chair and then use the knee to push the elbow.

When the introitus or the vagina is tight, it is advisable to tell the patient to bear down while the fingers are being inserted into the vagina. Another aid is to avoid the clitoris and urethra as much as possible and to insert the fingers into the vagina by pressing down on the perineal body. Frequently pain can be avoided and co-operation obtained by using only one finger (the index), instead of two, in the vagina.

The uterus should be palpated to determine its size, shape, consistency, position, movability, and tenderness. The adnexa should be palpated one at a time to determine their size, shape, tenderness, movability, consistency, and

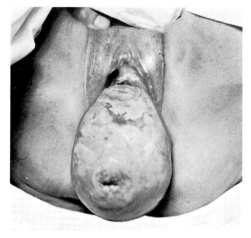

FIG. 4.—Complete prolapse of vagina.

FIG. 5.—Bimanual examination with two fingers of one hand in vagina and other hand on abdomen.

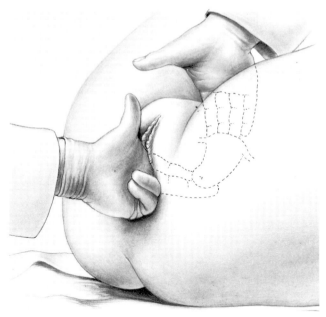

their relationship to the uterus. Normal tubes cannot be felt on bimanual examination. Normal ovaries can usually be outlined; they are generally slightly tender. Not infrequently one or both ovaries are situated in the culdesac, especially in cases of retroversion of the uterus. When the lower bowel is full, the presence of a tumor is frequently and erroneously suspected. An easy way to recognize feces is to push a finger into the mass through the vagina. If the mass is soft, dents, and remains dented, it is almost certain to be feces. In doubtful cases the patient should be told to take a cathartic and an enema and return for a second vaginal and rectal examination immediately after the enema.

If any growths are found, their size, location, movability, and pain should be noted. An excellent habit is to make a small drawing of any abnormality. Repeated sketches will reveal the growth of neoplasms. The size of growths should be stated in inches or centimeters, rather than in terms of objects, fruit, or nuts.

Anterior to the uterus, the bladder should be palpated. Also, it is a good habit to try to feel the pelvic portion of the ureters, especially in thin women. To feel the ureter, one must sweep the index and middle fingers in the vagina laterally from the cervix at the level of the internal os across the vaginal vault, at the same time making downward counterpressure with the hand outside. As the fingers are drawn forward, the ureter may be felt at the point where it passes from the broad ligament to its entrance into the bladder. It is a cordlike structure which may be rolled slightly from side to side. A normal ureter is always small and freely movable. Any thickening, enlargement, or irregularity indicates some disease of the ureter or kidney, or both. When the ureter is inflamed, it is very painful. Of course, if an abnormality in the ureter is detected, the patient should have a cystoscopic examination, with or without intravenous pyelography.

Before the fingers are removed from the vagina, the pelvic bones should be carefully palpated to obtain an accurate idea of the patient's obstetric possibilities. This is especially important for women who have never had children but who are anxious to become pregnant.

After the bimanual vaginoabdominal examination, a bimanual rectoabdominal exploration should be made. Before this is done the glove should be thoroughly washed. If gonorrhea is present or suspected, a different glove should be used for the rectal examination. The anal orifice should be carefully washed and dried before the index finger is inserted into the rectum (Fig. 6).

First, the anus is inspected and palpated for hemorrhoids, fissures, polyps, prolapse, and new growths. The tone of the sphincter muscle is determined, and then the pelvic organs are palpated. Frequently a pelvic tumor is better outlined through the rectum than through the vagina. The culdesac should again be palpated and also the uterosacral ligaments. The latter are much more

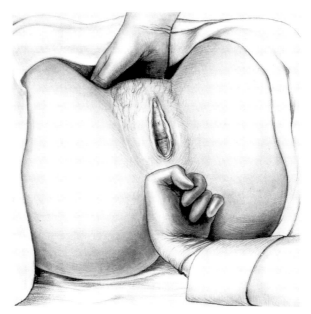

FIG. 6.—Bimanual examination with finger of one hand in rectum and other hand on abdomen.

satisfactorily investigated through the rectum than through the vagina. The rectovaginal septum is then palpated with the index finger in the rectum and the thumb of the same hand in the vagina (Fig. 7). After this the finger in the rectum is turned around, and the coccyx is palpated by gently compressing it between the index finger in the rectum and the thumb of the same hand, which is outside of the vagina.

Whenever a pelvic tumor is found or the presence of endometriosis or an enterocele is suspected, a combined vaginorectal examination should be made. This is accomplished by inserting the index finger in the vagina and the middle finger of the same hand in the rectum; with these two fingers and the hand outside, the outline of the pelvic organs and new growths is determined (Fig. 8). From this combined vaginal and rectal examination, much more informa-tion is elicited than from either a vaginal or a rectal examination alone. This is especially true if a tumor is present in the culdesac or in the rectovaginal septum or if an enterocele is present.

No bimanual examination is complete without inspection of the entire vagina and cervix. Therefore, a speculum is an indispensable instrument in gynecology not only for treatment but also for diagnosis. Speculums are of various types, such as the bivalve (Graves or duckbill), the trivalve, the tubular, and the spatular. Those used most commonly are the metal bivalve speculums. All

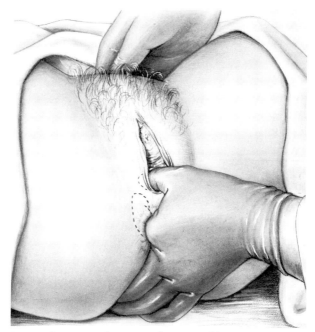

FIG. 7.—Palpation of rectovaginal septum and uterosacral ligaments. Index finger is in rectum and thumb of same hand is in vagina.

FIG. 8.—Bimanual vaginorectal examination. Index finger of one hand is in vagina and middle finger in rectum. Other hand is on the abdomen. This type of examination must always be done when there are masses in the culdesac, such as endometriosis, ovarian cysts and carcinoma.

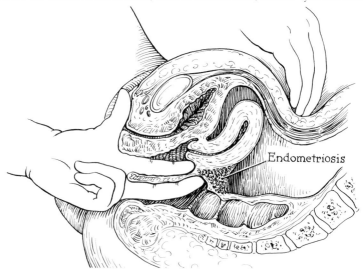

have a short anterior and a longer posterior part to conform with the anatomy of the vagina. Most speculums can be made self-retaining by adjusting one or more screws. Disposable speculums are available.

The speculum should be warmed and well lubricated before insertion and should be placed very gently in the vagina. If a bivalve speculum is used, the two blades should be closed and inserted in an anteroposterior direction into the vagina after the labia are separated with two fingers or the perineal body is held down gently with one finger. After the blades are in the vagina, they should be turned on the flat end with the short blade uppermost, and the tip of the posterior blade is pushed down into the posterior fornix. The two blades are opened, thus exposing the cervix (Fig. 9). The vaginal wall should be inspected all around by gently turning the speculum, and then the cervix should be carefully studied in good light. For this purpose the blades of the speculum are secured in position by tightening the screw or screws of the speculum. Special lighting attachments are helpful but not necessary. An ordinary electric bulb on a gooseneck stand back of the physician can be directed on the cervix to give all the light that is necessary. A few minutes should be spent scrutinizing the cervix. In patients who have a vaginal discharge, material can readily be obtained by means of a platinum loop, a glass catheter, or the gloved finger for hanging drop examinations for Trichomonas vaginalis or candida. Also, smears and cultures may be made. If polyps are present in the cervix, they may be removed easily through a speculum. When a suspect lesion is present in the cervix, it may be removed for microscopic study most easily by a special punch instrument or by means of scissors or

FIG. 9.—Use of bivalve speculum, with screws tightened to hold blades in place. **A,** front view; **B,** side view.

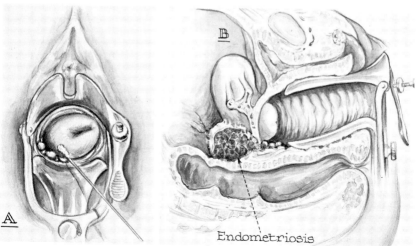

Endometriosis

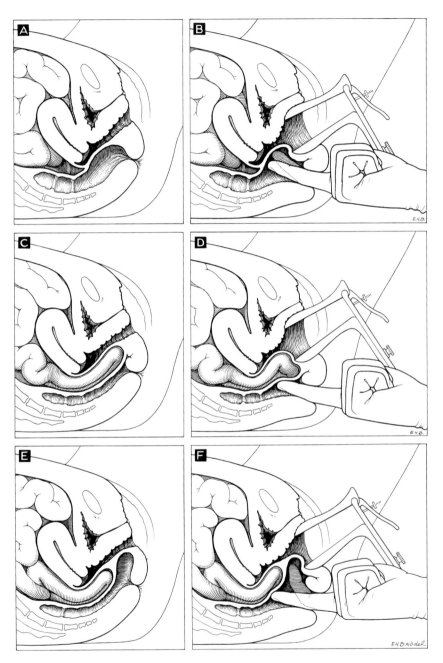

Fig. 10.—Legend on facing page.

a scalpel. The cervix is readily treated by the electric cautery or conization. (See the special chapters on all of these subjects.)

Waters described and illustrated an excellent technic for detection of an enterocele (Fig. 10). Another method of diagnosing an enterocele is to place a light in the rectum. This causes transillumination of the rectovaginal septum. The enterocele will not transmit light because it is not part of the rectum. But great care must be used when employing this procedure.

Sometimes, and especially when the uterus is unusually small, it is advisable to measure the length of the uterine cavity. This is done with a sterile uterine sound. When information is needed concerning the endometrium, this can readily be obtained by means of a tiny curet with or without a suction arrangement. (See Chapter 30 for endometrial biopsy.)

After a pelvic examination has been completed, the physician should dry the vulva and anus with a large piece of cotton. A moist vulva or anus is most uncomfortable, and, not infrequently, a physician who does not dry the vulva will discover that a patient has used one of his cloth towels or sheets for drying purposes.

Once in a great while bimanual examination will be so unsatisfactory that one will have to resort to an examination under general anesthesia.

Most physicians still hesitate to make a pelvic examination in a virgin. In fact, not even a rectal examination is attempted in most instances when an internal examination should be made. For the customary pelvic examination of a virgin, as, for example, before marriage or for pain in the lower part of the abdomen, a bimanual rectoabdominal examination is nearly always sufficient and satisfactory. However, there should be no compunction about making a vaginal examination when it is indicated in cases of vaginal discharge, abnormal bleeding, pelvic pain, and other pelvic symptoms. In girls who use vaginal tampons at the time of the menses, it is nearly always possible to insert a well-lubricated index finger gently without causing pain. With a little experience, as much information can be obtained by means of a one-finger examination as when two fingers are used. In girls with a very small hymenal orifice, it may be possible to dilate the opening gently so that it will admit one finger, particularly if considerable lubrication is used; otherwise a general

FIG. 10.—**A,** rectocele above firm perineal body. **B,** demonstrating rectocele. Withdrawal of speculum permits rectal wall to "fall away" from finger in rectum, which follows into sacculated rectocele. **C,** large enterocele without rectocele. **D,** demonstrating enterocele. On withdrawal of speculum, enterocele bulges into vagina, but rectal wall retains contact with finger in rectum, for enterocele separates and "fills" rectovaginal septum. **E,** enterocele and rectocele. **F,** demonstrating enterocele and rectocele. As speculum is withdrawn, enterocele herniates into vagina, but rectal wall maintains contact with finger in rectum, as in **D.** Further speculum withdrawal reaches site of rectocele; now rectal wall pulls forward away from finger, which must flex to maintain contact, as in **B.** (Courtesy of E. G. Waters, Am. J. Obst. & Gynec. 52:810, November, 1946.)

anesthetic should be given. Before an examination is made of any virgin, the physician should explain to the patient, and preferably also to her mother, that there is absolutely no harm in making a pelvic examination because the lack of an intact hymen is by no means a sign that coitus has taken place. In virgins a special tiny speculum or a Kelly urethral endoscope should be used. In no circumstance should force be used, for a spasm of the levator ani muscles and rigidity of the abdominal muscles will result and not only prevent the physician from outlining the pelvic organs but frighten the patient and cause her physical and mental anguish.

After the bimanual examinations have been made, the lower extremities are observed for varicose veins, edema, excessive hair growth, and deformities. After this, the patient is asked to stand so that her back may be examined. If there is uterine prolapse, an examination should be made with the patient standing with one foot on a stool or chair in order to determine the full extent of the prolapse. Straining will reveal the degree of prolapse or enterocele.

After the history is taken and the physical examination completed, it is necessary to make at least a few laboratory tests. At least once, every patient should have her urine examined, a complete blood count, and a blood Wassermann or Kahn test. The urine should be examined not only for albumin and sugar but also microscopically for pus, blood, and casts. In all cases in which urinary disturbances are present, a "clean" specimen should be obtained. This is practically identical with or even cleaner than a catheterized specimen and is obtained by the following procedure. The patient lies flat on the "unbroken" examining table with the legs flexed and abducted. Two clean, or sterile, basins are placed on the table between her legs. The vulva and external urinary meatus are cleansed as if the patient were to be catheterized. The labia are then separated by the thumb and index finger of one hand and a basin is held in the other hand. The patient is asked to urinate *very gently*, without force, and as the urine escapes it is caught in the basin. Immediately after the first flow is caught, the basin is quickly put down on the table and the second (empty) basin just as quickly pushed into place to catch the remainder of the urine passed. The second basin contains urine cleaner than a catheterized specimen. While the basins are being changed, the labia must be kept apart. A nurse can help considerably.

In every case of sterility, endocrine dysfunction, obesity, repeated abortion, and many other conditions, one or more tests of thyroid function should be carried out. These often yield unexpected information.

Whenever a vaginal discharge is present, not only should a smear be stained for gonococci but a hanging drop should be made to detect Trichomonas vaginalis or candida. In every case of urethral or cervical discharge, smears should be made of both the vagina and the rectum and stained with the Gram stain. If gonorrhea is suspected, some secretion should be cultured. All smears showing gonococci should be properly labeled and stored away. They may be needed as proof at a later date.

When necessary, other tests, such as blood chemistry, the Rubin test, hysterosalpingography, cystoscopy, intravenous pyelography, and so on, must be made. Roentgenograms may have to be taken. Whenever a cystic teratoma (dermoid cyst) of the ovary is suspected, a roentgenogram should be taken, because it may reveal bony tissue or the fat characteristic of a dermoid tumor. In some cases roentgenograms must be made to diagnose or exclude orthopedic conditions.

After the results of all the necessary laboratory tests and special examinations are added to the patient's history, the complete record is reviewed and a diagnosis made. In many cases the diagnosis will be incomplete or impossible, and then consultation must be had with other physicians. As soon as a correct diagnosis is made, treatment must, of course, be instituted. If the family physician is not equipped for, or capable of, properly treating a patient, he should turn her over to someone who can administer the necessary therapy, but he should not lose track of the patient. He should occasionally confer with the consultant.

4

Examination of the Breasts

THE BREASTS must be inspected and palpated as part of every physical examination of every woman regardless of age. An adequate examination includes several different steps and requires several minutes even when no abnormality is found. It is advantageous to develop a routine for examining the breasts, just as with the abdominal and pelvic examinations, because following an orderly routine guards against overlooking important details. Much of the data and all the illustrations in this chapter are from C. D. Haagensen's *Diseases of the Breast* (Philadelphia: 2d ed. W. B. Saunders Company, 1971).

SUPRACLAVICULAR AND AXILLARY REGIONS.—The procedure is begun with examination of the supraclavicular and axillary regions. The patient sits on the table facing the examiner, with her legs over its side. The supraclavicular regions (Fig. 11) and axillas are examined first. In the examination of the axilla (Fig. 12), it is essential that the pectoral muscles be relaxed. To achieve this, the examiner supports the patient's arm on one of his own. He then palpates with the tips of the fingers of his other hand. The gentler his palpation, the better he will feel lymph nodes lying against the thoracic wall. Lymph nodes high up in the axilla are difficult or impossible to feel. Not only the number but the consistency and movability of the axillary lymph nodes should be noted. They may be fixed to the underlying axillary structures or to the overlying skin. Palpation is unfortunately very inaccurate in revealing whether or not axillary lymph nodes contain metastases.

INSPECTION OF BREAST.—The next step is a critical inspection of the breasts themselves, first with the patient's arms at her sides and then with the arms raised high above her head (Fig. 13). The examination must be conducted in a good light, for nuances of light and shade and slight changes in contour of the breasts are of great importance and may be missed if the lighting is poor. The examiner compares the contour of the two breasts, following it from the anterior axillary fold to the mid-line on each side. An indentation or a bulge in this contour often betrays the site of a lesion. It is important to compare the height of the two breasts on the chest wall and their relative size.

It will sometimes be noted that one breast is slightly larger than the other, yet perfectly symmetrical with its mate. This mere disparity in size is often

34

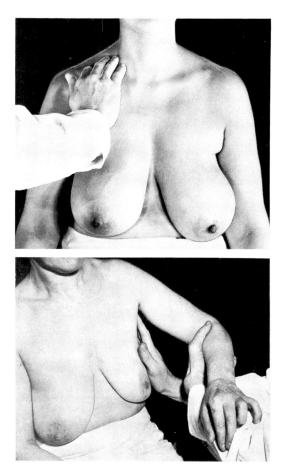

FIG. 11 (above).—Supraclavicular palpation.
FIG. 12 (below).—Axillary palpation.

only a developmental defect and, if not accompanied by other signs, is not significant.

The shape and size of the areolas and their comparative level are next studied. The shape of the nipples and the axes in which they point are compared. The surface of the nipples is carefully inspected in a search for crusting or erosion.

Palpation.—Inspection completed, the examiner is ready to palpate the breasts. This is best performed with the patient lying down. For adequate palpation, the breast should be balanced on the chest wall, forming an even layer flattened out upon the thoracic cage. To achieve this, the shoulder on

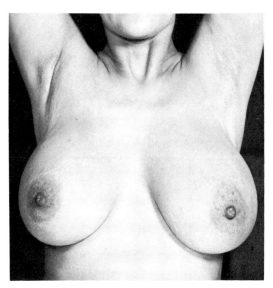

Fig. 13.—Inspection of breasts with arms raised above head.

the side of the breast being examined is elevated by means of a small pillow placed under it (Fig. 14). This throws the breast medially and flattens it out upon the thorax. If the breast is allowed to fall to the patient's side, folding on itself (Fig. 15), a small tumor within it may be masked by the thickness and density of the breast in this position.

Palpation of the breasts should be gentle, precise, and orderly. Palpation must never be so heavy handed that it distresses the patient. Such an experience may deter her from returning for subsequent vitally important re-examinations. Gentle palpation is also more informative than rough examination; indeed, the gentler the palpation, the more informative it will be. There is, moreover, a possible danger of causing metastasis by rough examination of a breast carcinoma. Palpation with one hand is usually more precise and gentler than palpation with both hands. When palpation of the breast is carried out in warm weather and the skin is moist, a little talcum powder on it diminishes friction and may add to the accuracy of tactile perception. The hands should always be warmed under running hot water before palpation.

The whole extent of the breast, as it lies flattened out and balanced upon the chest wall, should be gone over systematically with the flat of the fingers of one hand. Unless something is felt that arouses a suspicion of abnormality, each area need be palpated but once as the examiner's fingers explore, in orderly sequence, the whole extent of the breast beginning in the upper middle

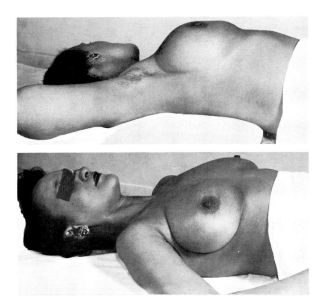

FIG. 14 (above).—Correct position for palpation of breast; shoulder elevated by pillow.
FIG. 15 (below).—Incorrect position for palpation of breasts; breasts fall laterally when shoulders are flat on table.

sector and proceeding clockwise to complete the examination of the upper outer sector.

In palpating the medial half of the breast, it is advantageous to have the arm raised above the head (Fig. 16), a position that tenses the pectoral muscle so that it provides a flatter surface upon which the medial half of the breast rests. In palpating the lateral half of the breast, however, it is helpful to have the patient's arm at her side (Fig. 17); in this position, the breast lies more caudad and is more accessible to palpation.

The breast tissue often extends over a wide area. A thin layer of it may reach the mid-line of the sternum medially, the lower edge of the clavicle above and the edge of the latissimus dorsi muscle laterally. Small subcutaneous tumors near these outer limits of the breast may be mistaken for benign subcutaneous lesions not associated with the breast when, in fact, they are carcinomas of the breast. The axillary prolongation of the breast extends high into the axilla in some women, and carcinoma arising in it is commonly mistaken for lymphosarcoma or adenitis of the axillary lymph nodes.

Palpation with the patient erect is an inaccurate method of examining the breast. The upper outer sector of the breast, where neoplasms are most frequent, is not conveniently accessible if the patient sits with her arm at her

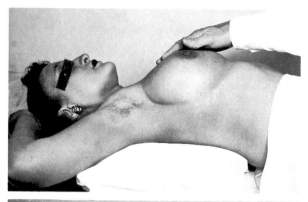

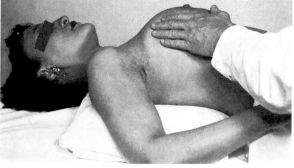

FIG. 16 (above).—Palpation of inner half of breast; arm raised above head.
FIG. 17 (below).—Palpation of lateral half of breast; arm at side.

side. If she sits with her arm raised, the tension upon the skin and subjacent fascia tends to mask abnormalities in the upper part of the breast.

Although palpation in the supine position is certainly the best method of detecting abnormalities in most parts of the breast, it is wise also to palpate the lower part of the breast and the subareolar region between the fingers of both hands with the patient sitting up if the breast is very large and thick. In the subareolar area, where the ducts converge to enter the base of the nipple, the breast structure is looser and less dense. In breasts that are thick and relatively firm, the comparatively dense breast tissue forms a sort of ledge around this softer subareolar region. The cephalad portion of this ledge is not infrequently mistaken for a tumor. On the other hand, a real tumor of small size situated in the softer subareolar area of a thick dense breast may be almost impalpable in the supine position, although when the breast is examined between the fingers in the sitting position the tumor is readily felt.

Careful palpation of the breast will reveal a carcinoma even when it measures only 4–5 mm. in diameter. The features that most often suggest carcinoma are hardness of the tumor and its relative fixation in the area of breast tissue in which it lies, so that it cannot be moved without carrying along the surrounding breast tissue. Most carcinomas are not sharply circumscribed; the edge of the lesion merges with the surrounding breast tissue that it infiltrates. This makes a carcinoma difficult to measure precisely.

But consistency, mobility, and circumscription are by no means reliable indications of the nature of a tumor of the breast.

RETRACTION PHENOMENA.—Greater reliance in diagnosis can be placed on the retraction phenomena that carcinoma almost always produces in the breast. When the examiner has completed his palpation of the breast, he should look for retraction signs. They constitute a whole series of clinical signs ranging from a small dimple in the skin over the tumor to shrinkage of the entire breast. They are due to the fact that, as carcinoma grows in the breast, it causes proliferation of fibroblasts not only within its own structure but into the surrounding breast tissue. This scar tissue, so to speak, contracts as it grows older, and since the breast is normally loose and fatty in structure, any or all of the tissues adjacent to the carcinoma may be pulled in toward it by the shortening strands of fibroblasts. This phenomenon is of fundamental importance in interpretation of the clinical signs the disease produces.

The fibrosis within the carcinoma and radiating out around it exerts an abnormal traction upon the fascial septa of the breast and pulls the skin inward to produce dimpling, deviates the axis in which the nipple points, or flattens and retracts the nipple when its duct system is involved by the disease. When the pectoral muscle is contracted, carrying the pectoral fascia cephalad, the sector of the breast in which the carcinoma lies is pulled upward abnormally and its contour distorted, because the carcinoma within it is abnormally fixed to the pectoral fascia.

Usually, retraction signs are not well developed. In small early carcinomas, they are often so subtle that they can be demonstrated only by certain maneuvers. When the arms are raised, elevating the pectoral fascia, the carcinoma and the overlying skin are pulled upward and inward to a greater degree than the surrounding normal breast, producing the telltale asymmetry.

Another maneuver that is useful in revealing retraction of the skin is for the examiner to lift the breast upward with his hand. When the carcinoma is in the upper half of the breast, this maneuver will often bring out a dimple in the skin over it. The mechanism of this phenomenon is a simple one. The skin over the carcinoma is tied down to it by fibrosis, while the skin over the normal surrounding breast lifts freely.

A variant of this lifting maneuver is gentle compression of the breast on both sides of the carcinoma as in Figure 18. Here again, a dimple develops over the lesion in the upper outer sector of the breast, while the surrounding skin bulges normally.

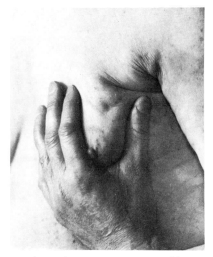

Fig. 18.—Dimple over carcinoma in upper outer sector of breast, demonstrated by gentle compression of adjacent breast tissue.

Another maneuver that is often helpful in demonstrating retraction signs in a carcinomatous breast is *pectoral contraction*. While in the sitting position, the patient relaxes and rests her hands on her hips, giving the examiner an opportunity to compare the relative heights of the lower edge of the breast and the level of the areola on each side, and to look for retraction signs over the tumor. The patient is then asked to press her hands against her hips, contracting her pectoral muscles, first on the normal and then on the diseased side. The normal breast is pulled upward slightly by this motion, but the carcinomatous breast often rises sharply as compared with its mate. The breast as a whole may be abnormally elevated, or merely the sector of the breast in which the carcinoma is situated. This abnormal elevation occurs because the fibrosis in the carcinomatous area attaches it to the underlying pectoral fascia. When contraction of the pectoralis major elevates the pectoral fascia, the carcinomatous area in the breast is pulled up with it.

Pectoral contraction also brings out other retraction signs—deviation of the nipple toward the carcinoma and furrows and dimples in the skin over it.

Another procedure of great value in demonstrating retraction signs in the breast is the *forward-bending maneuver*. The patient is asked to bend far forward from the hips, keeping her chin up and extending her hands forward to the examiner, who supports them on the tips of his own fingers as he sits before her (Fig. 19). In this position, normal breasts fall freely away from the chest wall and are perfectly symmetrical. But if a carcinoma is present in one of them, even though the growth is small, the fibrosis that accompanies

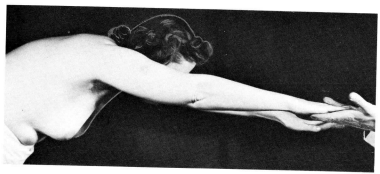

FIG. 19.—Forward-bending maneuver.

it will usually fix the diseased breast to the chest wall in some degree and produce an asymmetry that careful inspection from the side or from the front will disclose.

The examiner should pay special attention to changes in the areola and nipple. The horizontal levels of the areola and nipple are often elevated by a carcinoma in the upper half of the breast. Deviation of the axis in which the nipple points is a subtle retraction sign. The fibrosis in and about the carcinoma pulls on the duct system and tilts the nipple so that it points toward the carcinoma. When the carcinoma involves the area more or less directly beneath the nipple, the fibrosis shortens the whole duct system and pulls the nipple inward. This process may show itself merely as flattening and broadening of the nipple (see Fig. 20) on the side that is carcinomatous, in comparison with its mate.

Flattening or retraction of the nipple caused by carcinoma should not be

FIG. 20.—Flattening and broadening of right nipple due to carcinoma.

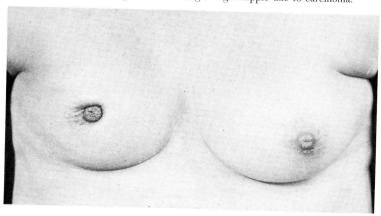

confused with mere inversion of the nipple, a condition seen in many women with no disease of the breast. Inversion of the nipple may be bilateral or unilateral. The patient will usually say that the inversion has been present for many years and that it interfered with nursing. Instead of protruding in the normal way, the nipple is hidden in a sulcus, from which it can usually be pulled out. The inverted nipple is not broadened, thickened and fixed, as is the retracted nipple of carcinoma.

There are few cases of carcinoma of the breast in which a careful examination fails to reveal any retraction signs.

EROSION OF NIPPLE.—Erosion of the nipple is an important sign of carcinoma. Even when it is only 2 or 3 mm. in diameter, it warrants a presumptive diagnosis of the Paget type of carcinoma. Not all erosions of the nipple, of course, are carcinomatous, for inflammatory and trophic eczema-like lesions do occasionally develop in the nipple and areola. But the percentage of nipple erosions that are carcinomatous is so high that biopsy of the erosion and microscopic proof of its nature are always necessary. The typical Paget erosion is a crusted or moist and granular area on the surface of the nipple. It dries up and seems to heal over from time to time but soon breaks open again, enlarging slowly but steadily. The nipple is flattened and finally destroyed by the process, which extends onto the areola and then over the skin of the breast. This type of carcinoma is relatively somewhat less malignant than other forms of carcinoma of the breast, and cure may be achieved even when the erosion has been present for years and has involved a large area of the skin over the breast.

DISCHARGE.—A discharge from the nipple is a sign of abnormality in the breast. This may be physiologic and harmless, or pathologic and an indication of inflammation or of epithelial proliferation. The character of the discharge is an important distinguishing feature.

A discharge that has the consistency and color of milk is usually just that. This kind of nipple secretion is usually bilateral. The few drops of milk that accumulate in the duct system of the breast do not usually escape spontaneously, but appear only when the breast is squeezed or the nipple is stimulated. Such a discharge from the nipple is harmless.

Low-grade inflammatory processes, developing in the subareolar portion of the breast close to the larger ducts, sometimes break into a duct that provides a channel for the escape of the exudate. This type of inflammatory discharge has the gross character of pus, and its nature can be confirmed by microscopic examination of a smear. Although recurring or persisting infection in the breast is notoriously difficult to eradicate, attempts to provide adequate surgical drainage should be made. When the abscess cavity is opened, it is wise to excise a small piece of tissue for microscopic examination, to rule out the possibility of unsuspected carcinoma.

A thin, yellowish, brownish, reddish, or frankly bloody discharge from the nipple is almost always a sign of epithelial proliferation. This kind of discharge usually escapes spontaneously and stains the patient's brassiere or nightgown. In an overwhelming majority of cases, it is due to an intraductal papilloma growing in one of the larger ducts in the subareolar region and not to carcinoma. The dilated duct containing the papilloma can usually be detected, by careful palpation, as a small cordlike or rounded tumor beneath or close to the areola. Pressure on it produces a drop or two of secretion from the opening of the involved duct on the surface of the nipple. Such a lesion should always be explored surgically, and the diseased duct or ducts excised. Microscopic examination will confirm the benign nature of the papilloma and rule out carcinoma. Mastectomy is not required for intraductal papilloma; local excision of the lesion suffices for cure.

If the papillary process is situated some distance out in the breast tissue, away from the subareolar region, or if it has grown to form a tumor of considerable size, it is wise to make a biopsy of the lesion before attempting to remove it, because such growths may be papillary carcinomas.

If, in a patient with a history of a yellowish, brownish, or bloody discharge from the nipple, careful palpation does not reveal any tumor or any point where pressure elicits the discharge, the physician should re-examine the breast after a week or two, cautioning the patient against squeezing the breast in the meantime. During this interval, the secretion will have an opportunity

FIG. 21.—Extensive edema of skin in carcinoma of breast.

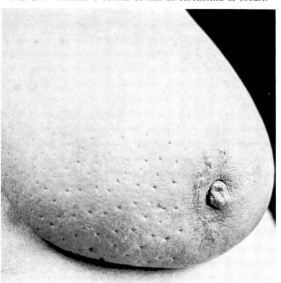

to accumulate in the diseased duct, and re-examination may localize it. The physician must keep track of the patient and re-examine her until he finds the lesion. Papanicolaou smears should be made and repeated at regular intervals, at first every 3 months, then every 6 months.

In rare instances, the discharge may be a sign of carcinoma. In the New York Presbyterian Hospital series of cases of carcinoma of the breast, there was a discharge from the nipple in only 1.03%. Although the chance that a nipple discharge indicates carcinoma is therefore small, this symptom can never be dismissed lightly.

Another group of clinical signs is produced by abnormal circulatory relationships in the breast. Carcinoma growing in the breast causes an increase in the blood supply to the part. This occasionally produces hyperemia of the skin, which is abnormally warm and sometimes reddened. The subcutaneous veins over the upper part of the breast may be visibly dilated. Infrared photographs bring out this dilatation in a striking manner.

Edema of the skin of the breast caused by blocking of the subdermal lymphatics is an important sign of carcinoma in an advanced stage. Lymph accumulates within the skin, until the skin is several times its normal thickness, and causes abnormal separation and deepening of the orifices of the cutaneous glands (Fig. 21).

Cystic Disease of the Breast

Another term for this, and the one commonly used, is chronic cystic mastitis. This term is, however, confusing and implies inflammation, which is not a characteristic feature of the condition. Whereas, in most cases, cystic disease of the breast is benign, in about 20% of all carcinomas of the breast, the origin is cystic disease. However, what percentage of cystic hyperplasias end in carcinoma is unknown, but when malignancy does occur it is usually in the late forties and early fifties. The time that the process takes to culminate in carcinoma is about 30 years.

Cysts that are due to cystic hyperplasia first come under clinical observation as (1) a single cyst, (2) multiple cysts, or (3) a localized nodularity in the breast. The age of patients with these lesions is about the early thirties, although the disease has been found in the late twenties.

SINGLE CYSTS.—When a single cyst reaches large proportions, it is hard and tense. The walls are smooth and sharply defined. It is freely movable, and fluctuation may be detected in it. Unless cysts are inflamed by trauma or infection, they are not adherent to the surrounding structures, the nipple is not retracted, and the axillary lymph nodes are not enlarged. Uncomplicated cysts contain a clear, straw-colored fluid. Cysts complicated by benign and malignant epithelial neoplasms may contain blood or serosanguineous fluid which, on microscopic examination, may show benign or malignant epithelial cells. A large cyst can be regarded as evidence that many small cysts are in the process of formation in this neighborhood. In the early stages of cyst formation, the patient may complain of pain, which usually ceases when the cyst has become clinically obvious. The probable cause of pain is the gradual distention of the tissues.

MULTIPLE CYSTS.—The clinical signs of multiple cysts depend on how early in the process the disease is observed. In the earliest stages, there is multi-nodularity among which are small, round, smooth, slippery swellings which are elastic on palpation.

LOCALIZED NODULARITY.—A localized collection of cysts is due to cystic hyperplasia occurring in a main duct, its branches and acini, or only in terminal ducts and their branches and acini.

It must always be remembered that upon the cystic epithelial hyperplasia may be superimposed an epithelial neoplasm. A definite clinical diagnosis of carcinoma in relation to cystic changes can be made only after the carcinoma has produced its characteristic clinical signs.

Next to physiologic mammary hyperplasia commonly called "chronic mastitis," cystic disease is the most common lesion of the breast. From a critical review of the most reliable reports in the literature, there seems to be general agreement that in women with cystic disease of the breast an expectation of breast cancer is greater than the expected incidence of the female population of comparable age.

The safest *therapeutic approach* of an apparently single cyst is wide excision of the involved area of the breast, but precautions must be taken to prevent possible dissemination of carcinoma because the latter may be present even when least suspected.

Women with cystic disease should undergo a thorough clinical examination of the breast at least every 3 months. Medication may be necessary for the relief of pain. This can be accomplished usually by ordinary anodynes and small doses of androgens.

In recent years *mammography* has come to be used increasingly for the detection of malignancy of the breast. This modality is actually soft-tissue roentgenography of the breast, because nothing is injected into the ducts or breasts. Mammography was first used clinically in 1929 by Warren. There is divided opinion regarding its usefulness and reliability. It may help in cases of (1) symptoms and signs of breast disease, whether disease is evident or not; (2) breast changes sufficient to have led to previous therapy; (3) strong family history of cancer of the breast; (4) repeated surveys of the opposite breast after mastectomy; (5) breasts difficult to examine manually; (6) women with cancerophobia; (7) adenocarcinoma with primary site undetermined; and (8) in cases in which a base line for future comparison of breast structure is needed. Mammography is most accurate in the adipose breast of the older woman, in the age group in which cancer of the breast is usually found.

Treatment of Carcinoma of the Breast

The diagnosis of carcinoma having been proved, a surgeon must decide how to treat the lesion. If the patients with far-advanced and inoperable lesions are excluded from the calculation, about one half of those operated on remain well for at least 5 years. In patients without axillary metastases, thoroughly radical operation is today achieving a 5-year clinical-cure rate of 90%. After 5 years have elapsed, recurrence is infrequent. One can therefore say that a woman whose disease is attacked before axillary metastases have developed has an excellent chance not only of 5-year cure but of permanent cure. The 5-year cure rate for patients with axillary involvement is about 50%.

It is generally agreed that the best results of treatment of carcinoma of the breast are still obtained by means of a carefully performed Halsted operation or modification of it, with removal of the breast, both pectoral muscles, and the axillary lymph nodes.

Postoperative radiation.—If carcinoma is found in any lymph nodes following radical mastectomy, radiation therapy either by x-ray or cobalt should be carried out. If the lymph nodes are free from metastases, there is no need for radiation.

Hormone therapy.—Between 30 and 50% of postmenopausal women who have superficial soft-part involvement as well as metastatic disease in the lungs and pleura will obtain relief from estrogen therapy. The response of metastatic bone disease is less favorable, occurring in only 10–20% of cases. Palliation is effective for about 18 months, but, in a small proportion of cases, benefits have lasted for several years. The common side effects of estrogen therapy are anorexia, nausea, and vomiting, which occur in about 50% of women. These symptoms often disappear after 7 to 10 days, especially if the dose is reduced. If oral estrogen medication produces disagreeable symptoms, hypodermic medication may be necessary. There is danger, however, of precipitating cardiac decompensation in old women with cardiovascular disease.

The commonly used *estrogens* for the relief of pain from carcinoma of the breast are: (1) diethylstilbestrol, 5 mg. orally t.i.d.; (2) ethinyl estradiol, 1 mg. orally t.i.d.; (3) conjugated estrogenic substance, 30 mg. orally daily; (4) estradiol benzoate, 5 mg. intramuscularly 3 times a week; (5) estradiol dipropionate intramuscularly, 5 mg. twice a week; and (6) estradiol valerate, 30 mg. intramuscularly every 2 weeks.

Androgens should be prescribed if estrogens produce side effects even when administered hypodermically. The usual doses of androgens are: (1) testosterone propionate, 100 mg. intramuscularly 3 times a week; (2) testosterone cyclopentylpropionate, 200 mg. intramuscularly 3 times a week; (3) fluoxymesterone (Halotestin), 10 mg. orally t.i.d.; (4) testosterone enanthate (Delatestryl), 200 Gm. intramuscularly every 2 weeks; and (5) methyltestosterone, 100 mg. orally daily.

In some instances it is advisable to give *corticosteroids*, as follows; (1) Prednisone, 30 mg. orally daily; (2) cortisone, 100–300 mg. orally daily; and (3) Decadron, 2–6 mg. orally daily.

CHEMOTHERAPY.—In advanced stages of carcinoma metastases, the following nonhormonal chemotherapeutic agents may be used: (1) 5-fluorouracil (5-FU), 15 Gm. per kg. daily for 5 days, then 7.5 mg. per kg. every second day 4 times, and repeat in 6 to 8 weeks (50% remissions); (2) triethylenethiophosphoramide (Thio-TEPA), (*a*) 30 mg. once, then 0.3 mg. weekly, based on the white blood cell count of 3,000–6,000, or (*b*) 0.6–1 mg. per kg. divided over 4 days, then no therapy for 10 days, then 0.4 mg. per kg. weekly 4 times, 0.4 mg. per kg. every 2 weeks 6 times, then the same dose every month (40% remissions); (3) cyclophosphamide (Cytoxan), 100–300 mg. daily or 20 mg. per kg. daily intravenously twice (50% remissions); and (4) a combination of androgen plus Thio-TEPA (high degree of remissions).

Richard G. Cooper reported that by employing a five-drug combination treatment he induced tumor regression in 90% of his patients with metastatic adenocarcinoma of the breast as compared with only 30% regression in women with standard therapeutic treatment. For the first 10 to 12 weeks the Cooper regimen is as follows: (1) 5-FU IV weekly at 12 mg./kg.; (2) methotrexate IV weekly at 0.6 mg./kg.; (3) vincristine IV weekly at 0.35 μg./kg. (but only for four to six weeks within this period, depending on the time of onset of neurotoxicity); (4) prednisone orally and daily, starting at 0.75 mg./kg. and in decreasing dosages until patient is taking a maintenance dose of about 5 mg. a day; (5) cyclophosphamide orally and daily at 2 mg./kg. For the second 10 to 12 weeks the Cooper regimen continues: (1) prednisone as above; (2) cyclophosphamide as above; (3) 5-FU and methotrexate as above, except every two weeks rather than every week.

5

Prophylactic Gynecology

Since a large proportion of minor and major gynecologic ailments arise from the process of childbirth, it is not amiss to discuss postpartum care, because proper control of patients after delivery is prophylactic gynecology.

Physicians generally examine their maternity patients at the time of their first visit and subsequently take the blood pressure and weight and examine the urine at more or less definite intervals. Because of this routine, many abnormal conditions, notably eclampsia, are avoided. On the other hand, for most physicians, postpartum care consists of a little attention in the hospital for a few days after delivery and then a so-called final examination in the office at the end of 6 or 8 weeks. Furthermore, this examination is usually cursory. Some pathologic conditions are overlooked, and the result, for some women at least, may be some degree of persistent invalidism.

Properly speaking, postpartum care begins in the third stage of labor. The amount of blood lost in the placental period, especially after a long labor, is a determining factor in convalescence. Ergonovine given hypodermically immediately after the anterior shoulder of the baby is born will help to reduce the amount of blood lost. As soon as the placenta has been released from the uterine wall, it should be expressed. After the placenta is delivered, all lacerations of the perineum and cervix should be repaired, and, of course, if an episiotomy was done, it must be sutured at this time.

Since exhaustion is a factor in the type of recovery, in cases of prolonged labor one should assist delivery of the child in primigravidas when the head is visible, either by performing an episiotomy or by combining an episiotomy with an outlet forceps operation. The episiotomy is repaired immediately after the placenta is delivered. If a patient is actually exhausted, it is safer to postpone the repair of lacerations or an episiotomy for 24 or more hours because the added anesthesia may unfavorably influence the patient's condition. Regional anesthesia should be used for the delivery of many obstetric patients, especially those with toxemia and respiratory infections and those who are to deliver a premature baby or twins.

The Puerperium

The puerperal period begins after delivery of the placenta, and it does not end until all the organs of reproduction have returned to their normal status. This period usually lasts from 6 to 8 weeks but may require much longer. It is generally divided into a strictly lying-in interval, which lasts from 3 to 6 days, and a further interval of 4 to 7 weeks, during which the patient gradually resumes her usual activities and at the end of which she returns to her physician for the so-called final examination.

The Lying-In Period

Immediately after delivery, the mother requires rest; this should be secured preferably with the aid of a sedative. Visitors should be barred and the baby should not be brought into the patient's room for at least 3 hours after birth. In the hospitals that have rooming-in, the mother and baby are in the same room for psychologic and other reasons.

Involution takes place not only in the uterus but also in all the tissues of the pelvis, in the ureters and in the abdominal wall. Conditions that may hinder involution are infection and relaxation of the pelvic tissue from lacerations. If permanent pathologic conditions remain, the patient complains of pain, leukorrhea, and abnormal bleeding.

Vulvar pads are not at all necessary but if used should be applied loosely; otherwise, they might carry infection by damming up the lochia and by forcing fecal matter up on the vulva. The pads should be changed after each urination and bowel movement and whenever soiled from any other cause. Douches should never be given.

The patient should be encouraged to urinate as soon as she is refreshed; every effort should be made to avoid the necessity for catheterization. There is no harm in having a patient go to the toilet, especially if it is connected with her room. This should be tried before a catheter is used. If catheterization is necessary, it should be carried out under strict aseptic precautions. Even after the patient begins to void spontaneously, she should be catheterized once a day immediately after a spontaneous urination, until less than 100 ml. of urine is obtained. This is to drain off the residual urine, which may become infected. Women who are catheterized should be given one of the sulfonamides or a combination of them for 5 or 6 days, as a prophylactic against infection.

For a painful episiotomy wound, a heat lamp or sitting in a tub of hot water for 30 minutes several times a day is most helpful. There is no harm whatever, but there is considerable relief from sitting in hot water.

There should be a bowel movement daily or every second day. Proper diet, Metamucil, and milk of magnesia may help to secure this result.

The diet should consist chiefly of liquids on the first day, but after this a regular diet may be given. With few reservations the patient may have almost any kind of food she desires. A diet rich in proteins may be conducive to an abundant supply of milk.

Women who have had toxemia during pregnancy should be watched carefully after delivery because, in about one fourth of eclamptic patients, the convulsions begin for the first time during the early puerperium. Hence patients who have had any signs or symptoms of toxemia during pregnancy should have, during the lying-in period, a bi-daily blood pressure reading and a daily examination of the urine. Patients who have had pyelonephritis during pregnancy should also have a daily urinalysis during the lying-in period. A sulfonamide or antibiotic should be given for a few days to prevent a recurrence.

Sedatives should be given for after-pains, which seldom last more than 48 hours. If severe after-pains occur in a primipara, one should suspect the retention of blood clots or placental tissue in the uterus or the presence of an infection. Sedatives with hot milk should also be given to secure sufficient sleep because insomnia is frequently a forerunner of puerperal insanity. Toxemic patients especially should be watched for signs of insanity.

All patients with infection should be isolated immediately. Fluids and nourishment should be forced to build up the patient's resistance. The sulfonamides and antibiotics are necessary in serious cases. The perineum should always be inspected when fever develops, and if stitches are present they should be removed. A vaginal examination should be made, but with extreme gentleness and cultures made from the cervix.

Bleeding that occurs during the lying-in period is usually due to subinvolution, retention of secundines, and/or infection. The treatment consists of rest in bed and the administration of ergot or ergonovine by mouth. The uterus should be curetted if the bleeding is severe.

The normal patient is encouraged to move freely in bed from the first day on. I urge nearly all of my patients to get out of bed the day after delivery, even those who have had a cesarean section or a gynecologic laparotomy, especially if they cannot urinate while they are in bed. Many of my patients who cannot urinate while in bed may get up a few hours after a delivery or an operation for this purpose. I have not observed any bad results from this procedure, which I have used for more than 35 years. However, a patient who bleeds considerably should not get out of bed until the bleeding ceases.

During the first day up, the patient walks to the bathroom as often as necessary. Beginning on the second day up, she may walk as much as she pleases. The patient may leave for home any time after the baby is 4 days old.

Recuperative Period

On her return home the patient may walk up the steps slowly. She should remain in bed for about 15 minutes. She should not go out for a ride or walk until the child is a week old. Baths should be taken daily. During the recuperative period, a tactful attempt should be made to keep away oversolicitous friends and relatives. After the second week, the patient should leave her home for 1 or 2 hours each day. Normal activities are resumed gradually. Social functions should be held to a minimum.

During the first few weeks, the patient's mental condition should be watched, because the strict routine of caring for a newborn baby, especially in a small apartment, may be too much for some women, especially primiparas. Fear of immediate conception may also play a role. Half of the obstetric psychoses appear for the first time during the puerperium. Hyperthyroidism, pulmonary tuberculosis, and cholecystitis frequently flare up after childbirth, hence they should be watched for.

The patient should return for an examination when the baby is 6 to 8 weeks old. At this time the physician should determine the condition of the breasts, the abdominal wall, the perineum, the bladder and rectal supports, the size and position of the uterus, the condition of the adnexa and broad ligaments, and the tone of the sphincter ani. The cervix should be not only palpated but also inspected with a speculum under a good light. Any lacerations, eversions, so-called erosions, cysts, leukorrheal discharge, and any other abnormality should be observed. If a troublesome discharge is present, it should be treated at this time.

Retroversion of the uterus is found in approximately 20% of all puerperal women, but this is about the same incidence noted among all unmarried women without a history of pelvic infection, pelvic tumor, or pregnancy. Hence uncomplicated retroversion requires no treatment.

If bleeding occurs during the recuperative period, it is usually the result of subinvolution. Rest in bed and ergot by mouth usually suffice to check this bleeding. However, if the uterus is retroverted, the bleeding may not cease until the uterus is elevated and a pessary inserted in the vagina. This treatment is rarely necessary.

The return of menstruation varies in different individuals. In those who do not nurse their babies, the menses usually return in 6 weeks, whereas in those who do nurse their children, the first period generally appears after the third or fourth month. In some women, however, it does not return until the baby is weaned. Since the first menstrual period is often profuse and prolonged, the patient should be warned about this to avoid alarm. Rest in bed will help.

If the cervix is red and granular and bleeds when touched or excessive or irritating discharge is present, the simplest and most efficient therapy is electrocautery. However, this treatment should be postponed until the baby is 4 months old. (See Chapter 13.)

It is important that all cervical pathologic processes be treated, otherwise the result may be chronic endocervicitis and cervicitis that ends in cyst formation, fibrosis, and hypertrophy. Annoying symptoms may follow. Furthermore, active treatment of the cervix after childbirth may prevent subsequent cancer of the cervix, because there may be some relationship between local trauma of the cervix and carcinoma even if the individual's constitution or endocrine glands play a role in this type of cancer.

Postpuerperal Period

Most physicians speak of the examination that is made 6 or 8 weeks after delivery as the "final" examination. This is unfortunate, because both the physician and the patient regard it as the last contact until a new pregnancy begins. Although a large proportion of women are in such good condition that they need not return to the physician until a new pregnancy occurs, many women unfortunately are not in this category. Some patients have subinvolution, cervical pathology, pyelitis, nephritis, heart disease, high blood pressure, and other medical complications which require careful observation and treatment. It is gross negligence not to continue to see these patients until their abnormalities are relieved as much as possible. Such observation and treatment usually must extend over a few months or even longer. Occasionally the examination made at the end of 6 or 8 weeks reveals no abnormality, whereas an examination made later does. Hence it is advisable to make another examination at the end of 6 months. Patients will be even better cared for if they are again examined when the child is 1 year old. In this age of prophylaxis, women should be educated to come for an examination, especially of the breasts and pelvic organs, at least once but preferably twice a year. Were this a universal custom, much invalidism and many deaths from cancer of the breasts, uterus and ovaries would be avoided. Women should be acquainted with this fact. Papanicolaou smears should be examined once a year in all women, young and old, pregnant or otherwise.

Oral Contraceptives

Also under the heading of Prophylactic Gynecology, I include the care of adolescent girls who use oral contraceptives. In spite of the fact that the great majority of these girls are in good health, a careful history must be taken to find out if the girl had or has any illness that is a contraindication to the use of oral contraceptives. Also, the same thorough examination must be made as is done in older women. This includes examination of the breasts, a bimanual vaginoabdominal examination, a specular examination of the cervix, a rectoabdominal examination, and, of course, Papanicolaou smears, made immediately after inserting the speculum. Such an examination must be made once a year, and this admonition should be emphasized. It is perhaps advisable to stop the use of the oral contraceptives for 2 to 4 months after a 2-year period to permit at least one ovulation to occur before resuming their use. Of course, during the time the oral contraceptives are not used, another form of contraception is mandatory.

There is absolutely no proof that the oral contraceptives lead to carcinomatous changes in the cervix. However, we must remember that young girls using the oral contraceptives generally have sexual intercourse with many different males, and this form of sex activity may lead indirectly to changes in the cervix, such as dysplasia and carcinoma-in-situ.

Teen-age and Unwed Mothers-To-Be

Teen-age and unwed mothers constitute a surprisingly large percentage of pregnant women, both in private practice and in public institutions. One third to one half of all high-school or teen-age marriages in the United States are associated with premarital pregnancies. Between 1960 and 1968, from 35 to 45% of the births in the United States resulted from unwanted pregnancies, according to a report issued by the Princeton University Office of Population Research. This is a remarkably high figure.

The increasing total number of out-of-wedlock births is not only because the rate is increasing, but also and especially because the total population is increasing enormously.

Problems arising from out-of-wedlock births are not new. They have been with us throughout civilization; but society has been increasingly aware of such social problems for generations, and now is beginning to face them.

Unwed mothers must be given special consideration because they are both young and pregnant. Many teen-age girls promptly drop out of school when they become pregnant, perhaps never to return for further education. These young mothers-to-be should continue some of their studies while they are pregnant and also after the baby arrives. Special courses can and should be arranged. Furthermore, they must not be rebuked or punished. They need and should have abundant empathy, help, understanding, and moral and material support.

In the hands of competent physicians in well-equipped and well-staffed hospitals, young pregnant girls have few physical problems. However, their bodies differ somewhat from older women. They gain more weight; the pelvis is smaller in about a fourth of the pregnant girls 16 years old or younger. However, the incidence of cesarean section is far lower, despite the small pelvis in many of them. The average duration of labor for young pregnant women is shorter than for older women. Premature labor and infant mortality are more frequent among younger women. The average weight of newborn babies of teen-age mothers is not different from that of other babies.

An Adolescent Guidance Program has been developed at Mount Sinai Hospital, New York, N.Y. The initial analysis was based on experiences with

135 pregnant teen-agers, mostly from broken homes, who had little awareness of contraception and were largely ignorant of the physiology of sex. These were the conclusions reached:

1. A comprehensive hospital-based program in a separate hospital unit improves the adolescent unwed mother's status.

2. Among adolescent pregnancies, antepartum and intrapartum complications are reduced, as are the normal anxieties of pregnancy, but intercurrent disease is high, especially iron-deficiency anemia, bronchitis, and inactive tuberculosis.

3. The pregnant adolescent increases the economic problems of the broken homes in the disadvantaged environment from which she comes.

4. Adolescents fail to recognize early pregnancy, and hide it later when they know.

5. None used contraception; 71% requested it in various forms after receiving instruction. Inadequate sex instruction was a factor in the occurrence of the pregnancy.

6. Patients were normally intelligent, but emotionally disturbed; pregnancy was more than a sexual accident.

7. The adolescent frequently returns to school, but her educational career is nevertheless affected.

8. Marital Health Clinics for those requiring it, especially adolescent out-of-wedlock pregnant women, would be helpful.

Office Pediatric Gynecology

In the past 30 years tremendous advances have been made in the physician's knowledge and understanding of the relation of parental and family environment and genital hypersensitivity of the young girl patient. Every physician who treats female children should be aware of the unique aspects of pediatric gynecology.

The sensory response by the majority of young girls to touch in the genital area is peculiar. Even a light touch with a cotton applicator almost always causes a response as to pain, fear, or anger, and seldom to the simple light touch that it is. Failure to respect this response may result in serious consequences in relation to therapy and later may have psychosexual repercussions. This sensory response is apt to be nonexistent at birth, is only slightly developed in infancy and early childhood, and is most highly developed between the ages of 4 and 9. It is often reasonably controlled after age 9. Its absence in the neonatal period and infancy makes thorough examination painless and easy.

Every newborn girl should be given a careful examination of the external genitalia, rectum, meatus, hymenal orifice, and vagina (gentle exploration with a blunt probe). Such an examination, aided by the little finger in the rectum, is entirely harmless and may be exceedingly helpful.

Routine Pelvic Examinations

The advisability of routine pelvic examinations of children from 4 to 11 years, is still moot, and there is no accepted standard for such examinations in adolescence and the later teens. A careful external examination to make sure of hymenal patency and genital normality, combined with a rectal examination, is sufficient except in the presence of serious indications.

As for complete pelvic examinations, much has been accomplished by those who have so examined many young girls aged 11 years and older. Certainly, if there are strict indications, there is no reason to avoid such an examination, which can, if necessary, be done under general anesthesia. Figures 22 and 23 demonstrate the differences seen in such examinations of young females and of adults. *Rectal examination*, as a matter of fact, is often not only less disturbing but actually more revealing, as described and depicted in Figure 23.

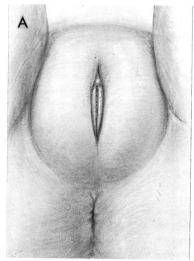

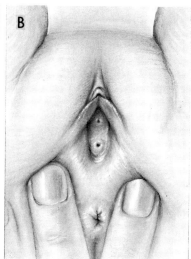

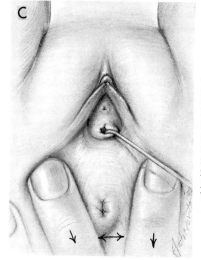

Fig. 22.—Visual examination of small children. **A,** in contrast to adult type, structures are prominent, protective hair is lacking, etc. **B,** first two fingers of left hand separate vulvar structures, producing pressure laterally and posteriorly (arrows in **C**). Child strains, pouting the cufflike hymen. Sharply curved probe aids in identification of hymenal orifice. (Figs. 22–24, 26, 27 and 29, from Shauffler, G. C.: *Pediatric Gynecology* [4th ed.; Chicago: Year Book Medical Publishers, Inc., 1958].)

EQUIPMENT AND SUPPLIES.—A convenient minimal set-up for attention to young patients may be arranged on a special tray. The usual gynecologic table is satisfactory. The physician should sit immediately adjacent to the exposure. Older girls can use the regular stirrups and young ones can be held satisfactorily by a trained attendant. Many physicians prefer to have the child in the knee-chest position. Instruments should be under cover until used, as their display, especially of metal ones, may frighten the child. Certain special

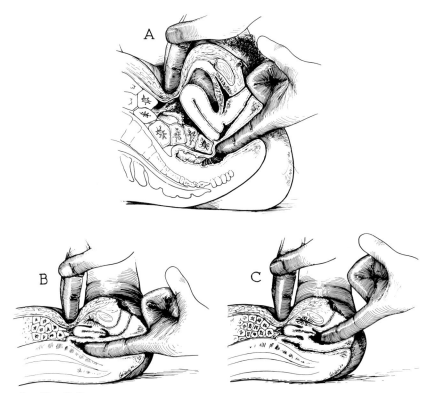

FIG. 23.—Different spatial relationships and size of organs on pelvic examination of adult, **A,** and infant, **B** and **C. A,** rectal examination in adult, showing greater ease of differentiating structures because of size, mobility, depth of culdesac, etc. **B,** rectal examination in infant, showing closely packed, firm tissues and organs, and deeper relative penetration from below. **C,** vaginal examination in child; difficult in infants and younger children and less instructive than rectal examination.

preparations are important. (Quoted with many changes from G. C. Schauffler, *Pediatric Gynecology* [4th ed.; Chicago: Year Book Medical Publishers, Inc., 1958].)

1. Cotton or wool applicators for smears should be carefully and tightly wrapped, as any loose cotton in the vagina may cause discomfort and require vaginoscopy for its removal. A small glass catheter with saline in the tip serves for obtaining material for bacteriologic examination. It may be fitted to a syringe by tubing, or a fine-pointed, rubber-bulb syringe may be used to obtain a saline inoculum for instillations or vaginal lavage.

2. Smooth rounded metal or glass instruments cause less discomfort than cotton or wool applicators. Thus, a fairly large probe, glass catheter, or sound can be passed without difficulty, whereas a tiny, tightly wrapped applicator

may be irritating. All metal and glass instruments should be warmed before use.

3. Gloves and an aseptic technic are, as always, essential.

4. Vaginoscopes of two sizes (no. 30 and 22 of the Boehm female urethro-scope) are adequate for visual vaginal examination of young girls; in older ones, the Huffman infant Graves-type speculum (Mueller) may be used. There is a larger size for teenagers. When special instruments are not available, a nasal speculum is satisfactory. Special wire wings to extend the blades are particularly helpful. Apparatus with a fine-bore cannula or small catheter for irrigation and syringes for suction of secretions or lavage through the urethro-scope should be available. A cystoscopy grasping forceps is useful for removing foreign bodies through the urethroscope and under vision.

ROUTINE VISUAL EXAMINATION (Fig. 22).—An established routine and con-fidence grounded in thorough knowledge of anatomy are essential for even a superficial examination. Failure to identify the urethra and the hymenal orifice has resulted in mistaken invasion of the urethra and even the injection into the urethra of medication intended for the vagina. Furthermore, unskilled attempts to pierce an imperforate hymen or minute hymenal orifice jeopard-izes the physician's status with the patient and her parents.

Valuable evidence relative to the nature of secretion or discharge may be destroyed if bathing or local cleansing of the vulvar area is not forbidden within 6 or more hours before examination. Parents should be instructed to bring soiled garments for inspection; also, the crotch of the garment the child is wearing should be examined.

The Vulva

The vulva is exposed as indicated in Figure 22; the differences from the appearance in maturity are seen in Figure 24. Generally pouting, fatty labia, reasonably protective, are the rule, although in undernourished children there may be little such protection. Inefficient genital and rectal hygiene, careless toilet hygiene, and a child's general rough-and-tumble existence account for many local irritations and rashes. Vulvar irritations are occasionally associated with pinworms, and the urine of diabetes may cause an otherwise unexplained vulvitis. Also always to be considered is chronic congestion from masturbation or manipulation by another person. Too often a primary infection is diagnosed, when actually the foregoing sources are causative. In fact, primary and secondary vulvar infections are rare. Small areas of ulceration, comedones, or true furuncles may occur in the vulva, as elsewhere.

Injuries in the genital area bleed easily and profusely but seldom for long. Healing proceeds with astonishing rapidity, and the restoration of normal contour seems to be akin to the reparative capacity of tissues at childbirth.

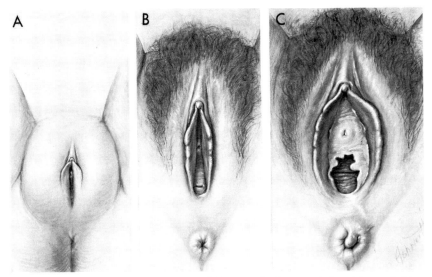

FIG. 24.—A, prepuberal habitus; B, virginal habitus (artificial exposure); C, multiparous habitus (artificial exposure).

Hematomas, which may become massive owing to the cavernous nature of the venous distribution, form rapidly. The prompt application of pressure with cold packs is helpful. Sometimes it may be wise to evacuate large hematomas by small incisions, particularly if there is pus from subsequent infection. If there is serious concern about the bleeding, deeply inclusive, nonabsorbable mattress-type sutures may be tied loosely and removed in 24 hours.

Tumors of the vulva before adolescence are rare. Carcinoma botryoides of the cervix often rapidly involves the vulva and may be first noted there. Actually, malignancy, like any new growth, is rare.

The hypoestrogenic phase of childhood has been recognized as the background for some puzzling and troublesome vulvar irregularities. The epithelium of the vagina and of the vulva is similarly affected. Aside from the irritation caused by discharge from this type of "senile vaginitis," there is an inherent fragility and lack of resistance, which is occasionally manifested as chronic vulvar dystrophy, and transverse agglutination of the labia.

Lichen sclerosus et atrophicus, which is not rare in children, reflects the low estrogenic concentration of childhood, just as it does in senility. Use of estrogen ointment or diethylstilbestrol by mouth is indicated, together with emollient washes and meticulous hygiene supervised by doctor and parent. Pruritus is seldom present in children. The condition is self-limited by puberty, or even earlier.

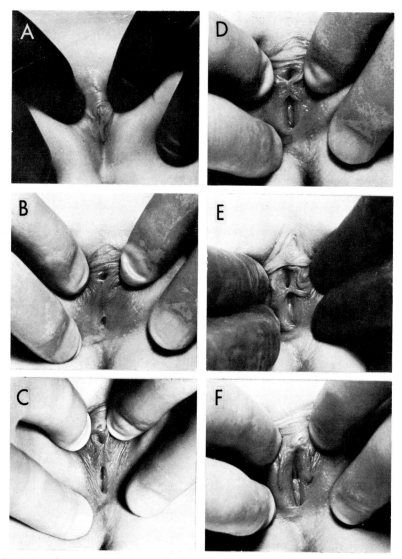

FIG. 25.—Therapy in typical case of adhesions of labia minora in girl, aged 5. **A,** before treatment; **B,** after 10 days of therapy; **C,** after 14 days; **D,** after 18 days; **E,** after 21 days; **F,** complete resolution after 24 days of therapy. (Courtesy of B. H. Williams and C. J. Cramm, Jr., South. M. J. 50:573, 1957.)

Transverse agglutination of the labia is best explained as epithelial fragility in the apposed and often frictional surfaces of the labia majora. The condition is often called adhesive vulvitis, but vulvitis is a misnomer because often primary infection is not present. The condition is ascribed to estrogen deprivation during infancy and childhood. This theory is borne out by study of epithelial smears and the effectiveness of estrogen therapy and by regression of the condition with the normal upsurge of estrogen during adolescence. Failure to separate eroded areas and lack of satisfactory hygiene allow bridging by serum and actual transverse agglutination, perhaps even in a more actual sense than adhesions of the foreskin (Fig. 25). This condition has led to the diagnosis of absence of the vagina or some other genital anomaly. It has been managed successfully with stilbestrol by mouth and with local application of estrogen with or without traction separation. Many minor instances of this condition are self-limited in the same sense that an adherent foreskin may be. However, urinary difficulties and other local complications frequently necessitate traction separation, under local anesthesia.

Williams and Cramm resolve the adhesions by daily topical applications of 5,000 units of an estrogenic ointment (Menformon Dosules); this procedure is continued for as long as necessary (Fig. 25). The child should be seen at intervals of 3 or 4 months for at least a year.

The Clitoris

If the normal or pathologic clitoris were not involved in masturbation or other psychosexual concerns of childhood, it would remain *terra incognita*. Even in masturbation, the clitoris is involved less specifically than general opinion indicates. Its injury, irritation, or infection requires the same considerations as vulvar injuries at later ages. Adherent foreskin with smegma retention is occasionally bothersome.

Simple hypertrophy of the clitoris (not an intersex anomaly) in the presence of an otherwise normal female habitus may occasionally require plastic surgery for esthetic reasons (Fig. 26). Special attention must be paid to other intersex characteristics (see Chapter 29).

The Hymen

The several types of hymen and hymenal orifice are shown in Figure 27, and differences from the adult appearance in Figure 24. Sentiment regarding the hymen has blocked rational management of genital irregularities for far too long. It is not the flat occlusive diaphragm described in many texts. On the contrary, it is a cufflike, generally fairly thick, fleshy, vascular membrane which protrudes its orifice when the child strains, coughs or cries.

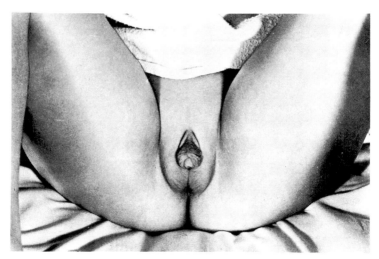

FIG. 26.—Simple hypertrophy of clitoris of a girl, 6, not associated with demonstrable intersex trends. Partial circumcision and conservative partial wedge resection were done for esthetic reasons.

The hymenal orifice, usually at or near the center of the hymen, has an amazing number of variations (Fig. 27). Knowledge of its exact location is imperative if the vagina is to be examined. Its unusual characteristics may occasionally suggest underlying congenital anomalies; for example, a symmetrical bilateral arrangement, as in **D** of Figure 27, may indicate a double anomaly of the uterus or the vagina.

The significance of an imperforate hymen should be recognized, for attempts to introduce instruments may have unhappy results. Although its correction in childhood is not necessary, knowledge of its existence is important before adolescence. Thus, examination of all babies neonatally will prevent trying, sometimes tragic, episodes in later life from hematocolpos and hematometra because of gynatresia. Simple dilatation, even with rupture of the hymen, is seldom permanent or satisfactory for an imperforate hymen. A wedge or square segment must be excised out to the circumference.

The Vagina

During infancy and childhood, the depth of the vagina varies from 1 to $1\frac{1}{2}$ in., with a potential distensibility to $\frac{1}{2}$ in., to a postpuberal size of 2–3 in. along the anterior wall and sometimes as much as 3–5 in. along the posterior wall. The infantile cavity is tiny, rugose, and cryptiform. Its complicated walls preclude patency, acting much as wet paper, and even when folded, stick

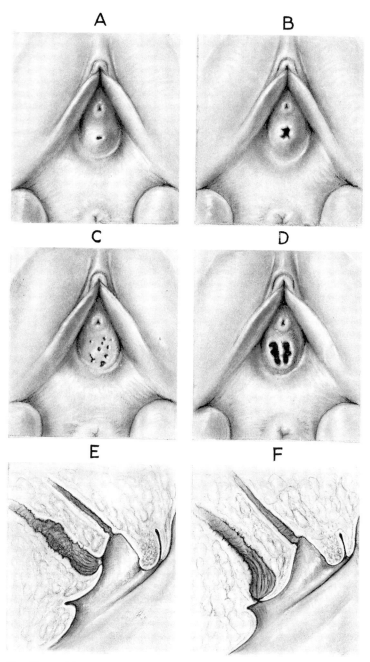

FIG. 27.—Types of hymen in immature subjects. **A,** punctate; **B,** normal; **C,** cribriform; **D,** septate; **E,** sagittal—long thin posterior lip; **F,** sagittal—long thick anterior lip.

together. Thus it is easy to understand why the vagina in early childhood is an almost ideal "harbor of infection."

The neonatal vaginal epithelium, under maternal hormone influence, has the thick, succulent, squamous characteristics of estrogenic smears, with a comparatively alkaline pH and prevalent Döderlein bacilli. The subsequent hypoestrogenic phase of childhood is characterized by decreased epithelial proliferation, a thinning at times almost to the point of subfunction, a tendency to an acid pH, and receptivity to various, often acidophilic, bacteria. This hypoestrogenic status accounts for the conditions mentioned earlier in relation to the vulva. A condition in otherwise normal children may be scarcely distinguishable from "senile vaginitis" which is not primarily due to bacterial invasion, frequently causes stubborn vaginal discharge and consequent vulvar irritation, and is too often diagnosed as "nonspecific vaginal infection."

With the beginning of adolescence, as estrogen levels rise, the epithelium becomes thicker and sturdier, occasionally causing a white curdlike vaginal discharge, mistakenly called premenstrual, which is essentially normal. The bacterial flora begins to change because of increased estrogen levels, external influences (manipulation), instrumentation, and use of tampons. In general, the vagina, though virginal, may be expected to have become mature considerably before actual ovulation.

Precocious changes in the vagina toward the adult status are definitely affected by the early approach of young girls to adult practices: use of tampons, experimentation or actual sex practice, examinations or instrumentation, and even pregnancy.

The VAGINITIS most frequently noted is caused by the hypoestrogenic status just described. There is an irritating, stubborn, thinnish vaginal discharge with mild to severe vulvitis, a thin-appearing, reddened, occasionally telangiectatic vaginal wall, and unrecognizable bacteria. For treatment, estrogen, 1 mg. diethylstilbestrol orally is indicated, preferably at bedtime for 14 days, or less if symptoms disappear. Diethylstilbestrol has fewer side effects in children than in adults, is cheap and its results are reliable.

The insertion of estrogen ointment, 0.5 ml. in infants and 1 or 2 ml. in older children, is facilitated by special tips° for tubes; also, appropriately sized suppositories are available. Local application can seldom be carried out satisfactorily at home. Initial treatment should be uninterrupted for at least 2 weeks. Combined treatment with sulfonamides or antibiotics orally may be advisable if the presence of any organism is proved or suspected by cultures or sensitivity tests. Several courses of treatment may be necessary, because this vaginitis is exceedingly stubborn. Reassurance and local hygiene may, however, be all that is necessary. Infectious vaginitis, except gonorrheal, is almost never clearly identified.

° Sheffield Tube Company, New London, Conn.

Gonorrheal vaginitis is almost nonexistent, except in outpatient clinic practice in large cities. It is effectively treated with antibiotics or sulfonamides orally and is far less troublesome than the nonspecific type just described.

The drug of choice for gonorrheal vulvovaginitis in children is penicillin, 10,000 units of crystalline procaine penicillin in aqueous suspension per pound of body weight up to 1,200,000 units a day on 3 successive days. This course may be repeated. If given orally, the doses are 100,000–250,000 units 4 times a day before meals and at bedtime. (The best method of detecting gonorrhea is by culture on Transgrow. See Chapter 11 for treatment of gonorrhea in adults.)

Trichomonas infection is uncommon before puberty, even in teenagers, except when vaginal changes have occurred because of use of tampons, precocious sex experimentation, and the like. Treatment is the same as in adults (p. 83). Oral medication with Flagyl (Searle) is apparently as effective and as harmless in young patients as in older ones.

Foreign bodies in the vagina are common. Except for lost tampons, they are found most often in girls aged 3–7, most of whom are normal youngsters with an overdeveloped exploratory bent, the kind of child who would insert

Fig. 28.—Causes of genital bleeding in childhood.

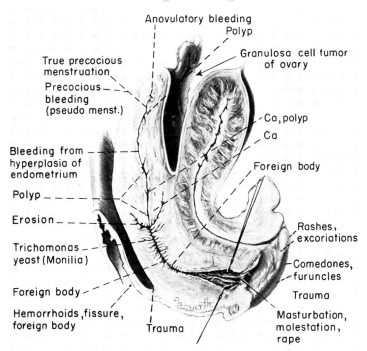

objects into the nose, ear, or rectum. However, few of these children will admit, especially prior to proof, that they have been up to such mischief. Therefore, the physician should be wary and thus avoid making the too frequent misdiagnosis of infectious vaginitis or possible malignancy.

A bloody component in a persistent or recurrent vaginal discharge is, especially if accompanied by an unpleasant odor, almost pathognomonic of vaginal foreign body. A resultant vulvitis may be confusing; if pain is present, it is most often the result of the foreign body piercing the delicate tissues of the vagina. Other causes of genital bleeding during childhood are shown in Figure 28.

Diagnosis is greatly facilitated by an examination made with a warm metal sound in the vagina and a finger in the rectum. The foreign body can generally be palpated with the sound as it passes up the vagina. On a tightly wrapped applicator, portions of fibrous material or colored substances such as red crayon, lipstick, and the like may adhere. Roentgenograms, only when essential, may reveal opaque foreign bodies. Vaginoscopy is frequently simple and helpful, and vaginal irrigation may wash out portions of soft material, seeds, and so on. Surgery is seldom required for removal of hard objects, and anesthesia is usually unnecessary. The aftermath depends on the trauma involved and whether infection has supervened; the general prognosis is excellent.

The Cervix

Up to puberty the cervix is a tiny, clam-necked structure. Things to remember about the immature cervix are: (1) that it is extremely small, even in older children; (2) that its vaginal portion shares in the cryptiform convoluted character of the rest of the vagina; and (3) that the endocervix up to midpuberty has none of the complicated epithelial structure of the adult cervix or endometrium. Fluhmann has demonstrated that the immature endocervix does not have glands and that an initial pseudoglandular structure develops from the troughlike convolutions similar to those in the vagina. This is important, because persistent or primary infection in the immature cervix is even less likely than in the vagina. This is the reverse of the adult situation and explains why primary vaginitis predominates during childhood and primary endocervicitis after maturity.

So-called congenital erosions of the cervix do occur in immature individuals, especially older girls. The pathologic process involves the delicate, single-layered cervical mucosa—ectopic in the vaginal portion of the cervix, when it becomes exposed to unfavorable vaginal adult events such as use of tampons, self-manipulation, and examinations. In such circumstances the condition may become "activated," and therapy as for an adult may be required. It rarely is the cause of bleeding or vaginal discharge.

The Uterus and Ovaries

The gross characteristics of the immature uterus are shown in Figure 29. Its lag in growth during childhood and its amazing "catching-up" phase during puberty have not been sufficiently appreciated. The uterus may be 3 cm. or smaller, up to age 11 or 12. If, on examination, such a uterus is not felt and no tumors, tenderness, fixation, or other abnormalities are noted, the patient is, by defensible inference, normal. Even when the child has been anesthetized, findings on pelvic examination may be unsatisfactory and relatively inferior to those on rectal examination. Naturally, this situation changes as the child grows into maturity.

Fig. 29.—Gross development of uterus to maturity. **A** and **E**, infantile habitus. Cervix comprises two thirds, corpus one third of total length. **B** and **F**, uterus at 3 years; **C** and **G**, at 10 years. Infantile habitus prevails. **D** and **H**, adult uterus. From 10 years to maturity, corpus increases in relative size (two-thirds) while cervix decreases (one-third).

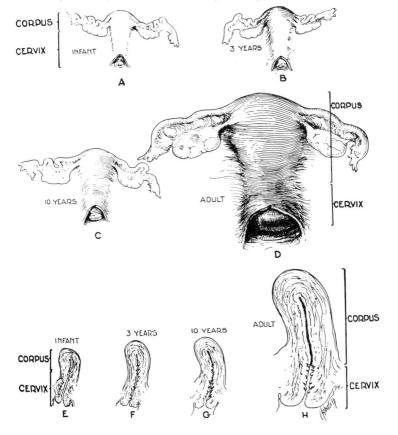

Changes in the uterus during childhood, exclusive of those of beginning menstruation, are not numerous. Precocious bleeding is due occasionally to estrogen-producing tumors but more often to sex precocity, which includes so-called constitutional sex precocity with cyclic bleeding with or without ovulation at incredibly early ages and the pseudoprecocities due to tumors of the ovaries or adrenals or to certain cerebral abnormalities (see pp. 72 f.).

It is important to remember that cyclic and regular precocious bleeding is more apt to be important than irregular uterine bleeding, which, however, is not to be neglected.

Endometrial biopsy or curettage should never be withheld if there are serious indications. The possibility of cancer is always to be borne in mind, especially as girls become older.

Immature ovaries are almost never palpable. If an ovary is palpable in a child, it is abnormally large. Cysts, cystic or malignant teratomas occasionally develop in immature ovaries, rarely functional tumors such as the granulosa cell tumor.

Cryptomenorrhea and Vaginal Agenesis

Vaginal obstruction at the outlet, although it may not become obvious in childhood, is exceedingly important once ovulation is established, and its early discovery is essential. Imperforate hymen is, of course, the most frequent cause, although partial agenesis of the lower part of the vagina is occasionally responsible. If the internal genitalia are normal, the establishment of menses without an available escape channel is exceedingly dangerous.

Anomalies of the hymenal orifice, simulating an imperforate hymen, may cause confusion in children and even in teenagers, so in any case of doubt, careful examination, under anesthesia if necessary, should always be conducted.

Vaginal agenesis, although it is not likely to be symptomatic until menstruation is established, is estimated to occur about once in 8,000 females. It is, interestingly, one of the more independent developmental anomalies in this area, with the young patient almost always a healthy, normal, female-appearing girl in all other respects. Although associated genital anomalies of the intersex type are rare, genitourinary anomalies occur sufficiently often to call for special genitourinary examinations when the condition is diagnosed.

Formerly, the diagnosis of vaginal agenesis was rarely established until the individual approached or passed the age of beginning menses. However, modern pediatric examination now often discloses this serious anomaly much earlier. Obstetricians and pediatricians should carry out routine investigation of female genitalia at birth, by simple and harmless exposure of the hymen and gentle sounding of the vagina neonatally.

These girls often have no uterus. Ovaries are usually present, occasionally normal and functional. Problems before and at the beginning of menstruation are therefore not emergent. But since these are otherwise functionally adequate and potential females, early attention must be given to the psychosomatic aspects of a proposed later operation to create a vagina satisfactory for coitus. The psychologic factors of such a situation are of the utmost importance, especially since as young women, they will not have the complete sexual impetus which is contingent on the prospect of childbirth. They must, therefore, prior to and for a considerable period after operation, be carefully conditioned and observed.

Double Anomalies

Double anomalies of the vagina and uterus should be discovered, if possible, before puberty. Much needless concern and numerous unnecessary operations due to misdiagnosis could be avoided if such conditions were understood prior to sex maturity and particularly prior to marriage and pregnancy. Here again, the child or young girl with these anomalies is apt to be in all other respects a thoroughly normal and functionally competent female.

A double hymenal opening, at any age, should suggest the possibility of vaginal septums, double vagina perhaps, or double cervix, double uterus, or other of the countless associated double anomalies (Fig. 30). Any septal irregularity of the vagina, even if it involves only the vault, and whether or not it is midline, longitudinal, or oblique, calls for careful investigation. The clinical management of vaginal septums is usually simple, provided further studies have ruled out double cervix or double uterus or both.

The first evidence of such anomalies may come at the first coitus, although even double vagina may not be obvious even to the marital partners. If there are subjective or coital impediments, surgical excision, which is seldom difficult or complicated, should be performed.

The more common and more serious complications of the double anomalies, especially double uterus, involve pregnancy. However, the most frequent and major concerns related to these anomalies are due to failure to diagnose them or to misdiagnosis. A second uterus is frequently mistaken for a leiomyoma, adnexal tumor, or ectopic pregnancy. Proper diagnosis is not difficult by the use of double sounding, and especially by hysterosalpingography (Fig. 31).

Sex Precocity

True sex precocity may include not only early uterine bleeding, either anovulatory or ovulatory (menstrual), but early maturation in the secondary sex characters and often in the attitudes and urges of femaleness, which may require special attention from a psychosomatic point of view.

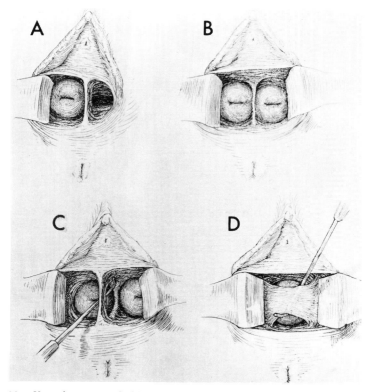

FIG. 30.—Vaginal septum in double anomalies. **A,** eccentric longitudinal septum with single cervix, double uterus. **B,** midline longitudinal septum with double cervix, double uterus. **C,** midline septum, fenestrated, with double cervix, double uterus. **D,** transverse septum not associated with double anomaly but caused by dyspareunia and dystocia. Exposure here is artificial, for clarification.

Precocious bleeding (before age 9) is the most common suggestive sign. Usually the children are otherwise normal. Interestingly, *cyclic* bleeding at this time, not irregular bleeding, is in contrast to irregular adult bleeding, and more important because it generally represents precocious ovulation. Irregular bleeding, on the other hand, unlike irregular adult bleeding, more often represents the less definitive precocities or some other cause of early bleeding, which must be excluded (see Fig. 28).

True sex precocity is generally designated (1) constitutional or (2) organic, although the terms isosexual and heterosexual are used by some. *Constitutional* precocity is by far the commoner and is characterized by more or less general precocious sexual development without apparent cause, as opposed to *organic* precocity, for which reasonable causes may be assigned. Apparently, in con-

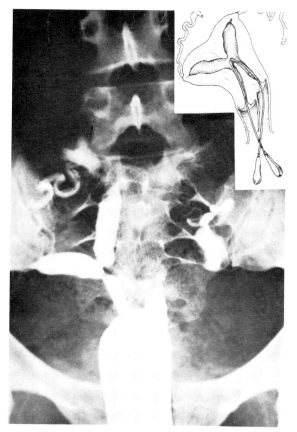

FIG. 31.—Hysterogram and drawing of double uterus.

stitutional cases, the hypothalamic-pituitary-ovarian axes operate efficiently, but on an advanced schedule, although there are usually related irregularities in target organs—uterus, ovaries, breasts.

These girls are generally taller at an earlier age than their contemporaries. Occasionally this is the first phenomenon to be noted. It is ascribed to the somatic early influence of the estrogenic growth impulse, whose effect is generally reversed in later years, so that these girls are apt, after the average age of puberty, to be shorter than normal, probably because continuing and accelerated estrogenic effect has caused early closure of the epiphyses.

Since the cause is unknown, treatment is not precise. However, it is encouraging that, provided environment and upbringing are satisfactorily directed, these children are likely to develop normally and to be capable of normal sex, marital, and maternal life later. Interestingly, too, the menopause in these individuals ordinarily starts at the average age. Therefore management involves continuous, conscientious efforts to see that the child is as well as possible attuned to her environment and does not develop psychotic stigmas as a result of maladjustment. Young girls who ovulate can become pregnant.

Organic sex precocity may be of the "cerebral type," ostensibly due to pressure from tumors or diseases in the region of the hypothalamus. Pituitary tumors and certain cerebral-meningeal disorders have also been blamed.

Granulosa cell tumor is one of the least common causes, but one most often suspected. It is frequently treated simply by removal of the affected ovary. However, because the 5–year mortality rate with this neoplasm is at least 25%, treatment should consist of total hysterectomy and bilateral salpingo-oophorectomy, followed by a course of deep x-ray therapy. In selected cases in very young girls, where the neoplasm is apparently confined in one ovary, only the involved ovary need be removed. There must be persistent follow-up for life because recurrences may be detected as long as 20 years after operation. Incidentally, girls under 15 and women over 40 have the lowest survival rates.

Estrogen medication before maturity, for whatever reasons, occasionally causes confusion in relation to precocity. It should be easily pinpointed as an artificial cause.

Aside from the true precocities, there occurs an inherent psychologic precocity—an exaggeration in the form of an accelerated and heightened sex interest at a very early age. Socially, this may assume exceedingly difficult proportions. In girls from 4 to 11, such a situation is often called to the physician's attention. The father or older brothers or any available male may be embarrassed by the child's overaffectionate advances. These girls frequently practice autoeroticism. All of this seems to have a purely psychogenic basis. Hormonal irregularities are not identifiable. It exists independently of parental and environmental influences. It may simply reflect a heightened and accelerated awareness of the sensual aspects of sex for which there is no rational explanation.

Genital Trauma

Trauma to the immature female genitalia is uncommon and is nearly always interpreted as being much worse than it actually is.

The most common injuries are, of course, external (vulvar)—a fall across the bar of a bicycle or a straddle injury from forceful contact with a sharp object. Ecchymosis is more common and generally more extensive than elsewhere in the body because of the venous character of the tissues. Although bleeding occurs easily and may seem alarming at first, it is fortunately apt to be self-limited or easily controlled. Early application of pressure to the area with a cold pack is often all that is needed. Abrasions or lacerations should be cleansed immediately with a mild antiseptic detergent. Although suturing may seem advisable, it is less often necessary here than elsewhere. When bleeding is considerable, widely placed, lightly tied tension sutures may be desirable, to be removed within 24 hours or sooner. If there is a deep wound produced by a metal or wood object, tetanus antitoxin should be given.

Deeper injuries are often the result of traumatic rape or attack (see following section). Young children obviously are more apt to suffer severe injuries than more mature youngsters. The initial injuries are likely to include rupture of the hymen and perhaps of the perineum or lacerations at other points in the introital circumference. Tears may enter the bladder or rectum or even invade the peritoneal cavity and injure the bowel.

In medicolegal or police cases involving assault, there are special obligations of the physician who first sees the patient. He may or may not notify the police at once, depending on the seriousness of the injury and the special circumstances. He will always do well, however, to secure specialized advice and not to assume any responsibilities beyond those that are necessary medically (see later).

Medicolegal Aspects

When sexual attack or rape is involved, immediate photographs of the injuries may be important legally. Washings in saline should be taken for identification of spermatozoa and possible gonorrheal infection.

Many physicians are not precise in their use of the various terms applied in sexual attack or molestation of immature females. Inexact statements to families or legal authority may cause considerable harm. Some of the terms are briefly defined here.

Sexual assault or *attack* is a general term meaning any actual or threatened, willful or offensive touching of the body (regardless of whether or not physical injury is sustained or actual contact is established). *Molestation*, a term which covers a multitude of sins, is unfortunately too frequently used. Because of its inexact connotations, it is wrongly considered to be synonymous with attack, assault, and even rape. Legally it is one of the lesser charges, even though minor injuries to the external genitalia or elsewhere are common.

Actually, complaints of this type are often mistakenly made to explain self-inflicted injury (forceful masturbation, forceful attempts to insert Tampax, etc.). The confusion arises because of unwillingness of the young patient to acknowledge the true cause. Increasingly, however, such injuries are due to precocious attempts at intercourse, often with the child's co-operation—later, of course, denied.

Rape is defined as actual sexual intercourse by violence, without the victim's consent. Even this definition is not exact in its connotations because coercion or persuasion of a female child to the performance of an act in which the aggressor assumes the passive role is vaguely undifferentiated under the term.

The question of *consent* enters at this point. Rape in general is considered a crime that requires the essential element of unwillingness, resistance, or attempted defense by the victim. However, in the case of females under the "age of consent" (different in various states, but average 15 years), this element of unwillingness or resistance is presumed by law, whether or not it has been present. The concept is based on the legal presumption that no child under the "age of consent" is capable of forming an adequate conception of the implications of the sexual act. So any evidence in such a case regarding willingness or compliance is inadmissible.

Contributing to the delinquency of a minor is again a too inclusive and too indefinite charge. Under this are most often mentioned heterosexual intercourse (extramarital), sodomy, fellatio, tactile stimulation of any erogenous zone of the body, exhibitionism, peeping, obscene talk, pornographic writing and illustrations. In the language of the statutes, these acts are "immoral." And any adult who induces overtly or by indiscretion their commission by a juvenile may be prosecuted on the charge. The definition of "a minor," incidentally, is not always clearly understood. The average age is 17 years or under, with some statutes making age distinctions between the sexes.

7

Diseases of the Vulva

DISEASES OF THE vulva are practically always diseases of the skin, because the vulva consists almost exclusively of skin and highly specialized structures. Since it is manifestly impossible to consider all vulvar lesions in this book, the commonest are briefly described.

By definition, the vulva is the external part of the organs of generation of the female, including the labia majora, the labia minora, the mons veneris, the clitoris, the perineal body, and the vestibule of the vagina.

DISEASES OF BLOOD VESSELS.—Diseases which affect the blood vessels include *varicose veins, hematoma, edema, elephantiasis,* and *angioneurotic edema.*

Varicose veins are the most common. They are usually associated with hemorrhoids or varicose veins in the lower extremities, and they occur much more often in pregnancy. Naturally, they increase in size when the patient stands up. They disappear when she lies down. Those that appear in pregnancy usually subside to a great extent after delivery.

A *hematoma* usually is the result of injury during labor but may occur in a nonpregnant person from rupture of a varix, a fall, or a blow with a sharp object. Treatment of a small hematoma is conservative, with local applications for relief of pain, but large hematomas must be opened and drained.

Edema of the labia is often associated with toxemia of pregnancy. In *angioneurotic edema* the cause must be sought. Usually it is an allergic reaction. *Elephantiasis* is usually due to obstruction of the lymph channels. If the swelling is not large, only local treatment need be used. However, if the mass is large, surgery is necessary.

DISEASES OF GLANDS.—*Bartholin's abscesses* and *cysts* arise from the Bartholin ducts and not from the glands. Generally only one abscess is present; the labium on the affected side is visibly swollen, inflamed, and exceedingly sensitive when touched. The patient usually has pain on walking, and coitus is almost out of the question. In most cases partial relief from pain can be obtained by the application of heat, but usually the abscess must be incised and drained. However, the abscess wall can be completely removed by Word's technic, marsupialization, or excision.

Small Bartholin duct cysts should be left alone. Large or painful ones should be removed by one of the aforementioned operations.

Inclusion cysts, often observed within the vagina, may also appear at the fourchette. These cysts are not due to obstruction of gland ducts but result from trauma of labor. They are usually small and may be either single or multiple. They, too, may be either left alone or removed surgically.

Sebaceous cysts are not uncommon. Small cysts need not be treated, but large ones should be removed. Great care must be taken to remove the entire capsule intact.

DISTURBANCES OF PIGMENTATION.—There is considerable pigment in the vulva, and this is particularly obvious in pregnancy. *Vitiligo* is infrequent. Since the cause is unknown, there is no specific treatment.

DERMATITIS.—Vulvar dermatitis varies considerably in etiology. Contact dermatitis (dermatitis venenata) may arise from true allergic sensitization or, more commonly, from primary irritation reactions. Offending materials include topical medications, antiseptics, and other chemicals. The process may be acute or chronic. Successful treatment depends upon elimination of the offending substance.

Various forms of *eczema* also affect the vulva. Treatment of these vulvar dermatitides depends upon the acuteness or chronicity of the process. Acute dermatitis is treated with bed rest, cool compresses, and soothing lotions. The more chronic processes are treated with creams or ointments frequently containing corticosteroids for topical use.

Psoriasis of the vulva is not common and is usually associated with psoriasis elsewhere. The lesions are usually brightly erythematous with a variable white scale and are symmetrically distributed. Treatment is not curative, but good results usually can be achieved through the use of topical corticosteroids.

Lichen planus is an inflammatory disease of the skin and mucous membranes. The characteristic skin lesions are angulated, flat, violaceous papules, whereas the mucosal lesions are usually white patches. Vulvar lichen planus is uncommon but must be differentiated from other white vulvar lesions, such as lichen sclerosis et atrophicus and leukoplakia (Chapter 35).

SYSTEMIC CONDITIONS AFFECTING THE VULVA.—The most common medical ailment that involves the vulva is *diabetes mellitus,* which produces not only an eruption and redness but also intense pruritus. Candida albicans infection is the cause of the pruritus in many cases of diabetes and therefore should always be looked for. Treatment should be directed to both the diabetes and the candidiasis (see Chapter 9).

ULCERS.—Vulvar ulcers are lesions of the skin in which there is local destruction of the whole thickness of the epidermis and part or all of the corium. There are essentially two types—*nonvenereal* and *venereal.* Among nonvenereal ulcers are so-called recurrent ulcers, ulcers due to bacterial infection, ulcers that appear during acute infectious diseases, ulcers from parasitic infection, and malignant ulcers. A well-known but rare type of ulcer is the ulcus vulvae acutum or Lipschütz ulcer.

VENEREAL DISEASES.—The lesions of syphilis are well known, as is also the treatment. Other venereal diseases affecting the vulva are chancroid, lympho-granuloma venereum, and granuloma inguinale.

Syphilis.—Primary syphilis in the female is often overlooked. Usually the lesion appears on the labia majora, the mons veneris, the clitoris, the four-chette, or the vaginal mucosa. The primary lesion or chancre is usually a flat, indurated, non-tender erythematous erosion. The vulva is a common site for the papules of secondary syphilis, condylomata lata.

Syphilis is detected by clinical signs and symptoms and also by one of the serologic tests for syphilis, such as the Kahn, Wassermann and VDRL tests. The disease must be treated adequately as soon as discovered. The following treatment is recommended for early syphilis: (1) benzathine penicillin-G, 2.4 million units total (1.2 million units in each buttock) by intramuscular injec-tion, or (2) PAM (procaine penicillin with 2% aluminum monostearate), 4.8 million units total, usually given as 2.4 million units at the first session and 1.2 million units at each of two subsequent injections, 3 days apart, or (3) aqueous procaine penicillin-G, 600,000 units daily for 8 days to a total of

FIG. 32.—Lymphogranuloma venereum.

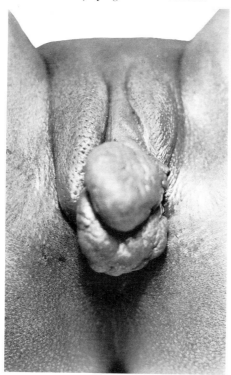

4.8 million units, or (4) alternate antibiotics. When penicillin sensitivity precludes the use of this drug of choice, erythromycin and tetracycline are the best substitutes. The recommended dosage is 20–30 Gm. of erythromycin or 30–40 Gm. of tetracycline given over a period of 10–15 days.

Lymphogranuloma venereum (Fig. 32) is due to a large virus in the Chlamydiaceae group. The primary lesion usually appears a few days after sexual exposure as a papule or a pustule on the vulva or, sometimes, in the vagina. In 1 to 3 weeks, there is lymphatic spread evidenced by the development of inguinal adenitis. The lymph nodes become painful and are matted together, and often there is suppuration with numerous draining sinuses. If the rectum is involved through the lymphatics, a stricture develops. There is often obstruction of the lymph channels with elephantiasis. The intradermal Frei test is specific for lymphogranuloma venereum, and it remains positive throughout life. For the Frei test, 0.1 ml. of antigen is injected intradermally on the forearm. A positive test is indicated by a papule 0.5 to 2 cm. in diameter surrounded by a circular reddened area. The maximum reaction appears in 48–72 hours. Several weeks may elapse after the onset of the disease before a positive reaction is obtained. Treatment of lymphogranuloma venereum is with tetracycline, 500 mg. every 6 hours for 15–30 days.

Granuloma inguinale (Fig. 33) is a chronic infectious granulomatous disease due to the gram-negative pleomorphic bacillus Klebsiella granulomatis (Donovania granulomatis). It is particularly common in the Negro race. The

FIG. 33.—Granuloma inguinale.

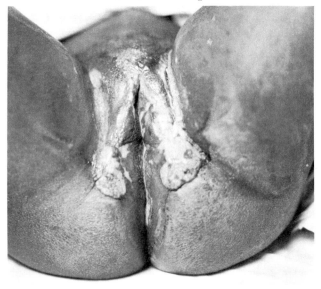

primary lesion is a circumscribed granulomatous nodule on the vulva, vagina, or cervix. The spread of this lesion is by direct extension and not through the lymphatics. The skin and mucous membranes are chiefly involved. The lesion is usually a red, exuberant granulomatous surface with serpiginous margins. The pathognomonic characteristic is the presence of Donovan bodies within large mononuclear cells. Treatment is with tetracycline, 500 mg. every 6 hours for 10–15 days, or streptomycin, 1 Gm. intramuscularly every 6 hours for 10–15 days.

Chancroid is a venereal infection due to the Ducrey bacillus (Haemophilus ducreyi). The primary lesion is a pustule or a papule surrounded by a vivid areola of inflammation, which may occur in the vestibule, in the fourchette, or in the labia minora. This develops into a soft chancre, which becomes punched out, necrotic, and purulent. Characteristically, the lesion is tender or painful. Frequently, the inguinal nodes suppurate. Treatment is with a soluble sulfonamide such as sulfisoxazole (Gantrisin), 3–4 Gm. a day for 1 week and 2 Gm. a day for an additional 1 or 2 weeks. Streptomycin may also be used at a dose of 1–2 Gm. every other day for 10–14 days.

BENIGN NEOPLASMS.—In this group are fibromas, condylomas, myomas, granular cell myoblastomas, lipomas, myxomas, and caruncles, all of which are easily removed surgically.

MALIGNANT DISEASES.—The commonest is carcinoma, and the most frequent type is squamous cell carcinoma. Treatment is radical vulvectomy and bilateral lymphadenectomy. An exception to the high degree of malignancy of cancer of the vulva is the basal cell type. This generally responds to wide excision.

Carcinoma of the clitoris, of Bartholin's glands, and of sweat glands may also occur. All of these are highly malignant and require extensive surgical therapy.

There are two types of intraepidermal carcinoma, namely Paget's disease and Bowen's disease. In both, wide excision of the vulva must be performed.

BACTERIAL DISEASES.—These include furuncles, carbuncles, folliculitis, impetigo, and erysipelas, all of which must be treated as elsewhere in the body. For gonorrheal infections, see Chapter 11. Other infections of the vulva are acute and chronic urethritis, acute and chronic skenitis, and vulvo-vaginitis. All these infections are discussed in other parts of this book.

Tuberculosis of the vulva is rare and may have to be treated surgically. However, dihydrostreptomycin, isoniazid, and para-aminosalicylic acid may be curative (see p. 179).

DISEASES DUE TO FILTRABLE VIRUSES.—Diseases of the vulva due to filtrable viruses include *warts, herpes zoster,* or *shingles; herpes simplex,* and *molluscum contagiosum.* Toluidine blue may be used to stain lesions of the vulva.

The commonest wart is *condyloma acuminatum,* also known as a moist wart or a venereal wart, although the condition is not venereal. Treatment is discussed in Chapter 12.

8

Trichomonas Vaginalis Vaginitis

VAGINAL DISCHARGES may be classified as follows:

INFECTIOUS	NON-INFECTIOUS
Trichomonas Vaginalis Vaginitis	Excessive cervical secretion
Candidiasis	Foreign body, especially diaphragms
Haemophilus Vaginalis Vaginitis	Neoplasms
Venereal	Benign polyps
Gonorrhea	Malignancy
Syphilis	Chemical or burn reactions
Granuloma Inguinale	Irradiation
Postmenopausal vaginitis	
Vaginitis in childhood	
Tuberculosis	

Trichomonas vaginalis was first discovered by Donné in 1837. The most important clinical work on this protozoon was done by Hoehne who, by 1916, had treated more than 100 patients. I wrote the first paper in the English language (Am. J. Obst. & Gynec. 16:870, 1928).

Trichomonas vaginalis, which is a parasitic, flagellated protozoon and causes a characteristic vaginal discharge, is nearly always overlooked because it is impossible to detect in stained preparations unless one has special information concerning its characteristics. It is, however, easily found in a hanging drop. Unfortunately, a hanging drop examination is seldom made of a vaginal discharge, although such an examination should be done as routine preliminary to the treatment of every vaginal discharge. Only by such careful routine will the nongonorrheal discharge be accurately diagnosed.

Clinical Course

The clinical picture produced by Trichomonas vaginalis when it is pathogenic is rather uniform and striking. The patients complain of a profuse discharge which in about half the cases is associated with a burning or itching sensation in the vagina and on the vulva. In some cases the irritation is so severe that sleep is disturbed. The patients often scratch the external genitals, and an inflammatory reaction similar to intertrigo may result. Often the discharge has a disagreeable and penetrating odor, which remains in a room or physician's office quite a while after a woman has left it.

On external examination, the introitus is usually seen to be reddened. The entire vaginal mucosa all the way up to the vault is reddened and sometimes is fiery red. In the introitus, the redness is usually diffuse, but, in the vagina, it may be diffuse or patchy. Often the vaginal mucosa is a deep orange color and contains many petechiae, and usually it presents the appearance of an inflammatory condition. For this reason the clinical picture is called Trichomonas vaginalis vaginitis. The cervix often presents petechiae, the area of the external os is usually red and occasionally it bleeds readily even though there is no erosion. No inflammatory condition, however, is found beyond the external os. The vagina contains a large amount of greenish-yellow, foamy pus which looks like gonorrheal pus; but sometimes the discharge is thin and watery. Most of it is found in the vaginal vault; it may have an acid, alkaline, or amphoteric reaction but is usually alkaline. Some patients are nervous owing to the constant irritation, sleeplessness, and fear of having contracted venereal disease. Many go from physician to physician, and although they secure temporary relief, they are not cured. Quite a few women, but by no means all, are unclean in their personal habits. It must be emphasized that not all women who harbor trichomonads have a discharge. Some women have no symptoms despite the fact that the vagina contains numerous trichomonads. This organism is rarely found in virgins.

Detection of Organism

The best way to study the organism is by means of hanging drop preparations or by diluting a drop of vaginal secretion with a drop of normal saline solution on an ordinary glass slide. The drop of secretion may be obtained with a platinum loop from the vault of the vagina after exposure with a speculum. A simpler method is to make a vaginal examination, and, on withdrawal, a moderate amount of secretion will be found adhering to the gloved fingers; one or more drops of the secretion may be placed on cover slips or slides and a drop of saline solution added. If the latter method is used and the glove is dry when drawn on, the dusting powder should be washed off with soap and water before the vaginal examination is made. No antiseptic or lubricant should be used on the glove or speculum. For studying the organism, fields should be selected where there is relatively little discharge, namely, at the periphery of the drop of secretion. The drop usually consists of a large number of leukocytes and bacteria, many epithelial cells and many trichomonads. With ordinary high-power lenses, the parasites are readily seen because of their motility.

Trichomonas vaginalis varies considerably in size. Usually it is larger than

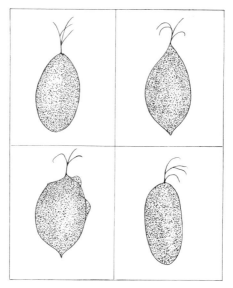

FIG. 34.—Various types of Trichomonas vaginalis.

a polymorphonuclear leukocyte but smaller than an epithelial cell. The organism also varies in shape. Usually the trichomonas is spindle shaped or pyriform (Figs. 34 and 35). The front end is rounded and from it protrude four flagella that rise from a common stem. In the fresh hanging drop preparation, the parasite is in constant motion. The movement of the flagella is somewhat similar to that of a fishing line when cast.

Trichomonas vaginalis nearly always lives in symbiosis with other organisms, usually bacteria, and most often the latter are gram-negative cocci which are smaller than gonococci. In most cases the bacterium found is Micrococcus aerogenes-alcaligenes. The gas bubbles present in the vaginal discharge of a large proportion of these cases are produced by these micrococci.

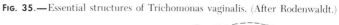

FIG. 35.—Essential structures of Trichomonas vaginalis. (After Rodenwaldt.)

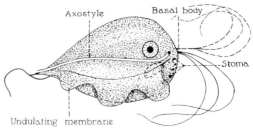

In some instances the trichomonads are associated with gonorrhea. In such cases, if only a hanging drop is examined, the gonococci will be overlooked. On the other hand, if only a stained smear is examined, the trichomonads will usually be missed. Hence in every case in which a vaginal discharge is present, both hanging drop and stained smear studies should be made.

Many pregnant women have Trichomonas vaginalis vaginitis, and some investigators believe that they have a much greater tendency toward a febrile puerperium than women without this condition. I have not found this to be true. There are no ill effects from treating patients during gestation. It is best, however, to avoid vaginal manipulation as much as possible in these patients during labor. In some cases, there is a spontaneous disappearance of the trichomonal discharge immediately after labor, but, in many of these, there is a recurrence of the discharge a few weeks later in a severer form.

Treatment

A drug that has made local vaginal treatment almost obsolete for many women is metronidazole (Flagyl). This remarkable drug may be taken by mouth in the form of tablets. About 90% of women will be free from trichomoniasis after taking 1 250-mg. tablet orally 3 times a day for 7 to 10 days. Some women cannot take the tablets because of nausea and a peculiar taste in the mouth. In some instances the husband must also be treated with the same tablets in order to prevent reinfection. Many gynecologists, particularly the French, consider trichomoniasis to be a true venereal disease; therefore both partners must be treated. Oral and vaginal use of tablets may be combined, but generally the oral therapy alone suffices. As far as we know, Flagyl produces no harm, but there may rarely be a decrease in the white blood cell count. In cases in which the drug has been used in pregnancy, it has not produced any apparent harm.

Although this type of vaginitis is readily relieved by local treatment, it is difficult to cure permanently. Most women have recurrences either early or late, and because of this, many therapeutic recommendations have been made.

The local treatment I use when women cannot tolerate Flagyl because of nausea, peculiar taste in the mouth, or other reasons follows. The vulva and vagina are cleaned with cotton balls wet first with green soap and then with tap water. The vagina is then thoroughly dried. A speculum is inserted into the vagina and a powder or liquid is blown against the cervix, all parts of the vaginal mucosa, the vulva, and the anus. *No powder or liquid should ever be blown into the vagina except through an open speculum. Insufflation should never be used during pregnancy.* Several deaths have occurred in pregnant women from embolism following insufflation. The powders I use are Floraquin and Tricofuron. This treatment is repeated every second to fourth day for 3 and sometimes 4 times. On the evenings of the intervening days, just before going to bed, the patient inserts a Floraquin tablet or Tricofuron suppository high up in the vagina. If menstruation supervenes, treatment is continued unless the flow of blood is profuse. After this course of treatment, the patient may take a douche every second day for 4 times if she finds douching helpful; douching is then discontinued. The usual douche prescribed follows.

Lactic acid—U.S.P., 85% . . . . 60 ml.
Distilled water to make . . . . 240 ml.
Directions: One teaspoonful in 2 qt. warm water used as a douche.

Instead of lactic acid, white vinegar may be used. In this event 4 table-spoonfuls of white vinegar should be added to the 2 qt. of warm water used for the douche. Lactic acid and vinegar are prescribed because it is essential to maintain an acid medium in the vagina.

I have also had considerable success with Vagisec both in local therapy in concentrated liquid form in the office and in a douche taken by the patient 2 or 3 times a week.

I advise against douching for so-called hygienic or cleansing purposes. I see absolutely no need for douches in healthy women except after sexual intercourse, if desired.

A matter of great importance, though unpleasant to discuss, is the cleansing of the anus after a bowel movement. Most women use an upward sweep toward the vagina and urethra, thereby bringing fecal matter and fecal bacteria to the vulva. Patients should be instructed to use a sweeping motion downward away from the vagina and toward the sacrum. The significance of this method of cleansing the anal region should be impressed on the patient, even though the intestinal type of trichomonas differs from the vaginal type.

Since recurrences of troublesome discharge take place in most patients and since these frequently manifest themselves immediately after menstruation, it is advisable to re-examine patients just before and just after a menstrual period. If organisms are found, another course of treatment should be given. Not only is there no harm in continuing therapy throughout the duration of the menstrual flow and immediately after it, but such treatment is a necessity in many cases. Patients who are likely to have recurrences are high strung, under tension, and emotional. The discharge and symptoms are aggravated or reappear when the women are upset emotionally. The constitutional make-up plays a role in the persistence or recurrence of the trichomonas infection.

When a patient is cured, it will be found that the parasites have disappeared, the character of the vaginal discharge has changed, the amount of discharge has been reduced to practically normal, the inflammatory changes in the

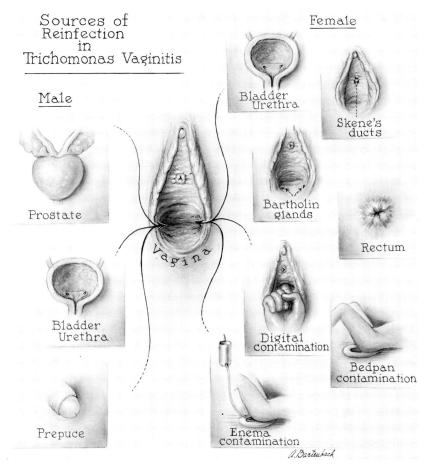

Sources of
Reinfection
in
Trichomonas Vaginitis

Female

Male

Bladder
Urethra

Skene's
ducts

Prostate

Bartholin
glands

Vagina

Rectum

Bladder
Urethra

Digital
contamination

Bedpan
contamination

Prepuce

Enema
contamination

a. Bartenbach

FIG. 36.—Possible sources of reinfection in Trichomonas vaginitis. (Courtesy of W. J. Reich *et al.*)

vaginal wall have subsided, and the symptoms, especially the itching and foul odor, have disappeared.

In cases that are difficult to cure, a search must be made for sources of reinfection, most of which are shown in Figure 36. In an occasional instance, the husband is the source of the persistence or recurrences of the troublesome discharge. Hence, in refractory cases, the husband's urethra and prostatic secretion should be examined for Trichomonas vaginalis. Trichomonas infection of the male genitals can be treated effectively, with Flagyl—1 250-mg. tablet orally 3 times a day for 7 to 10 days. To avoid reinfection of the patient, her husband, or her sex partner, condoms should be used during intercourse as long as trichomonads are present in either husband or wife.

Candidiasis

THE THIRD INTERNATIONAL MICROBIOLOGICAL CONGRESS in 1939 agreed that the name Candida should be applied to the group of fungi discussed in this chapter. The term *candidiasis* is used when the fungus is found in human beings. I shall discuss the fungi that affect the vagina; the term used for this condition is *vaginal candidiasis.*

The organism responsible for candidiasis consists of two parts, mycelia and conidia. The mycelia are long, fiber-like structures which are usually branched. The conidia are buds and usually are the size of a pus cell, but may vary considerably (Fig. 37).

In typical cases of candidiasis, the vulva is considerably reddened, edematous, and congested, and part of the surface may have a slight grayish cast because of epidermal necrosis. Since in nearly all cases there is considerable itching, the vulva may show excoriations from scratching. There may be urinary frequency, and dysuria and also dyspareunia. The pruritus associated with candida infections is more intense than any other type of pruritus of the vulva except perhaps kraurosis vulvae. The itching usually interferes with sleep in severe cases.

The vaginal wall and introitus are usually covered with tenacious, caseous material which resembles thrush in the mouth of newborn babies. In fact, the two organisms are identical. The walls of the vagina are intensely congested. This congestion is observed not only in the vaginal wall near the introitus and in the introitus itself, but also, in severe cases, on the labia minora and majora, around the anus, and even on the inner surfaces of the thighs for some distance from the vaginal orifice. In these areas the skin may be excoriated.

Mycotic infections of the vulva and vagina are more common in pregnant women and in women with diabetes than in normal nonpregnant women. Urine containing an abnormal amount of sugar favors the growth of mycotic organisms, but there is no concrete evidence that sugar itself is irritating. The vulvitis in diabetes is due to some agent other than the glycosuria, probably candidiasis, although there may be bacterial invasion. Of course, in diabetic women with yeast infections, both the diabetes and the local infection must be treated. In some pregnant women, the condition persists despite treatment but disappears spontaneously soon after delivery. It may return later. Other

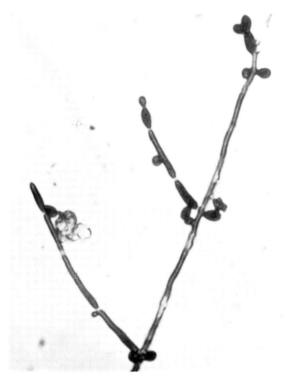

FIG. 37.—Candida. Note conidia (buds) and mycelia (fiber-like structures).

factors responsible for candidiasis are the use of some antibiotics and over-treatment of trichomoniasis.

Diagnosis

Candida infections can be diagnosed often by a hanging drop examination, but a much more certain way is to make a smear of a small portion of caseous material and stain for the fungi. A Gram stain suffices for this. The organisms are strongly gram-positive.

The most accurate means of detecting candidiasis is the culture method. A good culture medium is Sabouraud broth, but a simpler one, and one that can be used in a doctor's office, is Nickerson's medium. When caseous material containing candida is applied to this medium, the organisms grow in large black or brown, shiny, hemispheric colonies, with peripheral filaments on continued incubation. Before a culture is taken, the patient is instructed not to take a douche or use vaginal medication for a period of 3 days.

The simplest method of detecting candidiasis is to add a drop of KOH to some of the secretion contained from the vagina or introitus on the gloved finger and examine a hanging drop under a microscope.

If material is taken for cultures, it is best obtained through an unlubricated sterile bivalve speculum with a cotton-tipped, sterile applicator. The applicator is gently rolled over the Nickerson medium. The culture may be left at room temperature, in which case it rarely becomes positive in less than 48 hours. The culture should, however, be observed for 5 days before deciding that there is no candidiasis. If the culture medium is placed in an incubator at 32–37 C., results will be definite in 24–28 hours.

Treatment

The treatment of candida infections is simpler than that of Trichomonas vaginalis vaginitis. Thorough application to all parts of the vulva and vagina of a 1% aqueous solution of gentian violet nearly always gives spectacular and gratifying relief. This treatment should be carried out every second day for 2 or 3 times or until cure is accomplished. The patient must be warned that the dyes stain the clothing, so sufficient vulvar pads should be worn at all times.

Hesseltine recommends element iodine as found in one-fourth to one-half strength Lugol's solution or one-fifth to one-fourth strength tincture of iodine. Other satisfactory drugs for treating candidiasis are Gentersal cream (which contains 0.5% gentian violet and alkyl dimethyl benzyl-ammonium chloride) and nystatin (Mycostatin). The Gentersal cream (5 cc.) is inserted into the vagina morning and night for at least 14 days, including the days of menstruation. The patient is told not to take douches or have intercourse. Smears and cultures or both are repeated 3 weeks from the beginning of treatment. If the smears or cultures are positive, the treatment is repeated.

Nystatin (Mycostatin) is derived from Streptomyces noursei and is prepared in tablet form. Each tablet contains 100,000 units of nystatin. A tablet (sometimes 2 tablets are necessary) is inserted into the vagina every night, even during menstruation, for 10–14 nights. Relief from symptoms usually is obtained in 48 hours. Recurrences are treated the same way.

Another excellent tablet for the treatment of candidiasis is HYVA, which contains gentian violet. These tablets also are inserted at bedtime.

10

Haemophilus Vaginalis Vaginitis

ANY PATIENT whose ovarian activity is normal and who has a gray, homogeneous, malodorous vaginal discharge with a pH 5.0 to 5.5 that yields no trichomonads is likely to have Haemophilus vaginalis (H.V.) vaginitis. A wet smear preparation from the vagina of such a patient will contain the "clue cells" of Haemophilus vaginalis; in the stained smear, the bacterial flora will consist predominantly of heavy fields of short, gram-negative bacilli.

Probably more than 90% of vaginitides previously classified as "nonspecific" are caused by H. vaginalis. Following eradication of H vaginalis, the clinical findings of the disease disappear, and the vaginal secretions and bacterial flora revert to normal.

This vaginal infection was first described by Gardner and Dukes in 1954. In 1955, the same authors published a more detailed clinical and laboratory report, in which the name Haemophilus vaginalis was proposed for the bacterial agent.

Etiology

CAUSATIVE AGENT.—Haemophilus vaginalis (Fig. 38) is the sole etiologic agent of H. vaginalis vaginitis. The minute, rod-shaped, gram-negative bacillus is nonmotile and nonencapsulated and does not form endospores. It is a true parasite that grows only in the presence of serum and other accessory growth factors. H. vaginalis is a distinct species and can be separated from the other members of the genus Haemophilus serologically and biochemically, and, to a certain extent, by its growth and nutritional characteristics.

Sources of Infection

VENEREAL DISEASE.—Aside from an infinitesimally small percentage of cases, sexual intercourse is surely the method of transmission. The high rate of reinfection in patients whose husbands remain untreated and the recovery of the organism from the majority of husbands of infected wives are evidence of its venereal transmission. H. vaginalis is essentially nonexistent in premenarchal subjects.

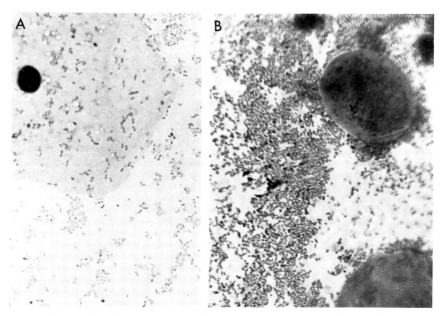

Fig. 38 **A** and **B.**—*Haemophilus vaginalis*, a short gram-negative bacillus usually observed in heavy fields. (Gram's stain × 1,200.) (From Gardner, H. L., and Kaufman, R. H.: *Benign Diseases of the Vulva and Vagina*. [St. Louis: C. V. Mosby Company, 1969].)

Prevalence

H.V. vaginitis is primarily a disease of the reproductive years. At present, an estimated 10 to 20% of women in this period of life harbor H. vaginalis.

Pathogenicity

H.V. vaginitis is a distinct disease of the vagina in which very uniform clinical and laboratory patterns are displayed. Further, the disease disappears abruptly upon eradication of H. vaginalis, the only organism consistently isolated from the vagina of patients with the entity.

INFECTION BY DIRECT INOCULATION.—Gardner and Dukes (1955) successfully inoculated disease-free vaginas with material from the vaginas of patients who exhibited the classical signs of H. vaginalis infection.

INFECTION IN HUSBANDS.—In a study reported by Gardner and Dukes (1959), the predominant organism in the urethras of 91 husbands of 101 infected wives was H. vaginalis. In contrast, in a study of urethral cultures obtained from 38 male medical students, only one was found to harbor the organism.

Clinical Features

H.V. vaginitis is the most benign of the common infectious vaginitides. In fact, the signs and symptoms are usually so mild that many clinicians fail to recognize it as a clinical entity, and the majority of patients do not complain of its manifestations.

OBJECTIVE SIGNS.—Leukorrhea is the most familiar objective sign of the disease. The consistency of the discharge is approximately the same as that of the discharge associated with trichomoniasis. It resembles a thin flour paste, being turbid and uniformly homogeneous, and has a tendency to adhere to the vaginal wall in a thin film rather than to pool in the posterior fornix. The odor of the discharge on a withdrawn speculum is characteristic. Usually it is less offensive than that of trichomoniasis. Frothiness of the discharge is apparent in 10 to 15% of cases. Most patients with H.V. vaginitis have a discharge within the range of pH 5.0 to 5.5. In contrast, the pH of normal vaginal secretions of practically all patients is within the range of pH 3.8 to 4.5.

Laboratory Findings

WET MOUNT PREPARATIONS.—Wet mount preparations should be examined under low-power and high-power objectives. Vaginal material from patients with H.V. vaginitis, when mixed with physiologic saline on a glass slide, exhibits a characteristic microscopic picture of the utmost diagnostic value. The appearance of many of the epithelial cells provides the strongest evidence of H.V. vaginitis—they appear to be stippled or granulated. Gardner and Dukes (1955) have referred to such cells as "clue cells" (Fig. 39). Their appearance is incident to adherent and uniformly spaced H. vaginalis upon their surfaces.

STAINED SMEARS.—The most striking feature of the gram-stained smear is the tremendous number of H. vaginalis organisms represented by small gram-negative bacilli, 0.3 to 0.6 micron wide and 1.0 to 2.0 micron long, with rounded ends. For general use, the gram-stained smear is probably the most reliable laboratory method for diagnosis of this disease.

CULTURE IDENTIFICATION.—Cultures are seldom required for differential diagnosis of vaginitis.

Treatment

Many patients with H.V. vaginitis are unaware of the infection until they experience the favorable changes that follow its cure. Patients who have the habit of frequent douching and those habituated to their own odors are unlikely to complain and seek treatment. While most patients should be

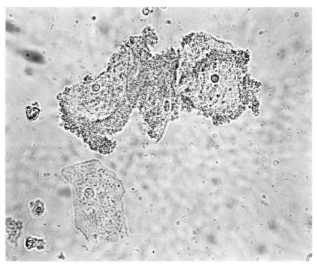

FIG. 39.—"Clue cells" of H. vaginalis vaginitis. Normal epithelial cell in *lower left.* Pus cells are few and lactobacilli are lacking. (Wet mount preparation.) (From Gardner, H. L., and Dukes, C. D.: Am. J. Obst. & Gynec. 69:962, 1955.)

treated upon diagnosis of the infection, certain asymptomatic patients should, perhaps, be allowed to continue in ignorance if cooperation between husband and wife is likely to be difficult. A lasting cure is often difficult to accomplish because of the very real problem of reinfection.

TOPICAL AGENTS.—Oxytetracycline (Terramycin) vaginal suppositories, when inserted into the vagina at bedtime for 10 days, are highly effective. The method is often successful after other topical agents but oral tetracyclines have proved worthless. A frequent unfavorable aftermath of intravaginal Terramycin is the development of vulvovaginal candidiasis. Concurrent use of vaginal nystatin (Mycostatin) tablets or other fungicidal agents, however, will usually protect the patient against this complication. Intravaginal sulfonamides are somewhat less effective than intravaginal Terramycin, though they are advantageous in that they do not tend to promote secondary candidal or bacterial infections. Sulfonamides available for intravaginal use include triple sulfa (Sultrin) cream and tablets, sulfisoxazole (Gantrisin) cream, and sulfadiazine (Gynben) vaginal suppositories and cream. These preparations should be inserted twice daily for a minimum of 10 days. Furacin vaginal suppositories and cream contain the antibacterial agent nitrofurazone. This agent gives results comparable to the sulfonamides.

SYSTEMIC AGENTS.—Ampicillin, 500 mg. administered every 6 hours for 5 days, has proved to be the most effective systemic agent used to date, but many strains are resistant to it.

Oral tetracyclines are partially effective, some strains responding rapidly and others not at all. The tetracyclines should be administered in a minimum dose of 250 mg. every 6 hours for 5 days. Oral sulfonamides in the usual dosage have been almost uniformly unsuccessful as a treatment for H.V. vaginitis. Penicillin, although reportedly effective, is of little value, most strains of H. vaginalis being highly resistant to the drug.

Treatment of Sexual Partner

Since more than 90% of men whose sexual partners are infected with H. vaginalis also yield the organism, they constitute a continuous source of reinfection. For this reason, the male sexual partner must be treated simultaneously with the patient if reinfections are to be prevented. Treatment schedules that have proved most successful in men are: ampicillin, 500 mg. every 6 hours for 5 days; Panalba, 250 mg. every 6 hours for a minimum of 5 days; and Terrastatin, 250 mg. every 6 hours for a minimum of 5 days. These schedules, however, are not uniformly successful.

11

Gonorrhea

GONORRHEA IS A contagious disease caused by the gonococcus, a biscuit-shaped diplococcus that is gram-negative. The gonococcus attacks chiefly mucous and serous membranes. At first the infection is local, but it soon spreads, usually by direct extension. It is the commonest communicable disease in the United States. Except in children, gonorrhea is contracted practically always by sexual intercourse. Of course, this is not true of gonorrheal conjunctivitis.

The gonococcus lives only in human beings. It shows a predisposition to invade columnar epithelium, living on the superficial surface and between the epithelial cells. Abrasions are not necessary for infection to take place. The incubation period varies between 3 and 10 days. Once the gonococcus has invaded the tissues it is difficult to eradicate.

One of the chief characteristics of a gonococcic infection is its tendency to become latent. The organism remains viable in the tissues but temporarily inactive. It may become actively virulent as a result of local hyperemia (such as coitus, menstruation, childbirth or trauma). The latent organisms may either induce a new attack in the host or be transmitted to another person in whom they will incite an acute infection.

Gonococci are easily demonstrated in acute cases. However, the longer the disease has been chronic, the more difficult it is to identify the organisms. In chronic cases the gonococcus is most readily found in or about the urethra and the cervix. The order of infection is: (1) urethra and cervix, (2) Skene's and Bartholin's glands, (3) endometrium, (4) endosalpinx, (5) ovaries, and (6) pelvic peritoneum. In infants and young girls before puberty, the main sites involved are the vulva and vagina. Outside the genitalia, the gonococcus usually invades the rectum and the conjunctiva, but almost any part of the body may be involved.

Diagnosis

The diagnosis of gonorrhea should be based on a history of exposure to persons known to have gonorrhea, transmitting the infection to another person, clinical evidence, finding of gonococci in stained smears, cultures, and such complications as ophthalmia and arthritis. It is wise to make a blood Wassermann or Kahn test of every patient with gonorrhea to make sure that syphilis is not also present.

The progress of gonorrhea may be divided into three stages: (1) the stage of infection, (2) the stage of pelvic invasion, and (3) the stage of pelvic degenerative lesions. A patient may be seen by a physician for the first time during any one of these stages. If the patient is observed during the stage of infection, there is a history of exposure. This may be through recent marriage, sexual intercourse with a new partner, or extramartial relations on the part of the patient or her husband. During this stage there is burning urination with frequency and urgency and also a vaginal discharge. On physical examination one finds an inflamed, swollen, reddened, gaping urethral meatus, swollen Skene's glands, an inflamed vulva, and an inflamed, granular cervix. All of these structures are bathed in a purulent discharge. Stained smears at first may fail to show intracellular diplococci, but in a few days they will reveal intracellular gram-negative diplococci. Therefore when smears are negative they should be repeated at least once.

In the stage of pelvic invasion, there will be a history of exposure some time before the patient's visit. The symptoms may include menstrual disturbances, particularly dysmenorrhea and excessive flow, pain in one or both lower quadrants, some fever, and persistent leukorrhea. Examination in the second stage will reveal tenderness of the uterus and adnexa and perhaps masses in the adnexal region. There may be some evidence of urethral involvement, and the cervix may be eroded and covered with a profuse purulent discharge. Cervical smears will usually reveal gonococci. The patient may be severely ill.

In the stage of pelvic degeneration, the patient has for a long time had pain in the lower part of the abdomen, persistent leukorrheal discharge, pain in the back, menstrual disturbances, and absolute or "one-child" sterility. She may perhaps have undergone one or more operations for the relief of pain and removal of adnexal masses. Examination will reveal tenderness in the lower part of the abdomen and perhaps scars on the abdomen. The urethra, cervix, and other structures usually look normal. Gonococci are rarely found in this late stage.

Smears

In all suspicious cases, it is wise for the physician to make smears and examine the slides himself. The patient should not take a douche or use vaginal medication for at least 24 hours before the examination and should not urinate for 2 hours prior to the examination. With the patient in the lithotomy position, the openings of the Bartholin's ducts should be inspected and the glands palpated, and also the urethra, including Skene's glands. The latter glands are situated on the floor of the urethra and their exits are just inside the external urinary meatus (Fig. 2). The external urinary meatus should be cleansed and the urethra "milked" for a drop of secretion (Fig. 3). The drop should be spread on dry, clean glass slides for staining. The films should be thin, and at least two slides of the drop should be made. Then the cervix should be exposed by means of a bivalve vaginal speculum and all mucus and discharge gently but thoroughly removed from the external os with dry cotton. After this the cervix should be squeezed with the speculum blades to milk the cervical "clefts." Secretion from the cervical canal should be obtained with a platinum loop, the round end of a metal catheter, or a medicine dropper that has its tip well drawn out so as to obtain a small amount of secretion. One drop of secretion from the cervix should be spread on two slides. The source of each slide should be marked because occasionally the disease is present in Bartholin's glands or the urethra but not in the cervix. Slides showing gonococci should be saved. Some cervical secretion should be saved for culture. Cervical material should be obtained even though the patient may be bleeding.

It is best to use Gram's stain for the slides because the vagina usually contains some organisms that are morphologically similar to the gonococcus

Fig. 40.—Gonococci. Diagnosis is made on finding more than 10 typical gram-negative diplococci intracellularly on same slide and 2 or more within same cell.

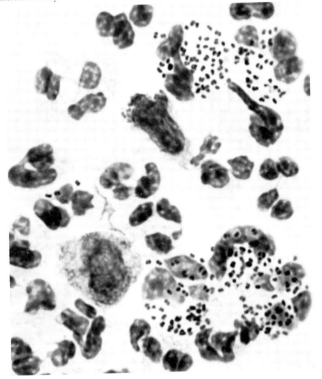

and cannot be differentiated by ordinary staining methods. Gonococci are gram-negative. Smears should also be made from the rectum.

The following method of using the Gram stain is recommended.

Dry the slide and apply crystal violet for 1 minute. Wash with water. Apply Gram's iodine for 2 minutes and wash with water. Decolorize with acetone. Dash on and wash with water quickly. Apply safranine for 1 minute. Wash with water and dry.

If desired, one of each pair of slides may be stained with alkaline methylene blue or Loeffler's stain, and then, if organisms similar to the gonococcus are found, the second slide of each pair can be stained with Gram's stain. The diagnosis of gonorrhea is based on the finding of gram-negative, kidney-bean- or coffee-bean-shaped diplococci that are intracellular but extranuclear. There must be more than 10 typical gram-negative diplococci intracellularly on the same slide and 2 or more within the same cell (Fig. 40).

If smears are negative and there is still clinical evidence or a suspicion of gonorrhea, more smears should be made the next day. These smears may be positive because the manipulation of the preceding day may have caused sufficient reaction to bring organisms to the surface. The most favorable time for the appearance of gonococci is during and just after a menstrual period. Other times are the postabortal period and the late puerperium.

Cultures

In acute gonorrhea it is easy to make a diagnosis, not only clinically but also by means of stained smears. In chronic cases, however, the diagnosis is usually difficult. When stained smears reveal the true diagnosis, usually no further tests need be made, but in suspected cases, when smears fail to be conclusive, cultures must be made. Cultures are far more accurate than smears. Cultures should also be made from the rectum because gonorrhea is not rare in the rectum. Transgrow is one of the best media for detecting gonorrhea.

There has been a great increase in the incidence of gonorrhea and syphilis, especially in young individuals, both male and female. This is due to the increased frequency of promiscuous sexual intercourse in teen-agers and also to the widespread use of the contraceptive pill which, while it prevents pregnancy, does not protect against venereal disease.

Treatment

PROPHYLAXIS.—It is important to inform patients who have gonorrhea about the great infectiousness of the disease, both to themselves and to others. They should be told how essential it is to wash the hands repeatedly and carefully with soap and water each time the genitals are touched. The great danger of infection of the eyes must be explained. Patients must also be informed that it is dangerous for little girls to sleep with them.

General care.—The patient's general resistance must be built up and sexual stimulation and sexual intercourse absolutely avoided. It is best for women to remain in bed during the menstrual period in the acute and subacute stages. Use of alcohol must be avoided. For pain, local heat or cold may be used or mild anodynes taken.

SYSTEMIC THERAPY.—The drugs of choice in cases of gonorrhea are penicillin and ampicillin. With the increasing numbers of penicillin-insensitive gonococci, ampicillin may become the drug of choice for gonorrhea.

A patient with gonorrhea should be given a single dose of 4.8 million units of procaine penicillin G by injection, one half in each buttock. This is to be preceded by 1 gm. of probenecid orally 1 hour before injection.

About 10–20% of patients have post-gonoccal urethritis, regardless of the treatment. In these cases there is associated asymptomatic urethritis with pyuria without culture evidence of N. gonorrhoeae in the secretions and urine sediment. This form of urethritis seems related to non-gonococcal infection. These patients are best treated with oral tetracycline for 7 days. The dose of tetracycline hydrochloride is 500 mg. orally every 6 hours.

Patients who are sensitive to penicillin and ampicillin may be treated effectively with a single oral dose of 1.5 Gm. of tetracycline hydrochloride.

Local treatment may be applied to the urethra and cervix if deemed necessary.

A Bartholin's duct abscess may follow a gonococcic infection. In the early stages of such an abscess, the patient should rest in bed and have hot applications to the vulva. As soon as pus is definitely detected, the abscess must be incised and drained or other operation performed.

Gonorrheal cervicitis is often difficult to cure because of the character of the mucosa of the cervix. In acute cases, there is a profuse purulent discharge, but, in chronic cases, there may be very little discharge except just before and just after the menses. A satisfactory way of clearing up cervical discharge is with diethylstilbestrol or penicillin. If the former is used, 1 mg. should be given every night for the first 20 nights of the menstrual cycle. This should be repeated 3 times. Penicillin therapy is the simplest because a single injection of 600,000 units in oily suspension is satisfactory in many cases.

The best treatment of chronic cervicitis associated with extensive erosion and/or nabothian follicle cysts is by means of the nasal tip cautery or conization. However, it is important not to cauterize the cervix too deeply nor too high in the cervical canal. Of course, electric treatment should not be used in acute or subacute cases or if the adnexa are involved.

When a gonorrheal infection extends beyond the cervix, it involves the uterus and fallopian tubes. Purulent material usually escapes from the fimbriated ends of the tubes and produces the typical clinical picture of gonorrheal pelvic peritonitis, which consists of high fever, pain in the lower part of the abdomen, urinary disturbances, and other symptoms. The treatment of these conditions is conservative, with antibiotics in most instances. Should surgical intervention become necessary, it must, of course, be carried out in a hospital.

Gonorrheal involvement of the rectum is more common than is believed. Symptoms of gonorrheal proctitis are usually mild and sometimes absent. Regardless of this, in acute and subacute cases of gonorrhea, the physician should never make a rectal examination for fear of introducing gonococci into the rectum. Nor should enemas be permitted unless they are absolutely necessary, in which case the external genitals and the anal region must be carefully cleansed first. Gonorrheal proctitis must be treated with penicillin and tetracycline, just like gonococcic infections elsewhere. It is worth while making routine smears of material from the rectum of all women with gonorrhea, especially when the source of reinfection cannot be found.

Pregnancy

Gonorrhea and pregnancy are frequently associated. In some cases, the disease precedes the pregnancy; in others, the disease is acquired at the time of conception, and, in still others, gonorrhea is contracted after pregnancy has started, even near full term.

Pregnancy may adversely affect pre-existing gonorrhea. The abundant congestion of the pelvic tissues may stimulate the growth of gonococci, thus lighting up an old infection. Gonorrhea rarely initiates an abortion, but it can cause considerable puerperal morbidity.

The symptoms during pregnancy are a profuse purulent discharge from the urethra and cervix and painful urination. The skin of the labia may be excoriated.

Treatment in acute cases includes rest in bed. The same antibiotic treatment is carried out as in nonpregnant individuals.

Criteria of Cure

Evidence of cure depends on clinical signs, bacteriologic tests and cultures. Examinations and clinical and smear studies should be made 2 weeks after treatment is carried out. After this there should be a monthly check-up, preferably during or just after each menstrual period. Also, examinations should be made after deliberate digital or medicinal (silver nitrate) trauma of the cervix or urethra. If after 3 months, 4 clinical and smear examinations have been negative, cultures are made, and, if these are negative, the patient can be considered cured. Only then are coitus and pregnancy considered safe. If, however, during this period of observation, evidence of reinfection develops, treatment must be resumed and the entire test of cure is repeated.

When evidence of infection appears after the 3 months of observation, the disease is more likely a reinfection than a recurrence.

In every instance of gonorrhea in a woman, the consort should be examined. If he has the disease, he should, of course, be treated. Otherwise the patient will be reinfected by the marital partner from time to time.

Physicians should remember that cases of gonorrhea and syphilis must be reported to their local health authorities.

12

Condylomata Acuminata

CONDYLOMA ACUMINATUM is a papilloma with a central core of connective tissue in a treelike structure covered with epithelium. The stroma is usually vascular and shows evidence of chronic inflammation with lymphocytes and plasma cells. Condylomata acuminata frequently, perhaps usually, are not of venereal origin and therefore should not be called venereal warts. There is a type of condyloma that results from syphilis; it is flat and is called *condyloma latum*.

The *cause* of condylomata acuminata is the same filtrable virus that causes the common wart, verruca vulgaris. Hence the disease is infectious and autoinoculable. Condylomata are commonly encountered during pregnancy and in women with gonorrhea. They occur chiefly on the vulva and perineum but may be found on the vagina, urethra, cervix, buttocks, and pubis (Fig. 41). They are usually multiple and vary in size from 1 mm. to 8 cm. They often grow together and may form large masses.

Treatment

An effective drug for treating small condylomas is podophyllin, a resin that has pronounced, delayed local irritant action. A 25% podophyllin ointment or 25% podophyllin in compound tincture of benzoin is applied to each condyloma by means of a cotton or glass applicator (Fig. 41). Because podophyllin is highly irritating, the surrounding normal skin must be covered with petrolatum, as shown in Figure 41. There is no immediate reaction but pain may ensue 6 or 8 hours later. After 3 to 6 hours, the medication is washed off with bland soap and water, preferably in the bathtub. During the next 12 hours there may be a pronounced local inflammatory and edematous reaction. The lesions usually begin to involute between the second and fifth days. More than one application may be necessary.

Graber, Barber, and O'Rourke say that the main objections of patients who are treated with podophyllin are burning and discomfort in spite of protective petrolatum coating, the number of treatments necessary for large lesions, and the failure of the medication to remove all the lesions if the disease is extensive. Podophyllin is toxic and highly laxative. If the lesion is extensive, there is absorption of the drug into the blood stream. In the pregnant patient, the

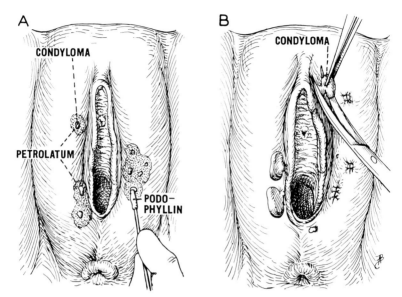

FIG. 41.—Condylomata acuminata. **A,** treatment with podophyllin. **B,** treatment by surgical excision. (From Greenhill, J. P.: *Surgical Gynecology* [4th ed.; Chicago: Year Book Medical Publishers, Inc., 1969].)

absorption of podophyllin into the maternal circulation may affect the vessels in the decidua with resulting vascular spasm and embarrassment of the fetal circulation and oxygenation.

Anything more than minimal disease should be treated with electrocoagulation, which takes care of the disease promptly and completely in one treatment. There is little postoperative pain, and no scarring or distortion of the vulva. The electrodessication is produced with a coagulating current. However, the dead tissue left behind is a nidus for infection. If the surgeon coagulates the tumor and then uses a thin curet or even a sharp uterine curet to remove the tumor, the depth of the electrodessication can be controlled exactly so that neither too much nor too little tissue is destroyed. The few small bleeders on the surface underlying the lesion can readily be controlled with an electric spark. The entire area is covered with Vaseline gauze. If the lesion is not too extensive, the procedure can be carried out in the office under local anesthesia. Large conglomerate cauliflower-like masses are best operated on in a hospital under general anesthesia.

Condylomata acuminata of the vulva in *pregnancy* deserve special consideration. The lesions are small-to-medium size, and outside of the vagina they can be treated by the method just described during the first half of pregnancy. In the latter stages there is great danger of hemorrhage because of the increased vascularity of the perineal area. Cleanliness and the use of local therapy to control vaginal discharge are about all that can be suggested. In the presence of large condylomata with sloughing and ulceration, death may occur from sepsis. Cesarean section is indicated in this situation.

Recurrences often follow treatment and are usually due to: (1) small lesions overlooked at the time of first treatment, (2) dissemination from the original lesions, and (3) reinfection from the original source, such as the vagina or rectum. An aid in preventing recurrences is the use of a germicidal soap on the external genitals twice a day, followed by a dusting powder containing equal parts of thymol iodide, bismuth, and talc.

13

The Uterine Cervix: Its Disturbances and Their Treatment

THE CERVIX is small, but despite this it is one of the most important organs from the point of view of both health and actual danger to life. It is best for the physician always to think of every lesion of the cervix as a potential forerunner of cancer.

The commonest disorders of the cervix are: (1) cervicitis and endocervicitis, (2) "erosions," (3) cysts, (4) polyps, (5) leukoplakia, (6) lacerations, and (7) carcinoma.

Frequently, two or more of these conditions are present at the same time. To understand properly the treatment of these conditions, one must know something of the anatomy, physiology, pathology, and bacteriology of the cervix and its adjacent structures.

Cervicitis, Endocervicitis, Erosions, and Cysts

The cervix differs from the corpus of the uterus in both structure and function. The endometrium of the corpus consists of a stroma interspersed with tubular glands which are lined with cuboidal epithelium. The uterine endometrium is in constant flux, undergoing the cyclic changes initiated by the ovarian hormones. The cervical mucosa is composed of high columnar epithelium.

Fluhmann and Dickmann found that the basic epithelial structure of the cervix uteri is one of multiple clefts, some recognizable grossly and others of microscopic dimensions. Contrary to general belief, there are no compound tubular racemose glands. It is likely that the clefts are derivatives of the mucosal folds that arise in the fetal cervix uteri. The term "compound clefts" suggested by Hertig to describe these formations seems appropriate.

The cervix is particularly susceptible to bacterial infection, especially by the gonococcus, whereas the corpus endometrium is rarely infected except by the gonococcus and the tubercle bacillus, and by these infrequently.

The organisms chiefly responsible for infection of the cervix are the gonococcus, the streptococcus, the staphylococcus, and Escherichia coli. Gonococcic infection may occur in an apparently normal cervix, but other infections of the cervix usually follow some kind of trauma, such as that of childbirth, instrumental dilatation, curettage, improper cauterization with chemicals or electric apparatus, the wearing of a stem pessary, and some operations on the cervix. Infections of the cervix may also occur by the hematogenous route (tuberculosis). Some erosions have an endocrine basis.

When the cervix is infected, the mucosa is edematous and often everted. As a result of the infection, the columnar epithelium is forced out of the cervical canal onto the portio, or vaginal portion of the cervix. There it replaces the squamous eqithelium which is normally present, and thus the so-called erosion arises. An erosion, therefore, is not really an ulceration, as the name implies, but new epithelial and cleft tissue—in reality, a hyperplasia. However, a true erosion with loss of squamous epithelium may result due to maceration from infected mucopurulent discharge. An erosion may be present all around the external os or only part way around. Usually with this condition there is an excessive secretion from the cervical epithelium. In many cases the mucosal folds become occluded or obstructed, and the secreted mucus gives rise to cysts. These are the nabothian cysts or follicles. Although many of these cysts are visible, some are situated deep in the cervical tissue and cannot be seen. They increase the size of the cervix, which is already enlarged, and may interfere with its circulation and muscular contraction. These changes are frequently responsible for the bleeding that occurs occasionally just before and just after menstruation and also for many cases of mucopurulent vaginal discharge. In numerous cases of cervicitis, there is an associated inflammation of the parametrial tissue and the uterosacral ligaments. The latter structures are then tender to the touch.

The chief symptom of chronic cervicitis is leukorrhea, which is present in every case. The type of discharge varies considerably. Other symptoms may be backache, bearing down feeling in the pelvis, dull pain in the lower part of the abdomen, and urinary disturbances, especially frequency and urgency of urination. In some cases there are dysmenorrhea and menorrhagia. Some women with severe chronic cervicitis and endocervicitis complain of painful intercourse. A rather frequent consequence of chronic cervicitis is sterility, as evidenced by a number of women who become pregnant after the cervicitis is cured. Occasionally the cervix acts as a source of irritation to other organs, such as the bladder.

Treatment

The treatment of chronic cervicitis and endocervicitis, erosions and cysts is both preventive and curative. Prevention of gonorrhea will eliminate a large proportion of cases, and proper obstetric care will prevent an additional extensive group. Prophylactic measures during labor consist of waiting for

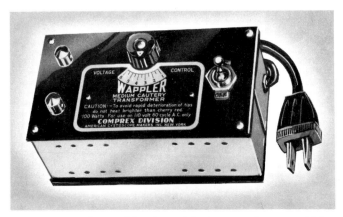

FIG. 42.—Cautery transformer. (Manufactured by American Cystoscope Makers, Inc.)

spontaneous complete dilatation of the cervix before delivery is attempted and immediate repair of all cervical lacerations.

Nasal Tip Cautery

One of the simplest and most successful office procedures for chronic cervicitis is the use of a nasal tip electric cautery (Figs. 42 and 43). Treatment with this instrument is practically painless; it is simple and inexpensive and will cure nearly all cases of chronic endocervicitis, erosions, and nabothian cysts.

No anesthetic is required. With the patient in the dorsal position, a bivalve speculum is lubricated and gently inserted into the vagina. The cervix is exposed and cleansed with a piece of dry cotton on a forceps. The cervix need not and should not be grasped with a tenaculum. If there is only a localized area of erosion, the cautery tip is placed on this area, and the current is turned on (Fig. 44). After the tip has become red hot, it is pressed gently into the cervical tissue for approximately $\frac{1}{16}$ in. across the total length of

FIG. 43.—Types of nasal tips for cauterization of the cervix.

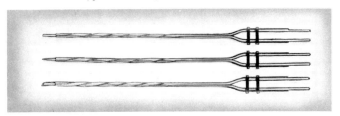

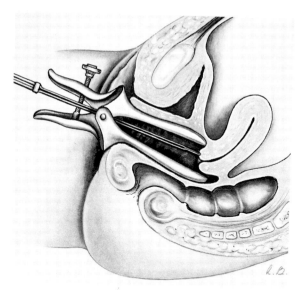

FIG. 44.—Placing of nasal tip on cervix for cauterization.

the eroded area. This usually requires only a few seconds and is all that is necessary. If, however, there is inflammation all around the external os of the cervix, a number of linear cautery incisions are necessary. Usually, there have to be two incisions on both the anterior and the posterior lips and one incision at either angle of the cervix. The incisions should be nearly 1 cm. apart. When more than four incisions are to be made, it is best to divide the treatment into two visits at intervals of 14 days. Nearly always, the patient may continue her activities immediately after treatment. The linear incisions must never extend into the cervical canal, certainly never as far as the internal os, and they must not be made too deeply. These precautions must be observed to avoid a stricture of the cervical canal. The incisions must not be too close together or there will not be enough islands of epithelium left in the cervical canal to permit re-epithelization (Fig. 45).

When nabothian follicle cysts are present, they can be punctured with the hot cautery tip. The cautery tip used for this purpose is slightly different from that used for linear cauterization, although the same type of tip may be used for both purposes (Fig. 46). As soon as the cyst wall is punctured, mucus escapes. All the mucus should be removed by reinserting the hot tip a few times. Then the entire cyst wall should be cauterized in order to destroy it completely.

The patient should be warned that she will have a profuse discharge for days or even weeks after a cautery treatment and that it may be blood tinged

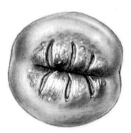

A. Three linear cauterizations on each lip

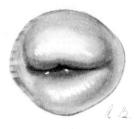

B. Healed cervix after cauterization

FIG. 45.—A, three cautery incisions on each lip of cervix. **B,** cervix after incisions have healed.

at times. Occasionally there is profuse bleeding, which will require the use of an anticoagulant or packing with hemostatic gauze. Backache may follow the treatments. It is best for the patient to avoid sexual intercourse for a few days after each treatment. Some women find it helpful to take a daily douche because of the discharge that results from the treatments, but this seldom should be recommended.

The electric cautery should never be used when the infection in the cervix is acute. Nor should the cautery be used in the presence of any acute infection of the genitals, external or internal, because the infection may spread.

Polyps

Cervical polyps vary from a few millimeters to more than 3 cm. in length; they are pedunculated, roughly pear shaped, soft, smooth, and reddish or

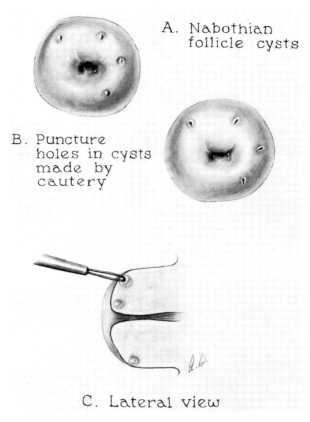

A. Nabothian follicle cysts

B. Puncture holes in cysts made by cautery

C. Lateral view

Fig. 46.—Use of cautery for puncturing nabothian follicle cysts. **A,** cysts; **B,** cysts after puncture with cautery; **C,** lateral view of cautery tip in cyst.

purplish. The pedicle arises nearly always from the cervical canal but occasionally from the external surface of the cervix or the endometrium. In the vast majority of instances, only a single polyp is present, but occasionally two or three are found at the same time. They seldom recur after removal. Microscopically, polyps are found to be a hyperplastic condition of the cervical mucosa. They have a large number of small blood vessels, especially near the surface. Most polyps are edematous and inflamed, and some contain cysts identical with the nabothian follicles found in the cervix.

The chief symptoms of polyps are metrorrhagia and leukorrhea, but most women with cervical polyps have no complaints.

Diagnosis of polyps is simple. On bimanual examination, a polyp is readily felt, and certainly when a speculum is inserted in the vagina, the red or purple polyp at once becomes prominent. Occasionally only the tip of the polyp is visible at the external os, most of it being high up in the cervical canal.

It is difficult to prevent the formation of polyps because their exact etiology is not known. However, it is most likely that polyps are the result of a polypoid hyperplasia of the cervical mucosa, which follows any condition leading to chronic passive congestion of the lower part of the uterus.

Treatment of mucous polyps is easy to carry out. The pedicle can be grasped with forceps and gently twisted in the same plane until the polyp comes away (Fig. 47, A, 2). After this simple procedure, there is rarely any bleeding. If

FIG. 47.—A: 1, cervical polyp; 2, removal by continuous twisting of curved forceps; 3, removal by ligation of pedicle and subsequent section of pedicle; 4, removal with tonsil snare. **B:** 1, cervical leiomyoma or huge cervical polyp; 2, removal by cauterization of base. **C:** 1, small sessile cervical polyps; 2, removal with tiny sharp uterine curet.

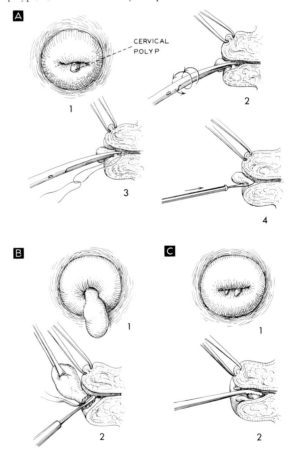

there is, the electric cautery tip may be applied for a few seconds. The same treatment may be applied for almost all polyps, although for the large ones and those that arise high in the canal, there may be a little difficulty in placing the clamp on the pedicle. A curved clamp is better than a straight one for this purpose. When there is a long thick pedicle, a curved clamp should be applied about 0.5 cm. above the origin of the pedicle. A surgical gut ligature should be tied between the clamp and the cervix, and the pedicle cut between clamp and ligature with a knife or scissors (Fig. 47, A, 3). Some polyps may be removed with a tonsil snare (Fig. 47, A, 4). Sessile polyps, which have no pedicle but rest directly on the cervix, are best removed with a tiny sharp curet (Fig. 47, C, 2). Even though malignancy occurs only about once in every 600 polyps, it is advisable to have every polyp examined microscopically. Hence, in removing polyps, care must be exercised not to crush them, and they should be placed in a bottle of fixing solution immediately after removal. Polyps are frequently associated with leiomyomas of the uterus.

Sometimes a readily accessible, pedunculated small leiomyoma can be removed in the office. It may be twisted off at its pedicle, but it is safer to place a ligature around the pedicle and then to cut the pedunculated leiomyoma away (Fig. 47, A, 3), or it may be removed by cutting across its pedicle with a cautery (Fig. 47, B, 2). Of course, antiseptic precautions must be observed.

Lacerations

Lacerations need not be treated unless they are deep and appear to interfere with conception or seem to be responsible for abortions. In such cases a simple operation should be performed. Lacerations themselves are not harmful.

Carcinoma

See the section on early diagnosis in Chapter 38, "Invasive Carcinoma of the Uterus."

14

Dyspareunia and Frigidity

THE TERMS "dyspareunia" and "frigidity" are often used interchangeably, but this usage is incorrect. Dyspareunia signifies difficult or painful sexual intercourse. It nearly always involves vaginismus, or spasm of the muscles surrounding the vagina. Vaginismus may occur without dyspareunia, as, for example, when a vaginal examination is made.

Dyspareunia

In most cases of dyspareunia, there is a large psychic factor. Nearly always the patient abhors sexual intercourse and, as the result of involuntary spasm, keeps out the penis. Examination under general anesthesia usually reveals ample space for coitus unless, of course, the dyspareunia is associated with an intact hymen, which is not common.

Sometimes dyspareunia is due to physical factors such as a rigid hymenal ring, an irritating vaginal discharge, vulvitis, chronic endocervicitis and cervicitis, senile vaginitis, too tight repair of a childbirth laceration, excessive narrowing of the introitus and vagina at the time of a plastic operation, presence of a tumor, kraurosis vulvae, Bartholin's duct cyst or abscess, urethral caruncle, pelvic tumors, or fissure in ano. In some cases the fault lies with the husband who, because of his lack of knowledge of the proper technic of intercourse, his clumsiness or inconsiderateness, causes pain.

Examination of a patient with dyspareunia is usually unsatisfactory unless a sedative or even a general anesthetic is given. When a patient complains of painful coitus, it is wise to obtain her confidence by a tactful and sympathetic conversation. Most patients will tell the real cause of their troubles, marital and otherwise, to a physician who is sympathetic and understanding in his approach. The information obtained is generally useful in helping the patient to recognize her fears and anxieties. Understanding these, she can often overcome the dyspareunia.

A thorough physical examination is indicated even if it appears obvious that psychic factors are responsible for the condition. The exception is when the first conversation with the physician has helped the patient so much that she feels confident she can have intercourse without difficulty. Such cases are unusual. If no abnormality is found, one can deal with the patient's mental reaction. Of course, if a physical cause for the dyspareunia exists, it should be removed. Thus, if an intact hymen is present, it should be ruptured and stretched with the patient under general anesthesia; irritating vaginal discharges should be cleared up; caruncles should be removed; and a tight perineum should be stretched digitally during anesthesia. In rare instances a perineoplasty must be done for a tight vaginal orifice. (See Greenhill, J. P.: *Surgical Gynecology* [4th ed.; Chicago: Year Book Medical Publishers, Inc., 1969].)

Many such patients tend to contract the introitus and vagina when an attempt is made to introduce a finger or speculum into the vagina. They may be helped considerably by being made aware of the emotional needs for the involuntary spasms of the perineal muscles. In no circumstance should forceful measures be used to eradicate the symptom. The physician must remember that this symptom serves as a first line of defense in the patient's emotional status against deep-seated fears.

Frigidity

The subject of frigidity in women is of considerable interest to gynecologists, psychiatrists, and generalists. The general practitioner, since he is a sort of father-confessor, can readily familiarize himself with the distressing cause of unhappiness. In my experience more than one third of all women do not enjoy sexual intercourse.

True frigidity must be differentiated not only from dyspareunia but from *pseudofrigidity*. The latter has many causes. Common ones are fear of pregnancy, even with the use of contraceptives, and pain from a too-tight perineal repair. The "frigidity" usually arises soon after a baby is born, particularly if the labor was hard and prolonged. The immediate postpartum period is often very trying, with a new baby in the home. When coitus is resumed after a baby is born, the wife frequently associates sexual intercourse with the cause of all her pain, fatigue, anxiety, and loss of freedom. This condition is called *postpartum frigidity*.

Other causes of pseudofrigidity are impotence of the husband, premature ejaculation, intracrural intercourse, clumsiness, ignorance of the proper technic on the part of the husband, misunderstandings, quarreling, and ill health.

According to some Freudian adherents, *true frigidity* involves two organs—the clitoris and the vagina. They claim that the clitoris is eroticized as the result of masturbatory habits of the child. This also occurs in the emotionally infantile adult. The clitoris is the most easily discovered part of the female genitals and the one that first yields the most pleasure when stimulated. Therefore, in childhood the attention is usually focused on the clitoris, and there is little opportunity for vaginal excitation. In women fixed at the clitoric level of development, there is a complete lack of pleasurable vaginal sensitivity to stimulation. These repressed feelings lead to concentration on pleasure from clitoric stimulation and subsequent denial of the vagina as a site for pleasurable sensations. The vagina is psychologically unimportant until puberty; therefore, in the child, the clitoris gives sexual satisfaction, whereas in the emotionally mature woman, the vagina is supposed to be the principal sexual organ. In frigid women the transference of sexual satisfaction and excitement from clitoris to vagina, which usually occurs with emotional maturation, does not occur.

However, Masters and Johnson say that, from an anatomic point of view, complete sexual response cycles, whether induced by clitoral area, vaginal, or breast stimulation, provide identical pelvic reaction patterns. I have interrogated a large number of women and many are not satisfied with clitoric orgasms. The human female's responses are governed by a wide variety of psychic and physical variables, and orgasm cannot be reduced to anatomical factors per se.

However, the vaginal anesthesia present in many frigid women probably represents an inner denial of the "normal" pleasurable sensations derived from intercourse. To these women the husband may symbolically represent the father, and sexual intercourse with him is therefore not allowed to yield pleasurable sensations. Since sexual desires for the father were forbidden, sexual pleasure with the husband is impossible. Frigidity may be due to fear of punishment for violating sexual prohibitions, conflicting loves, love of father as opposed to love of husband, love of self as contrasted to love of husband, and love of other women as opposed to love of men, represented by the husband. Unconscious resentment and hostility with a wish for revenge on men, based on the castration complex, or a wish to avenge the mother for all the suffering she went through at the hands of the father may lead to real frigidity. Hence, the reactions of the envy of men and fear of damage to their genital organs play at least some part in the psychosexual maturation of every girl, and in many cases they are the dominating factors in the development of the psychopathology responsible for the symptom complex of frigidity. The dynamics have been described. (See Kroger, W. S., and Freed, S. C.: *Psychosomatic Gynecology* [3d ed.; Los Angeles: Wilshire Book Co., 1963].)

DIAGNOSIS.—How can a physician attempt to determine whether or not true frigidity is present? If a physical examination of both husband and wife reveals no structural reasons for frigidity, one may safely assume that emotional problems interfere with adequate sexual response. One way of attempting to make a diagnosis is to question the husband concerning the wife's response to coitus. A physician may point out to the husband that there is only one matter in which the wife is completely helpless, namely, control of the involuntary contractions of the pelvic and perineal muscles that occur at the end of the coital act. This is one of the criteria for determining the presence or absence of orgasm. A woman has absolutely no volitional control over the muscles involved in these involuntary contractions. The husband may feel these fine fibrillary contractions culminating a gratifying sexual experience on the deepest inserted portion of the penis. Any attempt at such simulation is impossible, provided, of course, the husband knows how to detect the contractions.

Another, though less reliable, indication is the absence of lubrication at the entrance of the vagina before and during coitus. This is only a presumptive sign of frigidity. Of course, the reverse is not true. The presence of adequate secretion does not exclude the presence of some form of frigidity. Many women have a leukorrheal discharge that may be mistaken for glandular secretions. It should be easy for a physician to diagnose pseudofrigidity that results from impotence on the part of the husband, lack of proper technic, premature ejaculation, coitus interruptus, and intracrural coitus. The necessary information can be obtained by questioning both husband and wife.

TREATMENT.—*Prophylaxis.*—Prevention of frigidity is far more important and surely simpler than treatment. (See Chapter 39, "Premarital Examination and Advice.")

Knight made the following recommendations to parents and educators concerning the prophylaxis of frigidity:

1. In general, a home atmosphere characterized by security, affection and tolerance, absence of parental disagreement before the children and consistent giving of affection and enforcing of discipline by both parents to all the children constitutes good prophylaxis against all later emotional and psychosexual disorders.

2. It is particularly important that parents and older siblings do nothing to influence a child of one sex toward behavior and feelings appropriate to the other sex. When the parents have wanted a boy, for example, and instead a girl is born, it is essential that the girl not be apprised of the parental hopes and regrets in this regard. Also, she should be permitted and encouraged to be normally feminine and not be "processed" into a tomboy because they would have preferred a boy.

3. No matter how difficult the delivery of this girl was (or that of any of the other children) or how near death the mother was during or after childbirth, this story of suffering and miraculous escape from death should never be related to the little girl.

4. The parents, especially the mother, should take a practical, unembarrassed attitude toward matters of bathing, toilet training, childhood masturbation or childhood sexual exposures and experimentation with playmates, so that prudery is not furthered. Parental indignation, intimidation and severe punishment for childhood sexual manifestations many times do more harm than the experiences themselves do.

5. It is probably desirable that children of both sexes be permitted to play about naked and bathe before each other during the first 8 or 10 years, but childhood

observation of the parent of the opposite sex in the nude or during excretory activities has a harmful psychologic effect.

6. Children should, if at all possible, sleep alone in rooms of their own. It is always deleterious psychologically for children to sleep in the same bed or same room with the parents, and especially to observe or overhear parental coitus.

7. Unembarrassed explanations and preparation for the menarche before it happens should always be made by the mother.

8. Education of the little girl toward chastity can easily be overdone. Repeated warnings against boys and men as nasty cruel beasts constantly seeking to take advantage of and ruin girls and women are much worse than no education at all.

9. Children's sexual curiosity expressed in questions should always be answered fully and correctly. Children pay more attention to the tone of voice and attitude of the parent doing the explaining than they do toward the information itself.

Curative treatment.—The consequences of frigidity are often tragic for women. They lead from dissatisfaction, depression, and hysterical symptoms to the most typical defense mechanism, namely, denial by the woman that she is emotionally ill, and the constant changing of husbands and male friends. Every new affair ends in the same fiasco. Except for psychiatrists, as mentioned, the family physician and the obstetrician and gynecologist have a closer relationship with the emotional problems of the patient than any other type of physician.

In nearly all cases it is advisable to have a conference with the patient's husband. Much may be learned from this talk, but it is important for the physician to enlist the husband's co-operation in helping to overcome the wife's ailment without making her feel guilty. In many cases of dyspareunia, the husband loses patience and becomes angry, and discord arises. His impatience increases with each attempt at coitus, and, unless an understanding physician interferes early, a serious marital rift occurs. Therefore it is essential to discuss the situation with the husband soon after the patient's first visit.

If the physical examination fails to reveal any abnormalities and the patient has in the past experienced pleasurable sensations from coitus, testosterone will give satisfactory results because it produces a positive nitrogen balance with some degree of euphoria. A satisfactory method of stimulating or increasing sexual desire is to have the patient use 10-mg. sublingual testosterone tablets, 1 kept in the cheek until it is dissolved, daily for 10 days, then 1 every second day 10 times, and then 1 twice a week for 5 weeks. The enlargement of the clitoris stimulates the libido. In most cases the effect is long lasting, most likely because libidinous drives are aroused. While male hormone therapy is generally successful in women who have experienced orgasms and have become frigid, it will not arouse sex desire in women who have always been frigid. Patients who are treated for frigidity with androgens must be warned about the dangers of virilism, because the virilizing effects will surely add to their unhappiness, especially if treatment is a failure or they are vain about their looks. No patient should receive androgen therapy for frigidity if she does not desire it.

Since the problem of frigidity is predominantly emotional rather than somatic, some may question the right of anyone but a psychiatrist to treat women with frigidity. It is true that most such women should be treated by means of a psychotherapeutic approach; but many frigid women, particularly those who are not too emotionally unbalanced, can be helped considerably by an understanding physician versed in brief psychotherapy, as behavioral conditioning and hypnotherapy. Through posthypnotic suggestions and auto-hypnosis, these women can readily achieve the orgasm they once experienced by redintegration—the process of revivifying past mnemonic data. This is accomplished by obtaining a thorough description of subjective responses during previous orgasms, and then, under hypnosis, suggesting that the same feelings (sensory imagery conditioning of previously stored memories) will occur during a future sex contact.

When a woman fails to receive gratification from early coital attempts she is apt to feel guilty. All that these women need is encouragement, reduction of their guilty fears, and the knowledge that sexual gratification may eventually be achieved.

In some women pseudofrigidity is present even though they experience acute sexual arousal. They are only temporarily inhibited by some situation or circumstance affecting their sexual lives, the correction of which leaves them free to establish or re-establish a pattern of gratification. Frequently, the patient is handicapped by her faulty attitude toward her difficulties. Having begun her act of sexual life only to meet disappointment and frustration, the reasons for which are more or less obscure to her, she is confirmed in her disappointment by time, and tends to assume an attitude of indifference, which soon gives way to hostility and resentment. She acquires an attitude of defeat, looks for escape consciously or unconsciously and is tormented by feelings of inferiority. Such women are the ones who are desperately in need of help, perhaps more so than the truly frigid woman, for they have some idea of what they are missing in the emotional fulfillment of their lives. They are the persons whom the family physician, or the gynecologist particularly, may be able to help if he succeeds in discovering the factors responsible for their problem.

Conflict may be caused by the atmosphere and environment in which sexual intercourse occurs. The woman may lack a feeling of complete security. Inadequate housing that causes a couple to live with parents may produce more than the ordinary personal conflict resulting from two families living under one roof. The self-consciousness and guilt associated with the sexual activities of two young people living their sexual lives under the eyes and within the hearing of the parents is almost inevitable; for these same parents have often, by means of previous taboos and threats, sought to control the early sexual drives of their children. The mere legal sanction of marriage is not sufficient to allay or completely change their attitudes. No matter how trivial these factors may seem to the husband or physician, if their correction cures the pseudofrigidity, they are obviously important.

Personal habits may provide another source of conflict. If the partner is not fastidious in the care of his person, by taking too few baths and poor care of the teeth, the woman may feel disgust and be unable to participate freely and happily in intercourse. Furthermore, the husband may wish to indulge in certain types of sexual play that the woman feels are abnormal. She may feel offended by his desire to experiment with oral-genital contacts or what she considers abnormal postures for intercourse. The husband may have a deep need for gratification of a desire to see his partner in the nude and may want some light in the room, whereas the wife's sense of modesty and decorum may be offended by these procedures, with resulting inhibition of all sexual pleasures. All or any of these conflicts may be indicative of neurotic personality patterns, but they are not necessarily permanent and may be corrected by proper education. Some minor conditions that may easily be corrected are lack of pleasure from coitus interruptus, intracrural intercourse, and a real or imagined difference in the size of the penis and the vagina. In nearly all cases in which a woman says the penis is too large or too small, it will be found that faulty attitude and incorrect technics are responsible for the lack of pleasure. In rare cases the vagina is actually too large or the muscles are too lax for a woman to perceive and feel the penis properly in the vagina. In such cases a perineorraphy, or much more simply, activation of the pubococcygeus muscle as recommended by Kegel (see Chapter 24), will eliminate the source of the trouble.

15

Psychosomatic Gynecology

PSYCHOSOMATIC medicine may be defined as the study of the reciprocal action of body and mind in total environment as these affect behavior. Physicians know that functioning of the female generative tract, especially hormonal activities, can readily be disturbed by specific or non-specific stresses from within or without the organism. Psychiatrists recognize that the factors, particularly emotional tensions, that are responsible for functional gynecologic conditions usually originate during early development of the personality.

Relationship of Personality Factors to Psychogynecic Symptoms

Personality is the sum total of the individual's reaction to biologic and sociopsychologic factors. The interaction of these factors with internal stimuli determines symptomatology. For example, functional dysmenorrhea cannot occur without involvement of the entire personality. This symptom reflects the unhealthy attitude toward femininity that is so predominant in our society. At one time femininity, marriage, and motherhood were regarded as acceptable psychobiologic regularities of womanhood. For many women, this is no longer true. The woman who is at odds with her biologic self develops serious conflicts and tension, often leading to psychogynecic (psychosomatic and gynecologic) symptoms.

These symptoms usually are accompanied by unmistakable signs of emotional immaturity—a state wherein the individual, because of lack of self-confidence, is unable to face any crisis that disturbs her equilibrium. When an adult is confronted by threatening situations, there is usually an emotional return to behavior patterns characteristic of dependent periods in life, as infancy and childhood. During these states, responsibilities were unknown and nursing, thumb-sucking, and other forms of oral gratification successfully alleviated anxiety and helped re-establish emotional security. This "return-to-the-breast" reaction manifested by excessive oral intake illustrates how the adult can utilize regressive behavior patterns in an effort to allay oral tensions. However, the only result of the fleeting pleasure of overeating is more tension, painful conflict, and subsequent weight gain. The person, of course, is no longer consciously aware of the infantile patterns of reacting to stress and frustration by oral satisfaction.

Relationship of Personality Factors to Diagnosis

A careful review of the psychosomatic literature indicates that personality factors should be sought in the diagnosis of many conditions discussed in this book. These conditions include menstrual dysfunctions, the menopause, pruritus vulvae, urinary difficulties, sterility, and low back and pelvic pain. The same approach must be followed in cases of frigidity and dyspareunia due to vaginismus. Behind the psychogynecic manifestations of long-standing conflict and tension are the following prodromata: poor concentration, irritability, temper tantrums, mood swings, mild gastric upsets, vague pelvic discomfort, anorexia, headaches, easy fatigability, diffuse substernal pain, cardiac palpitation, restlessness, and, particularly, insomnia.

Psychosomatic illness is one of the most insidious of all human afflictions. It is the end-product of an emotional illness that evolved so imperceptibly that no one, least of all the patient, recognized it. Although physical symptoms may be the first and only manifestation of an incipient neurosis, it is imperative to rule out an organic etiology. Contrarily, the absence of physical findings does not necessarily indicate that the symptoms are of psychologic origin.

How can this differentiation be accomplished? First, did stress precede the onset of the symptoms? Are the symptoms connected with, or aggravated by, emotional upsets? Is there evidence of a previous personality disturbance? What was the behavior reaction to other environmental difficulties? Is there a history of acute or chronic illness, particularly one that may have interfered with sexual and social adjustment? If so, were the symptoms similar to the present complaints? What is the present life situation, and is there any evidence of psychosexual maladjustment? Are the complaints compatible with the physical findings? Finally, and this is most important, does the patient accept herself as a woman?

The way the patient responds to spontaneous questions will help bring out the above information. However, these questions must never be phrased in such a way as to bias the patient's reply. If the physician watches his tone of voice and choice of words, the patient will not be given a clue to the answers expected. The significance of unintentional verbal implications such as "slips of the tongue," sighs, jocularity, and hypochondriacal expressions should be noted. For instance, does the patient laugh off or minimize serious symptoms such as prolonged menstrual bleeding; or are fleeting abdominal aches and pains exaggerated? To be especially looked for are blushing or blanching, flickering or lowering of the eyes, and other changes in facial expression, tensing of the jaw muscles or fists, changes in intonation of voice, rapidity of speech, stuttering (the last occurs when highly charged emotional material is touched upon), and the quickness with which direct questions are answered. "Clamming up," confusion, and amnesia indicate an emotional block.

Even when the patient appears to be relaxed, rapid-fire questions are to be avoided, as the answers are apt to be glib ones. Multiple questions asked simultaneously also provide an opportunity for the patient to dodge one of the questions by focusing entirely on others.

The time taken for the formal history can be used to gain the patient's confidence. Routine questions should not be asked, because the patient usually feels that the physician who asks routine questions deserves only routine answers and has no right to know about her intimate or personal life. Beginning with the physical examination, the facts relative to the presenting complaints can be elicited. However, apparently significant facts should never be accepted at face value, since many patients not only lie but are confused and rationalize about their symptoms and complaints. If additional information is needed, interviews with other members of the family are necessary. A complete battery of psychologic tests are time savers and afford a comprehensive survey of the personality, even in extremely sick patients.

In handling disturbed patients, the physician should remember the following facts: (1) The emotionally upset person is the most difficult to handle. Therefore the physical examination should be conducted in such a manner as to avoid causing excessive anxiety. Since the emotionally upset patient is susceptible to chance remarks, the physician's approach should be as meticulous as his surgical asepsis. (2) The doctor should make the patient feel accepted, and above all he should avoid a prejudicial or dictatorial attitude. He must be warm, understanding, and objective. The patient will be more likely to "open up" if she feels that the doctor understands and is interested in what her experiences mean to her. Psychosomatic histories, especially when there is a profound sexual disturbance, often disclose a variety of frustrations, pain, unfulfilled wishes, disappointments, tragic situations, and ultimate catastrophe as the desire for divorce. Unquestionably, the physician who senses what these things mean in terms of psychic suffering will more effectively inspire faith and optimism in his patient. (3) Premature pronouncements or interpretations, as "You are going to be all right," must be avoided, since it is fairly obvious to the patient that the physician does not yet know why she is ill. (4) The physician should keep within his psychotherapeutic limitations and not attempt to uncover "hot" material unless he knows what to do when it appears. (5) He must take plenty of time to listen to the patient's troubles and not be interrupted by telephone calls or the frequent intrusion of an assistant or nurse. The information will come forth freely if the patient is relaxed. Many women feel more comfortable if they are allowed to smoke during interviews. At first the questions should be directed toward subjects that are nonsexual and least likely to disturb the patient. One must follow a sequence that leads to the gradual discussion of difficult subjects, leaving those matters which may cause embarrassment for later interviews. A sensitive and skilled physician will immediately drop a line of inquiry that causes an adverse reaction in his patient. Later, the interviews should allow the patient an opportunity to develop her own thinking, express her hopes and sorrows, and bring into the open the things she was unable previously to admit even to herself. Patients who have a genuine desire to get well will seldom cover up, deny, or fail to relate their secrets in a permissive atmosphere. (6) A good doctor-patient relationship is necessary, especially when the information is of an intimate or sexual nature. The physician, interested in these matters, should be able to discuss any type of sexual behavior objectively, without signs of disgust and without social or moral evaluation. Furthermore, all questions relative to sex should be asked without hesitation or apology and at the level of the patient's intelligence. If the patient senses that the physician is embarrassed and cannot talk freely about sex problems, she will usually answer evasively and dishonestly about these matters.

Psychodynamics

The term "psychodynamic" refers to the forces of the mind in action. It does *not* refer to a specific mode of psychotherapy. In this section, the interaction of ideas, impulses, and emotions responsible for the commoner psychogynecic entities will be discussed briefly.

Many women, wittingly or unwittingly, exaggerate the severity of their complaints to gratify neurotic desires. They seldom connect their physical discomfort and anxiety with a need for attention, dependence, or dislike of responsibility. Often they develop ailments in order to dominate those around them or use such ailments as self-punishment for their own hostility and aggression. The latter mechanism is frequently associated with psychogenic pruritus vulvae; the bottled-up hostility over sexual frustration is displaced to the genital zone, thus providing a ready-made alibi for the excessive scratching.

One often sees patients with polysurgical addiction, who make the rounds of physicians' offices seeking yet another operation. Previous operations usually include appendectomy, removal of ovarian cysts, suspension of the uterus, and correction of adhesions. Patients with polysurgical addiction are not aware of their deep-seated need for an operative assault. Because of their seldom-recognized guilt feelings, the surgery serves as punishment, as atonement, and finally as a license to commit new offenses. It is fortunate that most physicians sense such patients' demands and refuse to operate. However, when the conscience-stricken patient finally finds an obliging doctor, her demand for surgery is met. As a rule, the improvement is temporary after such obtuse therapy, and the unwarranted surgery always makes the neurotic patient worse. Many such women also request urethral and vaginal treatments for nonexistent disease. These demands are masturbation equivalents; sexual gratification is obtained in the guise of the physician's treatment, whereas self-manipulation of the genitals is taboo. The doctor must constantly realize that the patient may be only vaguely, if at all, aware of the connection between her symptoms and her emotional problem. Many such patients are also frigid. The psychosomatic aspects of frigidity, as well as dyspareunia due to vaginismus, are discussed in Chapter 14.

Functional amenorrhea may occur in women who consciously or unconsciously cannot accept womanhood. This condition is commonly noted in "tomboys." Stress secondary to emotional conflicts may also produce amenorrhea by altering the cortical stimuli to the hypothalamic nuclei responsible for releasing the proper pituitary gonadotrophic hormones. These women may have strong sexual drives, but because of deep-seated hostility toward males, or femininity, or both, they regard menstruation as something "dirty" and indicative of their own inferiority. In addition to hormonal assays and other laboratory tests, a study of the personality patterns and attitudes of amenorrheic patients is a prerequisite before any type of therapy is employed.

Pseudocyesis is another form of functional amenorrhea. It results from a powerful wish for a child. This entity beautifully illustrates how psychic forces are capable of altering physiologic processes—release of luteotrophins and suppression of follicle-stimulating hormone. The patient must never be told that she is not pregnant until her neurotic needs for maintaining the "pregnancy" have been made clear to her.

Functional uterine bleeding may occur as a defense against intercourse. More often, it is associated with fear of pregnancy, fright, and other anxieties. The psychosomatic mechanisms responsible for this entity have not yet been clarified.

Functional dysmenorrhea is generally a symptom of a personality disorder, even though hormonal imbalance may be present. Therefore, a thorough study of the woman's attitudes toward femininity is often necessary. Menstruation is a "badge of femininity," which may be worn in misery, pain, or pride, according to the attitude of the woman. Because the vast reservoir of the unconscious background contains the memories of painful experiences, a conditioned pain pattern, analogous to the pain of phantom limb in amputees, can be established in the cortex. Early conflicts associated with puberty and adolescence may give rise to the idea that pain and menstruation are synonymous, that menstruation is, in reality, "the curse." What makes it a typical emotional disorder is that, as a rule, there are no gross lesions, and monthly pain varies according to mood swings and spontaneous cure often occurs. The contradictory endocrine theories, the varied reports, and the frequent relapses with endocrine therapy all seem to confirm the psychosomatic nature of functional dysmenorrhea.

Regarding the climacteric, doubt exists as to the onset, the degree of relief afforded by hormones, the importance of psychologic factors, and the very nature of menopausal symptoms. To confuse the picture further, women with intense hot flashes may have vaginal smears indicating adequate estrogen production, whereas some others devoid of symptoms have complete absence of vaginal cornification. Evidence exists that a "third gonad" in the adrenal gland is capable of producing estrogens and androgens long after the ovaries atrophy. The vasomotor symptoms occurring during the menopause can be relieved by homespun psychotherapy. This consists of eradication of such fallacies concerning the change of life as loss of libido, unattractiveness, and premature aging. Such re-education and assurance, together with the judicious use of mild sedatives, tranquilizers, and antidepressants, as well as estrogens orally, will help make the patient independent of hypodermic medication.

Functional low backache and pelvic pain often have an emotional basis. These symptoms cannot be approached with the scalpel. For "vertebral hypochondriacs," worry is a "pain in the back." Their back symptoms express the language of the body, saying, "I have such a load (conflict) on my back—I just can't carry my troubles around any longer." The diagnosis of low back and pelvic pain of psychosomatic origin is admittedly difficult. There can, however, be no question of real versus psychic pain. All pain is real, regardless of the cause. For the differential diagnosis of low back pain, the reader is referred to Chapter 23.

Chronic vascular congestion of the pelvic organs, secondary to autonomic imbalance based on nonspecific emotional stimuli, accounts for a large proportion of office gynecology. Included are most of the conditions described in this book, as well as idiopathic leukorrhea, uterine hypertrophy, endocervicitis, so-called congested and cystic ovaries, and other entities commonly classified as endocrine and inflammatory.

In nervous women, infertility may be produced by tubal spasm secondary to emotional tension. This spasm, often erroneously mistaken for tubal occlusion, has been observed by direct visualization of the tubes under fluoroscopy or culdoscopy. These examinations as well as other recommended procedures should be carried out in all cases of psychosomatic sterility. The physician who treats infertility should recognize that some women, even those who ardently wish to become pregnant, really do not want a child. The attentive physician can deduce this desire from the patient's remarks. She may say, "I want children, Doctor, but will my heart stand it?" or "Doctor, am I too set in my ways to care for a child properly?" Some women do not want the trouble of rearing a child because it will interfere with their social life; others may fear the interruption of a career. Of course, the patient is wholly unaware of this rejection of pregnancy. Rejection occurs in women who have strong masculine drives or those who cannot face the responsibilities of motherhood.

When such women finally succeed in having a baby, they usually "take their spite out" on the unwanted child, thus adversely affecting its psychic development. Hence, successful treatment of infertility should always include an adequate personality appraisal and, if necessary, therapy directed toward acceptance of the maternal role.

Uncomplicated retroversion of the uterus is clinically insignificant. The phrase "tipped womb" should be eliminated from the physician's vocabulary. This iatrogenic diagnosis often connotes the possibility of serious disease, causing the patient to focus her attention on her pelvic organs.

Psychosomatic Treatment

Contrary to current medical opinion, psychosomatic treatment does not consist only of a purely psychologic approach. Such therapy is based on the fundamental principles of internal medicine as well as on an understanding of psychogenic processes. The therapeutic value of all interviews depends upon the patient-doctor relationship, which begins with the initial visit. The quality of this relationship is determined by the personality of the patient as well as by the personality and training of the physician and his attitude toward the patient and her problems.

Although psychiatric training is a valuable adjunct for every physician, it is not absolutely necessary to an understanding of the surface aspects of patients' problems and significant emotional experiences. The family physician is in a unique position, since he already is a sort of father-confessor and is constantly presented with the opportunity of understanding his patient as *one inseparable whole*, both in sickness and in health. Understanding should not be confused with cure, because in all fields of medicine the attempt to cure is often unsuccessful in spite of complete understanding. However, once a physician becomes aware of the patient's aspirations, conflicts, and tensions, common sense and a practical knowledge of human nature will allow him to evaluate the influence of psychic factors on gynecologic problems, and vice versa. Clinical practice, moreover, provides him with ample opportunity for differentiating normal and abnormal behavior patterns and deciding on the type of psychotherapy.

After it seems evident that no organic disease is responsible for the symptoms, no further medical measures are indicated, since they render the prognosis much less favorable and increase the difficulties of psychotherapy. Psychotherapy is directed toward breaking up the interaction of the neurotic patterns and somatic symptoms that characterize gynecologic dysfunctions. In this approach, recognition of the patient's motivation for seeking treatment is imperative. The patient may believe that she is suffering from organic disease and expect purely medical treatment, or she may ascribe the symptom of low back pain, for example, to excessive housework, without perceiving that her *attitude* toward her labors at home may be the real cause for her complaint.

The mere suggestion of psychotherapy often arouses resistance in the anxious patient. This reaction springs from an instinctive opposition to any attempt to bring deeply repressed, anxiety-producing material into conscious awareness. Such resistance is usually manifested by broken appointments, medical shopping, self-treatment, devaluation of the doctor's ability, haggling over a fee, procrastination in obtaining diagnostic tests, and resort to previously ineffective remedies. Exposing a defensive attitude and resistance should not prove too difficult for the experienced physician. To have this type of patient come for treatment, he must have a heart-to-heart talk with her and tactfully point out the reasons for her delaying tactics.

The patient will more readily discuss her emotional problems if given a simple explanation of how nervous feelings, fears, and depression can be productive of symptomatology. The doctor may cite the commonly observed psychosomatic symptoms, such as rapid heart action in response to excitement, slow heart action caused by intense fear, and loss of appetite during periods of depression. In the explanation he should avoid psychiatric terminology and should not use words that imply *mental* disturbance, such as "psychoneurotic." In a psychoneurosis, the influence of the doctor on the patient's attitudes and feelings is the principal therapeutic factor; to make light of the patient's suffering is a grave mistake and may damage the doctor-patient relationship irreparably.

If the cause of nervous tension is recognized, it should not be bluntly made known to the patient. Rather it should be discussed in such a manner that it finally becomes self-revealing to her. The need on the part of the patient to understand the responsible mechanisms may not in itself be important, but how she feels about her anxiety-producing situations, how she reacts to them emotionally, is of the utmost importance. This information also will shed light on her ability to bear emotional upheavals.

If the physician doubts his ability to treat the patient, he should refer her to a psychiatrist. Sometimes this is a ticklish situation for both physician and patient. He may feel that the consultation reflects on his ability. The patient may incorrectly get the impression that the physician thinks she is unbalanced. Proper preparation for psychiatric referral can be managed by discussing some of the patient's emotional problems (about which he now has some information) and noting her reactions to this discussion. When he has established good rapport (and this may take several visits), he may remark, "If your eyes needed to be tested, I would send you to an ophthalmologist. Likewise, there are physicians who specialize in treating emotional conditions." Naturally few patients wish to be suspected of being neurotic. The patient usually comes solely for relief of her physical symptoms, and, if diplomacy is not used, the physician will have a hostile ex-patient.

The physician untrained in psychiatry can use superficial psychotherapy, such as persuasion, suggestion, and reassurance, which are essentially supportive measures. Superficial psychotherapy, or supportive therapy, is a method directed toward modification of the emotional conflicts and their physical results by supporting the inherent strength of the patient's personality. It is designed to help the patient adjust to her difficulties on a *here* and *now* basis. There is no need to fish in the past, as such an approach yields only diminishing returns. Rather, it is advisable to elicit the problems and advise her how to cope with them. This type of therapy is rapidly gaining more adherents as confidence in the utility of psychoanalysis wanes.

If the patient has previously been well adjusted and is suffering only from nervous reactions due to pressure from some recent and unusually trying situation, supportive therapy is the one of choice. If because of anxiety and preoccupation with her symptoms, the patient remains disturbed, the doctor should lead her into an objective discussion of her emotional problems, so that she understands *how* and *why* she reacts as she does. Her ability to talk out her problems will be facilitated by sympathy and interest, which will help make her feel that someone is at last on her side. Such a healthy relationship between patient and physician establishes a beachhead on the periphery of her neurosis. This, together with the lessening of her fears, will enable her to know how she should *face* her problems instead of always running away from them. Thus, in many cases tension is reduced, and, at the same time, the patient's self-esteem and self-confidence are increased. Deeply disturbed patients, however, require the services of psychiatrically trained physicians, who may employ hypnotherapy, behavioral conditioning, and eclectic psychotherapeutic modalities.

16

Infertility and Sterility

ABSOLUTE INFERTILITY or sterility refers to a condition in which reproduction is impossible temporarily or permanently. Women in whom the uterus has never developed are absolutely and permanently sterile. However, women who undergo sterilization operations may be only temporarily infertile, because failures are not uncommon following such operations. Even after hysterectomy, women have conceived.

Relative infertility is midway between absolute sterility and absolute fertility, the latter condition being common in animals.

In general, about 12% of all married couples are infertile. Meaker listed nine conditions as requisites of absolute fertility: (1) The testicles must produce normal spermatozoa. (2) The male genital tract must allow the free passage of spermatozoa from the testicles to the urethral meatus. (3) The prostatovesicular secretions must be favorable to spermatozoa. (4) Ejaculated spermatozoa must be delivered to and received by the cervix. (5) The endocervical secretions must be favorable to spermatozoa. (6) The uterus must allow free passage of spermatozoa from the cervix to the uterine openings of the tubes. (7) The tubes must allow free ascent of spermatozoa and descent of ova. (8) The ovariotubal spaces must allow free passage of ova from the ovaries to the abdominal openings of the tubes. (9) The ovaries must produce normal ova. To these I would add: (10) The uterine endometrium must be in proper condition to permit embedding and growth of the fertilized ovum.

The causes of infertility may, therefore, be listed as: (1) deficient spermatogenesis; (2) obstruction and occlusion of the male genital tract; (3) unfavorable prostatovesicular secretions; (4) faults of delivery during coitus and reception; (5) unfavorable endocervical secretions; (6) uterine factors; (7) tubal obstruction and occlusion; (8) obstruction of ovariotubal spaces; (9) ovulation failure; and (10) defective endometrium.

1. Deficient spermatogenesis may be due to atrophy of the testicles, constitutional disturbances, or some endocrine abnormality. In obtaining a history from the husband, inquiry should always be made concerning mumps. In some cases of bilateral orchitis occurring as a complication of mumps, sterility results.

2. Obstruction and occlusion in the male genital tract frequently results from gonorrhea.

3. Prostatovesicular secretions are frequently unfavorable, but this fact is easily overlooked.

4. In analyzing faults of delivery during coitus, one must consider both the male and the female. Among the male faults may be mentioned malformations, impotence, and premature ejaculation. In the female, malformations and deformities also play a role. Dyspareunia is a factor in some cases.

5. The endocervical secretions may be chemically, serologically, bacteriologically, or mechanically unfavorable. Probably only the mechanical type is important in sterility. Little is known about the others. There is an alteration in the cervical mucus at the time of presumed ovulation, as first shown by Seguy, Vimeux, and Simmonet. During the time of ovulation the cervical mucus becomes more glairy and profuse and is occasionally blood tinged. It is at this time that spermatozoa gain access to the uterine cavity most readily.

6. Uterine factors that prevent passage of spermatozoa may result from submucous leiomyomas, uterine abnormalities, operations on the uterus, and extensive uterine synechiae (Asherman's syndrome).

7. Tubal obstruction and occlusion may result from conditions outside the tube, abnormalities inside the tube, developmental anomalies, inflammation, or muscular spasm.

8. Disturbances at the ovariotubal space may be more common than is believed. It has been shown that in some lower animals the fimbriated ends of the tubes surround the ovaries during the time of ovulation and pick up the ovum. If this is a universal occurrence, interference with this mechanism may result in sterility.

9. Ovulation failure may be due to hypoplasia of the entire reproductive tract. This results from a disturbance in the constitution during adolescence. Local conditions in the ovary may also interfere with ovulation, as may constitutional conditions, periovarian adhesions, inflammation, tumors, and exposure to radiation, either roentgen or radium, over a long period.

10. Defective endometrium may be due to submucous leiomyomas, destructive manipulation such as improper curettage, and inflammation such as tuberculosis. Tuberculosis has been found to be the cause of sterility in a high percentage of cases in some countries but not in the United States.

It is of fundamental importance to appreciate that in the ordinary case infertility is due not to one deviation from the normal but to a summation of several causative factors. However, only in a few instances can the blame be placed entirely on one partner.

Investigation of the Infertile Couple

The best results in the treatment of infertility are forthcoming when infertile couples are examined by a group of physicians composed of a gynecologist, a urologist, an internist, an endocrinologist, and a clinical pathologist. However, such a group study is possible for only a small minority of infertile couples. Usually the gynecologist or general practitioner must handle the infertile couple alone, and he can accomplish a great deal in most cases.

First, a complete history is obtained from both husband and wife. Then a complete physical examination is made of both partners. Special attention, of course, is paid to the genital organs. Semen should be examined before any extensive investigation of the wife is made. The period of continence to be prescribed before the semen specimen is obtained is determined by the frequency of intercourse to which the couple has been accustomed during the time they have been seeking conception. That is to say, if their frequency of intercourse during this time is twice weekly, the period of continence prior to submission of the specimen should be 3 or 4 days. The specimen should be obtained by masturbation if possible and delivered into a clean (not necessarily sterile) glass receptacle, great care being taken that none of the ejaculate is lost. If the manual method is impossible or distasteful, the specimen should be obtained by withdrawal after intercourse. A condom specimen never should be accepted. The specimen can be obtained at home and should be brought to the physician's office within 1 hour. The specimen should be tightly corked and never refrigerated. Unless the outside temperature is severe (under 30°F.), no special temperature precautions are necessary during transport.

For Catholic patients and others, Doyle recommends a procedure that is simple and acceptable psychologically and morally. This is the use of a plastic-lined cervical spoon which the husband inserts into the vagina. This spoon and a vinyl-coated cervical tampon aid sperm deposition and sperm survival for maximum utilization of the migration potentiality in cases where the husband has a low sperm count. The spoon is also useful for obtaining a physiologic post-coital semen specimen, available for motility and viability assay.

If the patient has had any febrile illness during 2 months prior to the semen examination and if the latter shows defects, another specimen should be examined several weeks later. The effect of hyperpyrexia upon spermatogenesis is important. Carl Moore and his co-workers showed that exposure of the testes of the rat, guinea pig, and sheep to temperatures above that of the scrotum results in degeneration of the germinal epithelium and consequent failure of spermatogenesis. MacLeod and Hotchkiss studied the effects of elevated body temperature on the total sperm counts in men and found that the effects followed closely the results of similar experiments on animals. For nearly 3 weeks after fever, the human sperm count remains at a relatively normal level. This indicates that the store of mature spermatozoa in the epididymis and ductus deferens not only is not affected by the temperature elevation but is of such magnitude that any injury to the germinal epithelium is not manifested immediately. The deleterious effect of the fever may last for 50 days. MacLeod showed that a relatively mild disease in the adult, such as chickenpox, might depress spermatogenesis to the point of absolute sterility and that the time sequence of the depression and recovery was similar to that found in simple hyperpyrexia.

Therefore, when defects in semen quality are found, it is important to know about recent illnesses. In any event, if a low sperm count or poor motility is found in the first examination, a second examination should be made.

Whereas examination of the semen gives a great deal of information about the male partner, it often may be misleading. It is conceivable, of course, that the spermatozoa may be alive in a jar and yet may not reach the uterine cavity. It is therefore important to know what happens in the cervix. Huhner is considered the first to have made systematic and routine examinations of the spermatozoa in the cervical canal by what is now called the Huhner test. However, J. Marion Sims, in 1868, described this test, so it should be called the *Sims-Huhner* test. It is simple to carry out (see p. 147).

In women the vagina is always acid and the cervix always alkaline. I have long maintained that the acidity of the vagina plays no role in sterility or fertility. The spermatozoon that fertilizes the ovum is nearly always one of the millions that are forced against the cervix at the time of ejaculation.

In certain animals, particularly rats, millions of live spermatozoa can regularly be found in the uterine cavity within 60 seconds of ejaculation. Either the spermatozoa are ejected into the uterine cavity through an open cervix or the spermatozoa are aspirated quickly, but, whichever takes place, the sperm gain access to the uterine cavity almost simultaneously with the ejaculation. On examining fecund couples, Sobrero and MacLeod found active spermatozoa in the cervical mucus within $1\frac{1}{2}$ minutes after intercourse. This seemed to bear out the idea that the sperm that are ejaculated directly at the cervix during an orgasm are the ones really responsible for fertilization. These workers suggested that orgasm may intensify cervical insemination, since it is apt to increase protrusion of the cervical plug. The healthy cervical secretion is most favorable for spermatozoa, because sperm will survive at least 3 times as long in cervical mucus as in their own seminal fluid at comparable temperatures.

A *semen penetration test* may be performed in the following way. A drop of semen and some cervical mucus are placed on a slide so that the surfaces become contiguous when covered by a glass cover slide. The result is positive if columns of spermatozoa can be seen microscopically in the mucus. The result is negative if the spermatozoa fail to penetrate the mucus. Satisfactory postcoital tests can be obtained over a wide range of the menstrual cycle and not, as is believed, only on days coincident with or close to ovulation (see Fig. 52).

EVALUATION OF SEMEN.—For complete evaluation of the fertilizing potential of a specimen of semen, six facts must be known: (1) volume of the ejaculate, (2) number of spermatozoa per milliliter of semen, (3) total number of spermatozoa in the ejaculate, (4) percentage of motile spermatozoa, (5) quality (vigor of progressive motion) of motility, and (6) percentage of cells showing abnormal morphology.

1. The ejaculate volume depends in part on the period of continence preceding the obtaining of the specimen, but after 3 or 4 days, the period of continence usually practiced by married persons, the average ejaculate volume is about 3.5 ml., with a range between 2 and 5 ml. A volume below 2.0 ml. after 3 or 4 days of continence should be considered low and possibly a factor in the failure of conception. It is not necessary to measure the pH of semen; the pH is physiologic at the time of ejaculation (7.0–7.3), but rapidly becomes alkaline (8.0–9.0) owing to loss of CO_2 on exposure to air.

2. There are many ways to determine the exact number of spermatozoa per milliliter of semen, the simplest probably being that of Hotchkiss. The diluent for counting is a saturated solution of sodium bicarbonate and 1% phenol. The white blood cell pipet and ordinary Neubauer chamber are used. If numerous spermatozoa are seen in the fresh drop under the high dry lens, a 1:20 dilution is made by drawing the well-mixed semen to the 0.5 mark on the pipet, which is then filled to the 11 mark with the bicarbonate-phenol solution. After thorough shaking, about half of the mixture is discarded and the remainder used for the count. The mixture is applied to the counting chamber in such fashion that the chamber is just filled. Precisely the same technic is followed in making sperm counts as in making blood cell counts. Five blocks of 16 squares, or one fifth of the red blood cell field, are used. All of the spermatozoa lying within this area and with bodies overlying the lines on two sides of the squares are counted. The total number of spermatozoa counted in the five blocks plus six ciphers gives the spermatozoa count per milliliter.

3. The total number of spermatozoa is, of course, determined by multiplying the number of spermatozoa per milliliter of the ejaculate by the ejaculate volume.

4. The percentage of active spermatozoa may be determined with reasonable accuracy by means of the Ehrlich ocular screen, in which the field of vision is divided into four quadrants. But, for ordinary purposes outside the research field, the percentage of active spermatozoa can be roughly estimated by simply examining a high dry field. It does not require appreciable skill to determine whether 30 or 50% of the cells are inert. If the semen of fertile men is examined thus within 3 hours after ejaculation, at least 40% of the cells should show a reasonable degree (see below) of vigorous forward motion. The average percentage found in fertile men after 3 to 6 days of continence is about 60%,

though this percentage is likely to be considerably lower after prolonged (10 days plus) continence. A percentage of 80–90% active is unusually high.

5. The assessment of quality of motility is largely a matter of experience and does not require elaborate equipment. However, since this is probably the most important single aspect of the semen examination, care should be taken as to the conditions under which it is measured.

Motile activity should not be assessed until at least 1 hour after ejaculation and preferably within 3 hours. The semen usually is coagulated immediately after ejaculation, and the spermatozoa are tightly enmeshed in the coagulum. Liquefaction should be complete within 30 minutes in most specimens, but it should be emphasized that some specimens retain a high viscosity for indefinite periods. This viscosity, however, is different from the coagulation that accompanies ejaculation and need not necessarily (indeed, it seldom does) act as an impediment to good motile activity.

It is extremely doubtful, according to MacLeod and Gold, that periodic examinations of motility beyond 5 hours after ejaculation have any validity. A single examination of motility within 3 to 4 hours after ejaculation would, in most cases, suffice and be quite representative of the potential fertility of any particular specimen. A rapid deterioration in motility within a few hours may represent changes in the seminal environment of the spermatozoa which under physiologic conditions they would not encounter. It should be remembered that the seminal fluid is not a physiologic environment for the spermatozoa beyond a period of a few minutes.

It should not be difficult for even the least experienced observer to determine whether spermatozoa exhibit vigorous, progressive motion or are either sluggish or erratic in their movements. The expression of such activity in terms of distance traveled per unit of time is exceedingly difficult and not at all practical. Nor is it feasible in clinical practice to subject the spermatozoa to various temperatures or other tests in order to determine their resistance. The motility should be determined at room temperature on a drop of semen placed between slide and cover glass.

Hotchkiss suggested the following standards for motility, which have been found satisfactory by many workers: grade 4, excellent, aggressive; grade 3, good, progressive; grade 2, fair to poor; grade 1, sluggish, with little space-gaining activity.

For morphological examination, a drop of semen is placed near the end of a glass slide and, with another slide at a 45° angle, a thin smear is obtained. This is air dried and fixed with 10% formalin for one minute, rinsed in water, and stained by the Papanicolaou technique.

An alternative method (Williams) is to prepare a smear and remove the mucus by means of a 0.5% chloramine solution (brief rinse), wash in water, air dry, and stain as follows:

1. 0.25% aqueous crystal violet for 3 minutes.
2. Wash briefly with water.
3. De-stain with 95% alcohol.
4. Wash in water.
5. Rose Bengal 1% aqueous solution for 30 seconds.
6. Wash with water and dry.

Examine the cells under an oil-immersion objective. The enumeration of 100 cells should be sufficient to determine the degree of abnormality.

In recent years, a certain pattern of sperm morphology has been recognized as representing the response of the human testes to a variety of trauma (viral illnesses, other infections, allergic reactions, liver disease and anti-spermatogenic agents). It is found particularly in the presence of varicocele where this anomaly is accompanied by severe oligospermia (under 10 million/ml.) and impaired motility. This pattern is distinguished by a high percentage of tapering forms (hyper-elongation of sperm heads) and of immature forms of the germinal line (spermatids). In the wet mount the latter often are mistaken for "pus" cells.

The sperm count has always been the chief index in considering potential fertility, but just as much if not more emphasis should be placed on the percentage of active cells in a semen specimen and the quality of motility shown by these cells. In recent years, there has been considerable controversy about the lower sperm count limit for a normal male. For many years the figure 60,000,000 per ml. stood out like a red light, but this figure is far too high. MacLeod and Gold, in extensive studies of semen quality in 1,000 men of known fertility and in 1,000 infertile marriages, found that the really significant difference in the sperm counts of both populations lay in the range between one and 20,000,000. In this category, more than three times as many infertile as fertile men were to be found. These authors have shown, furthermore, that above 20,000,000 there is no rise in the potential fertility of the male provided the cells show good qualities of motility and morphology. In other words, the sperm count is not the all-important factor in male fertility. If the spermatozoa of any given specimen show a good quality of motility and possess good morphology, true male infertility, so far as count is concerned, should be considered as beginning at a count level close to 20,000,000 per milliliter. *No man should ever be told he cannot have children simply because his sperm count is very low, even under 10,000,000 per milliliter.*

Other factors than sperm count must also be considered. One of these is morphology. MacLeod and Gold found that the sperm morphology of their fertile group of men was consistently better than that of their infertile group. A good "percentage active" figure is 75, and one between 50 and 60 is average. The critical level at which the sharp difference between the fertile and the "infertile" men becomes apparent is less than 40% active. The time taken to achieve conception decreases with increasing "percentage active" cells, because the chances of fertility increase with rising quality of motility. All primary aspects of semen quality (count, motility, and morphology) are important. Semen quality is poor as long as one quality is poor; it is adequate when there are no poor qualities and good when all three are good.

As mentioned earlier, the quality of motility shown by the spermatozoa may perhaps be the most important single factor. Certainly, good quality of motility is a most important compensatory factor if other defects in semen quality are present.

In summary, with regard to semen quality, the lowest standards that should be accepted are:

1. A volume of 2 ml.
2. A sperm count of 20,000,000 per milliliter or more.
3. At least 40% active cells.
4. A quality of motility above grade 2.
5. At least 60% normal forms.

OTHER FACTORS.—Another factor in the marital relationship that should be considered in sterility is the frequency of intercourse. Once a week is not a rate most conducive to conception, and it is surprising how many infertile couples think such a frequency is quite normal. MacLeod and Gold showed that a frequency of intercourse of 3 or 4 times weekly is far more conducive to conception than the lower frequencies.

If the spermatozoa are normal, as indicated by their number, morphology, and activity, the patency of the fallopian tubes is determined by the Rubin test (see Chapter 17). If the tubes are not patent, the test should be repeated later. If necessary, a radiopaque substance is injected into the uterus (see Chapter 18). Patients suspected of having thyroid dysfunction should have not only repeated basal metabolic studies but determinations of serum-precipitable iodine, blood cholesterol content, and thyroidal accumulation of I^{131}. I doubt that the basal metabolic rate alone is a reliable index of the need for thyroid medication. Even I^{131} uptake is not entirely dependable. The diagnosis of thyroid disturbance, either hyper- or hypothyroidism, should rest not on laboratory data alone but also on the total clinical picture presented. For patients with definite evidence of hypothyroidism, thyroid therapy is indicated, but not for others. If hysterosalpingography is to be employed using iodine-containing radiopaque substances, the test should be postponed until after the protein-bound iodine and the I^{131} studies have been completed on the wife.

PROSTAGLANDINS.—In spite of the extended and erudite studies on the complex chemistry of the seminal plasma during the past 30 years, no sound evidence to date has been produced that relates any single entity to male fertility per se. The single exception may be the high concentration of reducing sugar (fructose) in the secretion of the seminal vesicles, which plays an obvious role as a substrate for spermatozoan motility.

During the past 10 years, the prostaglandins (so named because of the original discovery of their presence in seminal plasma) have attained prominence due to their powerful pharmacologic properties in producing contraction of uterine (and all) smooth muscle and blood pressure depression. Prostaglandin E is by far the most active in these regards, and its absorption into the systemic circulation via the vaginal mucosa has been demonstrated. It would be easy, therefore, to assume that its presence in such high concentrations (a thousand times greater than that required to contract isolated smooth muscle) would, for example, induce contractions of the uterus and perhaps facilitate sperm transport. There is no positive evidence in any species investigated to date that any such physiological effect is produced.

Nor has any substantial correlation been found between subfertility states in the human male and the concentration of prostaglandins in the semen.

Immunologic Infertility*

The last decade has seen considerable interest manifested in the possible role of an immunologic factor as a cause for unexplained infertility. The concept is based on the fact that sperm have been demonstrated to be antigenic; that these antigens can produce antibodies under experimental conditions; that these antibodies in turn interact, resulting in reduction of fertility. However, the sequence of events is not nearly so simple, and much work is yet to be done before this concept, appealing as it may be, can be clearly elucidated and meaningfully used clinically.

It is also to be expected that the body under normal circumstances would provide a protective mechanism against expression of sperm antigenicity and that only when such a mechanism breaks down, or when the patient exhibits undue sensitivity, will the antigen-antibody reaction manifest itself. Consequently, the incidence of an immunologic factor as a real cause for infertility must be and, in fact, is rather small.

Thus at least 12 antigens have been isolated from human semen ejaculate, some originating from the serum, others in the male accessory structures that coat the sperm, and a few from the acrosomal membrane or the tail of the sperm itself. As yet, the specific antigen implicated in the causation of infertility has not been isolated. These antigens produce different types of antibody, i.e., agglutinating, immobilizing, cytotoxic, or complement-fixing. These are found in the circulation. However, immunoglobulins have also been found in the cervical secretions, uterine and oviductal flushings, and vagina, but with

---

° At my request, Dr. J. S. Behrman contributed this section on "Immunologic Infertility."

different IgG to IgA ratios. The IgA found in the local genital secretions is predominantly of the 11S variety and has been called the "secretory IgA." This 11S high-molecular immunoglobulin is composed of a 7S IgA similar to that found in the serum, plus a 4S transport (T-piece) piece produced locally. Furthermore, synthesis of this 11S IgA, or local antibody, by the entire reproductive system similar to the trachea, urinary tract, and salivary glands, provides the first line of defense against non-invasive pathogens that do not liberate exotoxins. This type of cervical antibody is complement linked and may cause agglutination or immobilization of the sperm in the cervical mucus. Hence, the presence of this secretory IgA in the secretions and the ability of the genital tract to synthesize and produce it locally may well be very important clinically.

Of great interest is that the local immune response is largely independent of any co-existing systemic response, and there is no significant correlation between the isohemoagglutinin levels in the genital secretions and the serum. This may explain the discrepancy reported by various investigators between the level of circulating antibody, the detection of cervical immunoglobulins, and clinical infertility. Thus, the isolation of this locally produced antibody to a specific antigen on the sperm, as yet undetermined, and proof that it is responsible for infertility, followed by elaboration of its mechanism and site of action, is the focal point of current research.

Another form of important immunologic infertility is the auto-immune sensitization of the male to his own sperm, wherein he produces and secretes via the accessory glands an immobilizing antibody that coats the tail and then results in tail-to-tail immobilization of the sperm in the ejaculate.

Clinically speaking then, any couple with primary infertility, who are apparently normal by all current methods of testing, are candidates for immunologic investigation. Another important indication for testing would be the patient with a post-coital Sims-Huhner test that shows massive agglutination or immobilization of sperm. It should, however, be realized that these cervical findings could also be a result of changes of vaginal pH, severe infection, or other causes in the male. A much more useful and simple test is the cervical mucus penetration test of Kremer. Here, clean ovulatory cervical mucus is drawn into 30 ml. × 2 ml. capillaries and fresh sperm allowed to penetrate the mucus for 30 minutes. Less than 10 mm. progression of the sperm in the cervix over the allotted time suggests a search for a possible immune factor, whereas progression of the sperm to the full 30 mm. almost certainly rules out any immobilizing antibody.

Reports by various investigators and our own laboratory at this time show that the incidence of agglutinating antibodies with titers higher than 1:32 in women with unexplained infertility is in the order of 10–14%. In these couples, condom therapy over a period of 3–6 months, with checking after each month, will show that the vast majority will reduce their agglutinating titer to undetectable levels and that when condom therapy is abandoned in our series, 48% become pregnant. The incidence of immobilizing antibody does not exceed 7%. In these instances condom therapy has not been proven of much help, nor has cortisone. As of this moment there is no useful treatment for this form of immunologic infertility, and investigation continues. The incidence of auto-immune disease or immobilizing antibody in the male is in the order of 3%. In this latter type of case, as reported by Fjällbrant in Sweden, not a single woman conceived. Cortisone has been unsuccessful, but suggestions that testosterone suppression of spermatogenesis for a period of 6 months or longer may be sufficient to remove the antigenic stimulus and thus reduce the level of circulating antibody have been made. Studies continue along these lines.

Treatment of Infertility

MALE.—Usually when there is hypoplasia of the testicles with absence of spermatogenesis, nothing can be done. If there is a history of excessive sexual intercourse, moderation should be advised. It is also important to give specific instructions to patients to be certain to indulge in coitus at the time of ovulation. The exact dates should be written down for them (see Chapter 26). Coitus should take place at least 3 times during the supposedly fertile week.

When there is a blockade of the epididymis and normal spermatozoa are present in the globus major, a surgical operation may overcome the obstruction. Surgery may also be helpful when a varicocele is present.

In cases of chronic passive congestion of the prostate and seminal vesicles, local treatment, attention to diet, exercise, and avoidance of excessive coitus are usually curative.

Impotence and premature ejaculation frequently have a psychic basis, and this must be taken into consideration in the treatment of these conditions.

It is now recognized that varicocele or the conditions that lead to it may severely impair spermatogenesis (see p. 134). Although the anomaly almost invariably is unilateral (in the venous circulation of the left testis), the effect is bilateral. In these cases, high ligation of the internal spermatic vein may result in dramatic improvements in semen quality. Varicocele, however small, should be sought whenever oligospermia and the pattern of sperm morphology is the distinctive type described on page 134 and when the individual does not present any other pathology.

In some cases in which the husband is almost certainly permanently sterile, it may be advisable to use semen from a donor. (See Chapter 19, "Artificial Insemination.")

FEMALE.—In some cases of *malformation and deformity* of the genital organs, a cure may be effected by surgery. For example, a rigid hymen may be stretched or incised, an anatomically constricted vagina may be widened, and obstructive bands in the vagina may be incised or excised. Dyspareunia may require local treatment, psychotherapy, or both. If local conditions cause the dyspareunia, they should be removed. Such disturbances may be tender carunculae myrtiformes, inflammation of the vulva or vagina, Bartholin's duct cyst or abscess, urethral caruncle, anal fissure, or kraurosis vulvae.

When there is a thick tenacious *cervical plug* at the time of ovulation, this must be removed. Such plugs can readily be removed, but temporarily, by suction with a syringe (without a needle) or by the application of liquor antisepticus alkalinus or dilute hydrogen peroxide. However, it is not easy to prevent the recurrence of these thick plugs, which may interfere with conception. Frequently, treatment of the cervical canal with electric cautery brings about a cure, but one must be extremely careful not to produce a stricture of the cervix. A few women have become pregnant after cauterization of the cervix. Much simpler procedures for the removal of abnormal cervical discharges are administration of (1) diethylstilbestrol (0.1 mg. orally every night for the first 20 nights of the menstrual cycle, repeated 3 times), (2) sulfonamides (1 Gm. daily for 10 days), and (3) penicillin (300,000 units in oily suspension hypodermically) or specific antibiotics after cultures and sensitivity tests.

Defects of the uterus are difficult to overcome. However, in some cases of hypoplasia, benefit has been claimed from the injection of massive doses of estrogenic substance to bring about a temporary increase in the size of the uterus. Of course, if ovulation does not take place, there is no corpus luteum and no progravid endometrium no matter how large the uterus becomes. Therefore the sterility is not affected by the estrogens.

In cases of *tubal blockade*, sometimes repeated insufflations of carbon dioxide gas or injections of radiopaque substance remove the blockade and conception follows. I believe that a Rubin test should be performed first. If the tubes are not patent, atropine sulfate or nitroglycerin is given (see Chapter 17), and if the second Rubin test fails to permit gas to go through the tubes, hysterosalpingography should be performed. Often the radiopaque substance will penetrate the tubes when the gas will not. At any rate, if the tubes are closed, the hysterosalpingogram will reveal the site of obstruction. The films may be shown to the husband and wife and the condition explained. The pictures usually indicate whether an operation is advisable and, if so, the type of surgery to be performed.

I have collected statistics from many gynecologists especially interested in plastic tubal operations, not only in the United States but in many other countries. The 2,113 plastic tubal operations that were assembled were followed by 405 pregnancies, an incidence of 19.1%, or one pregnancy following every five operations. There were only 313 living children, an incidence of

77.3% of the pregnancies, and a frequency of 15.1% of all the operations, or one living child after every $6\frac{1}{2}$ operations. The presence or absence of ectopic pregnancies was specified in 286 pregnancies, 70.6% of the pregnancies. In this group there were 45 tubal pregnancies, an incidence of 15.7%, or one ectopic pregnancy after approximately every six operations. If we assume that there were no ectopic pregnancies in the rest of the cases, the incidence of ectopic gestation is 11.1%.

Although the results are good, they are still far short of what they should be to justify indiscriminate plastic tubal operations. Furthermore, a high incidence of tubal pregnancies follows these operations. Also, it appears that nonsurgical treatment of closed tubes yields results that are almost as good as those of surgery. Tinkering with closed tubes even by nonsurgical procedures, such as Rubin tests under high pressure and hysterosalpingography, may lead to an increased frequency of tubal pregnancies.

I believe that candidates for tubal plastic operations should be sent to those gynecologists who are especially interested in this subject and are performing skilful operations, because the results of these investigators, while still not what they should be, are considerably better than those obtained by surgeons who perform plastic tubal operations only occasionally. The following conditions should be present before plastic operations on the tubes are performed. The patient must be in the child-bearing period, preferably less than 35 years of age. She must have at least one functioning ovary. Both tubes or the only remaining tube must be proved to be closed. There must be no other cause of the sterility but tubal closure. There must be no tuberculous infection in the genital tract. The patient must be a good surgical risk. Of course, the husband must be fertile and healthy.

Generally speaking, *ovulation failure* is difficult to overcome. Considerable success has been obtained with human pituitary gonadotrophins, clomiphene citrate, and other hormones (p. 279).

In some instances, as in women with the Stein-Leventhal syndrome, resection of portions of the ovaries is helpful.

Patients who have *hypothyroidism*, demonstrated by determinations of serum-precipitable iodine, blood cholesterol content, and thyroidal accumulation of I^{131}, must be given thyroid medication.

It has been amply demonstrated that at least 10% of "sterile" women become pregnant within a year after a bimanual examination. In addition, a larger percentage of women conceive within 12 months after a uterine sound is passed beyond the internal os. In fact, in Sharman's large series of 1,575 primary sterility patients, among the 893 women in whom tubal insufflation tests were done, the incidence of pregnancy within a year (17.4%) was slightly less than among the 253 women in whom a uterine sound was passed (17.7%). The group treated with hormones showed only a little improvement (19.6%), and the group for whom nothing was done had a 10.8% incidence of pregnancy. These figures belittle some of the extravagant claims made by the enthusiasts of hormone, vitamin, and thyroid therapy.

Ovulation

By ovulation we mean the formation and discharge of an unfertilized egg from a graafian follicle of the ovary. In many animals, including the monkey, the exact time of ovulation can be determined with ease, but in most women this is not yet the case. Knowledge of the exact day of ovulation is most helpful for many reasons, including assurance of the optimal day for coitus for some infertile couples, a means of preventing conception, and a guide in artificial insemination.

Some women know when they ovulate. They have pelvic discomfort which may vary from a mild ache to sharp pain and may have a slight bloody discharge which arises in the uterus. The Germans call this bleeding *kleine Regel*, or small or minor menstruation. The discomfort is called *mittelschmerz*, or intermenstrual pain. It is generally believed that pain in one iliac fossa at about the middle of the intermenstrual interval is initiated by ovulation. Hartman doubts the validity of this explanation, believing that the pain is due to pathologic processes in the uterus and its appendages, perhaps in response to excessive ovarian secretion, though the possibility remains that general swelling of the ovary causes intermenstrual pain.

There are objective ways of trying to determine the exact time of ovulation. They include the following.

1. PRESENCE OF A LIVE OVUM IN THE TUBE.—This indicates without a doubt that ovulation has taken place, but only a few such ova have been recovered. Furthermore, it is difficult to tell exactly when ovulation took place.

2. EXAMINATION OF THE OVARIES BY CULDOSCOPY, LAPAROSCOPY, OR AT LAPAROTOMY.—The presence of a fully mature follicle that looks as if it is about to rupture may indicate that ovulation is to take place, and the finding of a recently ruptured follicle or fresh corpus luteum may indicate that ovulation has just taken place.

3. EXAMINATION OF THE ENDOMETRIUM.—Usually the changes in the uterine endometrium indicate accurately what is going on in the ovary. Whereas in nearly all cases the finding of luteal endometrium by biopsy or curettage indicates that ovulation has taken place, it is often difficult to determine the exact day it took place. Even if this could be determined, it would not follow that ovulation would take place in subsequent months on the same day.

The time of ovulation even in the rhesus monkey has rarely been determined with an accuracy of less than 12 hours, and the time that may elapse between insemination and fertilization is unknown in primates.

The morphologic changes in the ovaries provide the only satisfactory criteria for determining the sequence of events during the cycle. This is especially true of the meteoric career of the corpus luteum. The target organs are less satisfactory, for they are subject to factors other than hormonal tides. This is true also of systemic changes, such as fluctuations in basal temperature. In abundant material from rhesus monkeys, the endometria have been classified on the basis of ovarian findings, and obvious differences have been found in endometria associated with similar ovarian conditions. Such differences are to be expected, since different regions of the same endometrium react differently to the same hormone concentration. Even when the endometria are arranged in as many as eight groups corresponding to the phases of the ovarian cycle, there are specimens that exhibit some features of one group and other features of the succeeding group.

4. REACTION OF THE UTERUS TO PITUITARY EXTRACT.—Knaus maintains that in the first half of the menstrual cycle the uterus reacts to pituitary extract but that this response is lost 48 hours after the follicle ruptures. However, some investigators deny that there is any difference in response of the uterus to pituitary extract before and after ovulation.

5. HORMONE STUDIES OF BLOOD AND URINE.—Kurzrok found a rise in gonadotrophin excretion 24 hours before ovulation, and D'Amour observed an increase in this hormone between the twelfth and the sixteenth day before the onset of bleeding. In many cases there was a second rise just before menstruation began. There were also two peaks of estrogen output that usually preceded the increase in gonadotrophin. Venning and Browne found that excretion of pregnanediol, an excretion product of progestin, rose to a plateau after ovulation and then fell abruptly just before the onset of flow.

6. FARRIS TEST.—This is based on the observation that, for about four days before ovulation, the urine contains a gonadotrophic substance, presumably of pituitary origin, which produces hyperemia of ovaries in immature rats. In this test 2 ml. of morning urine is injected subcutaneously into two immature female white rats of the Wistar strain. Each is killed by illuminating gas after 2 hours. The color of each ovary is compared with the graded shades of red in the Munsell color system. In the absence of ovulation, there is no hyperemia of the rat's ovary. If ovulation is abnormal, hyperemia occurs, but usually not on 4 consecutive days.

Corner, Farris, and Corner said that the urinary rat test indicates the time of ovulation in a high proportion of cases with sufficient accuracy for clinical use. However, not all investigators of the Farris test have been able to substantiate Farris' claims.

7. FERN-LEAF CRYSTALLIZATION OF CERVICAL MUCUS.—Papanicolaou proved that cervical mucus secretion, when spread and dried on a slide, crystallizes with arborization; this phenomenon is most pronounced at ovulation time and may be due to estrogenic activity. Rydberg referred to such crystallization as "fern-leaf" structure and showed that it could also be produced by mixing egg albumin and normal saline.

Compos da Paz described fern-leaf crystallization as a test for the diagnosis of cervical sterility, and Roland advocated its use to determine ovulation, estrogenic activity, and early pregnancy. The fernlike pattern of the cervical mucus is present in the first half of the menstrual cycle and during the ovulation period. It is absent after ovulation, during pregnancy, and after the menopause, at which time the mucus exhibits only cellular content. Only during anovulatory menstrual cycles with a normal estrogen level can fernlike crystallization of the cervical mucus be found at any time of the cycle. Fernlike crystallization is closely related to estrogen function. Progesterone does not cause its appearance; on the contrary, it seems to inhibit it. Fernlike crystallization is also related to the receptivity of the cervical mucus to spermatozoa. As the crystallization loses its characteristic features, the receptivity of the mucus diminishes. When the crystallization is absent, the mucus, as a rule, is hostile to spermatozoa.

8. BASAL BODY TEMPERATURE.—Many believe that, in normal women during the child-bearing period, rectal temperatures taken each day at the same time and under the same conditions vary characteristically during the menstrual cycle. If rectal or oral temperatures are plotted on a graph, a curve is obtained showing the exact day of ovulation. Rubenstein stated that the lowest temperature coincides with the day of ovulation, but others insist that the rise in temperature indicates ovulation. Rubenstein found that not only did the lowest body temperatures of the month coincide with the characteristic ovulative smear (Fig. 48), but the highest temperatures coincided with the characteristic premenstrual smear. Not all are agreed on the value of the basal body tem-

FIG. **48.**—A normal temperature curve during the menstrual cycle. Patient, 24; cycle 28–29/3–4. Temperature shift that occurs at, or about, the time of ovulation will precede menstruation by about 14 days regardless of length of cycle. In a 28-day cycle the temperature shift is 14 days after menstruation; in a 34-day cycle, 20 days after menstruation. Studies of corpus luteum and endometrium and hormone assays suggest that the interval between menstruation and ovulation may vary widely but that the interval from ovulation until the next period is fixed at about 14 days. Temperature graphs support this belief.

(As a convenience, special grid sheets are desirable. If not available, graphs may be prepared on ordinary graph paper lined five to the inch. If such paper is used, the best graphs are obtained by a scale of 1 in. for 5 days (horizontally) and 1 in. for 1 degree F. (vertically). Temperatures are taken under "basal" conditions with a clinical thermometer read in fifths or tenths of a degree F. (Figs. 48–51 reproduced through courtesy of Dr. Pendleton Tompkins.)

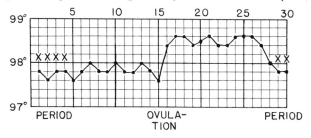

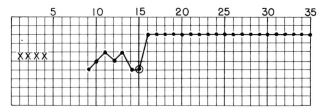

FIG. 49.—Woman, 25, cycle regular, 28/3, commenced a graph in hope of planning a visit to her husband in an Army camp at a time when conception would be probable. Her husband came home on a one-day pass (marked by the circle) just 14 days before menstruation was expected. The next day the temperature shift occurred, the temperature remained elevated (this elevation is maintained for many weeks after conception) and eventually the diagnosis of pregnancy was established. Coitus took place only in one 24-hour period during the month.

perature in determining the day of ovulation, but there is no doubt that in many women, perhaps one third, graphs properly plotted do reveal the day of ovulation, as proved by successful pregnancies planned according to the graphs (Figs. 48–51).

9. CHANGES IN CERVICAL MUCUS.—Pommerenke and Viergiver determined the length of the ovulatory phase in the normal menstrual cycle on the basis of the increased quantity and decreased cellularity of the cervical mucus secreted at this time. This phase of increased secretion was found to vary from 3 to 7 days in length and to occur later in cycles of longer length. The shift in basal temperature was found to occur, with rare exceptions, only during this phase of increased mucus secretion. The day of maximal mucus production usually occurred 16–12 days before onset of the subsequent menstrual period,

FIG. 50.—Another example of conception after infrequent intercourse (marked by circles). During the January-February cycle, intercourse occurred on the twelfth and eleventh days before menstruation, a little after the theoretical moment of maximal fertility and, as shown, a little after the temperature shift. The patient was advised to have intercourse a few days earlier in the next cycle and, on the basis of the first graph, to expect a temperature shift about March 1. That day a shift did occur, coitus took place, and the patient conceived. She was delivered November 23, 268 days after the temperature shift. (Theoretical duration of pregnancy, 266 days.)

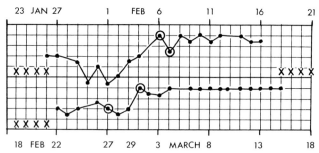

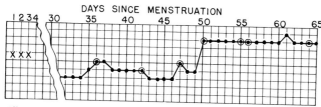

FIG. 51.—Illustration of use of temperature graphs in determining time of ovulation for a patient with periods "every 2 or 3 months." Graph was begun the thirtieth day after menstruation. The fiftieth day a sharp temperature shift occurred and coitus took place. The temperature remained elevated for over 3 weeks, and pregnancy was confirmed by the Friedman test.

regardless of the length of the cycle. A study of the cervical mucus cycle together with the basal temperature is suggested as a possible aid in planning pregnancies.

Table 1 summarizes the differences in certain properties of cervical mucus between the ovulatory phase and the pre- and post-ovulatory phases. The "ovulatory phase" is synonymous with the fertile period during which conception can occur.

Spinnbarkeit is the capacity of liquids to be drawn into threads and is maximal at the time of ovulation when threads 15 cm. long may be obtained. *Flow elasticity* or *retraction* is the ability of cervical mucus to return to its original shape after deformation by external stress or pressure. Both spinnbarkeit and flow elasticity change throughout the phases of the menstrual cycle and are optimal at the time of ovulation. *Plasticity* allows cervical mucus to

TABLE 1.—Cervical Mucus Properties During
Phases of Menstrual Cycle°

	Ovulatory	Pre- and Postovulatory
Daily quantity	200–700 mg.	60 mg. or less
Transparency	High (clear)	Low (opaque)
Light scattering	Low	High
Viscosity	Low	High
Flow elasticity	Maximal	Minimal
Spinnbarkeit	10–15 cm.	1–2 cm.
Arborization	Present	Progressive ferning preovulation; replaced by cellular pattern postovulation
Water content	96–98%	92–94%
Dry weight	Low	High
pH	Max. alkalinity	Usually alkaline
Leukocytes	0–4 WBC/hpf	Often > 5 WBC/hpf
Spermatozoal penetrability	1.5–2.0 mm./min.	0.1–0.5 mm./min.

° From Marcus, S. C., and Marcus, C. C.: Obst. & Gynec. Surv. 18:749, 1963.

be deformed continuously without rupture and is seen especially in pregnancy. *Tack* is the stickiness of mucus and is determined by drawing a cover slip away from mucus on a glass slide.

The physical characteristics of cervical mucus at about the time of ovulation are high transparency, low viscosity, maximal spinnbarkeit and flow elasticity, and low plasticity and tack. During pregnancy there are low transparency, high viscosity, minimal spinnbarkeit and flow elasticity, and high plasticity and tack.

Certain observations suggest that cervical mucus is not always homogeneous. The arborization of cervical mucus occasionally reveals different, well-defined formations in the same sample. Repeated measurements of the spinnbarkeit of the same specimen may sometimes give different values. In studies of in vitro invasion of a sample of mucus by spermatozoa, there may be certain areas of massive invasion while other areas demonstrate no penetration at all. These observations suggest that care must be exercised in the analysis and interpretation of a single sample of cervical mucus.

Perloff and Steinberger showed that cervical mucus and seminal fluid, placed in apposition in vitro, form phase lines with phalanges and canals projecting into the mucus. Arborization of phalanges develops, and spermatozoa are trapped in these repositories almost immediately, from which they gradually penetrate the mucus (Fig. 52). The phenomenon of arborization does not

FIG. 52.—Phalanx formation visualized by phase microscopy. **A,** formation of phase lines between cervical mucus **(M)** and seminal fluid **(S)** and beginning phalanx formation. **B,** elongation of phalanx into the mucus; blurred white areas result from rapid movement of spermatozoa. **C,** phalanx arborized and congested with spermatozoa. (Figs. 52 and 53, courtesy of W. H. Perloff and E. Steinberger: Am. J. Obst. & Gynec. 88:439, 1964.)

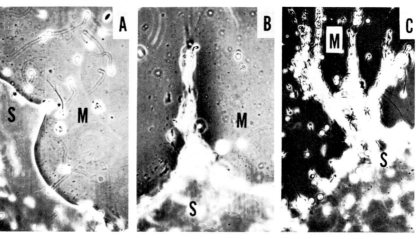

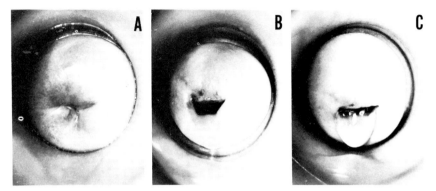

FIG. 53.—Cervical changes at ovulation. **A,** normal cervix, postmenstrually, with closed os and plug of thick, turbid, tenacious mucus. **B,** at ovulation, cervical os gapes and clear cervical mucus extrudes. **C,** slight pressure on cervical lips causes mucus to pour out of the os.

depend on the presence of motile spermatozoa, since it occurs equally well with azoospermic seminal fluid.

Spermatozoa move readily, not only from seminal fluid into cervical mucus but also back into azoospermic seminal fluid from spermatozoa-containing cervical mucus, indicating that no significant chemotactic or other directional influence is operating.

Immediately after menstruation, the cervical os is small and contains a plug of thick, turbid, tenacious mucus. With the approach of ovulation and increase in circulating estrogen, the os opens gradually, and the cervical mucus becomes more profuse, clearer, and shows increasing spinnbarkeit. At ovulation, the cervical os gapes, and large amounts of clear acellular mucus with marked spinnbarkeit pour forth (Fig. 53). Within 1 or at most 2 days after ovulation, as indicated by rise in basal body temperature, cervical mucus becomes scantier, thicker, and more tenacious, and the cervical os closes, returning to a postmenstrual appearance. Typically, development of the cervix requires from 3 to 5 days, but regression takes no more than 1 to 2 days, coincidentally with onset of production of progesterone, which counteracts the effect of estrogen on the cervix and its mucus.

Postcoital Tests.—Various technics are used to carry out the *Sims-Huhner* procedure. The initial test may be performed satisfactorily 6 to 8 hours after coitus. An immediate postcoital test may be indicated if the Sims-Huhner results are consistently negative during several ovulatory phases. In the post-coital test a vaginal speculum is inserted without lubrication and the first specimen obtained with a pipet from the posterior fornix (Fig. 54). A second specimen is obtained from the external os (Fig. 55), after which the endocervix should be wiped clean and a third specimen obtained from high within the

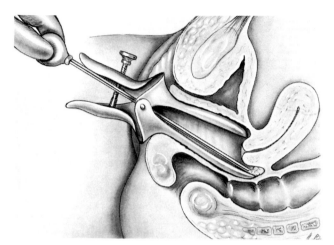

FIG. 54.—Aspirating semen from posterior fornix of vagina.

endocervical canal. The physician should note the volume of mucus, acidity or alkalinity, color, spinnbarkeit, flow elasticity, and viscosity. The specimen is then examined for spermatozoa and cellular content. A portion of the specimen may be allowed to dry for evaluation of the arborization phenomenon (see later).

A single postcoital test has only a positive value; that is, the finding of highly motile spermatozoa in the endocervical specimen constitutes a positive result. Failure to find living, highly motile spermatozoa on a single test has no prognostic value. The test must be repeated on alternate days at estimated midcycle in successive cycles. If no highly motile sperm are found in the

FIG. 55.—Aspirating semen from cervical canal.

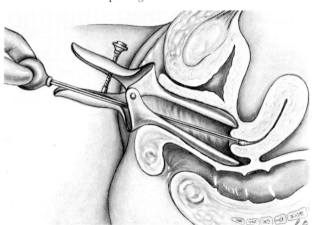

endocervical sample on repeated postcoital tests on varying days near the time of ovulation, the results may be considered abnormal. Two causes for the abnormal test include (1) poor timing of the test in relation to ovulation and (2) abnormal or hostile cervical mucus.

The *ferning* or *arborization test* may be of value in the infertility study for (1) determining endogenous estrogen activity, (2) evaluating the luteal phase, (3) approximating the time of ovulation, (4) diagnosing endocervicitis, and (5) evaluating response of the endocervical glands to exogenous estrogens.

Chronic cervicitis may contribute to the problem of infertility. Various organisms have been found to be spermicidal in vitro, including Escherichia coli and streptococci as well as Aerobacter, Paracolobactrum and Alcaligenes. Whether or not treatment of endocervicitis increases the chance of pregnancy is debatable.

10. VAGINAL SMEARS.—Papanicolaou showed that the vaginal epithelium of human beings, like that of many laboratory animals, undergoes cyclic changes during the month. However, not all agree that such changes can be detected regularly; therefore the study of vaginal smears, although of great value, has limited applicability.

D'Amour studied 20 menstrual cycles in five women, using concurrently four to six of the following sources of information: gonadotrophin assay, estrogen assay, pregnanediol determination, vaginal smears, basal body temperature, and subjective experiences. The purpose was to evaluate the validity of the tests on the basis of uniformity in the occurrence of positive responses and synchrony of their appearance. It was concluded that (1) subjective experiences are valueless as tests for ovulation; (2) basal body temperature fluctuations are not sufficiently regular or clear cut to be reliable; (3) uniformity of results of hormonal assays and vaginal smears confirm the validity of each, and a certain sequence of events appears typical of the normal cycle; (4) because of its sharpness and its apparent close association with ovulation, the gonadotrophin peak, occurring in the mid-interval, is most indicative of the exact time of ovulation.

In advising infertile couples, it is most important to tell them specifically the most favorable days in the month for conception. These days vary, of course, with the intervals between menstrual bleedings. Figure 87 (p. 209) should be used as a guide. The chart shows the most fertile days for menstrual cycles varying from 21 to 38 days, and these fertile days should be written down for each patient who is anxious to become pregnant.

Prevention of Infertility

The time to prevent infertility is before and during puberty. Boys and girls should be given full information concerning sexual relations and should be warned about all aspects of venereal disease. They should be taught how to lead normal, healthy lives, with ample outdoor activities. They should have proper diets, and they should dress properly, especially in winter. Above all, young girls should not be forced to study hard, take arduous music lessons, and work long hours indoors during puberty. They should not be exposed to severe physical or mental competitions at this time. As a prophylactic measure against trouble in later years, young girls should be taught the importance of rest, relaxation, and recreation. Adolescent girls should also be warned never to deviate from the habit of having a set time for a daily bowel movement; otherwise they will perpetuate the old expression that "woman is a constipated biped with a backache."

If a girl has not begun to menstruate by the time she reaches her fifteenth year, she should have a complete physical examination, including blood count, tests for thyroid function, endocrine study, inspection of the vulva and hymen, and a rectal examination. A hymenal orifice must be determined. Occasionally a one-finger vaginal examination must be made. For this, the well-lubricated, warmed little finger should be used. Sometimes abnormalities are found which, when corrected, lead to normal menstruation and subsequent reproduction. If no abnormalities are found, and this is the rule, nothing should be done until the amenorrhea has persisted for at least 2 more years.

Emotional Factors in Infertility

All physicians have had apparently infertile patients become pregnant after their first interview and even before bimanual examination was made. Many such women conceive following only a pelvic examination and an explanation of the tests that should be performed. Some become pregnant between the time of a bimanual examination and the time the husband's semen is to be examined, or soon after the semen study was made and the assurance that the husband is fertile. Frequently gestation occurs after a simple manipulative procedure. The women who become pregnant before any therapy is carried out constitute a high percentage of all supposedly sterile women.

Why do so many women who are anxious and even panicky about their inability to conceive become pregnant soon after a brief talk with a physician, a pelvic examination, or a simple manipulation, or even immediately after giving up remunerative employment? Was the infertility in these women psychosomatic? We must admit that in some instances of sterility the mind (whatever that encompasses) plays a dominant role.

AMENORRHEA.—Women who do not ovulate cannot, of course, become pregnant. In some women amenorrhea with absence of ovulation results from psychic trauma. The mechanism involved was elucidated in the last few years. In experiments on monkeys, Markee observed that bleeding was arrested in endometrial transplants during the late phase of menstruation, and he said:

"Fright at this stage causes within 15 to 25 seconds, re-opening of the arteriole, which for 5 to 15 seconds delivers blood that promptly clots." We know also that fear, perhaps of pregnancy itself, may delay or entirely suppress a menstrual period. In 1943, Loeser reported a study of four women in whom temporary arrest of endometrial development occurred as the result of "emotional shock." Biopsy revealed the endometrium to be at the stage of development it would normally have reached at the time of the shock, but no further development after the shock, suggesting that the shock caused an immediate arrest of development by interrupting the release of the proper pituitary hormones.

During World War II the vast majority of the women in concentration camps in different parts of the world, such as the Philippines, Hungary, Germany, and France, were amenorrheic. Severe psychic shock, worry, and fear, which, acting through the autonomic nervous system, caused complete suppression of ovarian function, were probably the causes of this war amenorrhea. Menstruation returned spontaneously in most of the women after release from the camps.

Additional evidence of the psychogenic origin of some menstrual disturbances is the fact that in hypnosis amenorrhea may be either produced or relieved.

HABITUAL ABORTION.—Psychogenic factors play a role in many instances of habitual abortion. Bevis treated 32 women who had had three or more previous spontaneous abortions by extra bed rest at the time their menses would have appeared, but with no other specific treatment. Without any hormonal therapy, 29 of these women (91%) reached the twenty-eighth week of pregnancy, and 26 babies (81%) were born alive and healthy. Bevis emphasized the high degree of confidence that his patients had in his investigation, and to this psychologic support, rendered unintentionally, he attributed a large part of the success he achieved. Bevis maintained that psychotherapy is the most valuable form of treatment for patients with a history of sequential abortions.

DIAGNOSIS AND TREATMENT.—The diagnosis and treatment of emotional aspects of sterility and infertility belong in the domain of analytically oriented psychiatrists. However, a sympathetic physician who shows an interest in his patient's problems can recognize the infertile patient who has emotional difficulties, and he can sometimes help his patient realize the cause of her sterility. When a physician is not qualified or is unable to help his patient, he should refer her to a psychiatrist.

17

The Rubin Test: Transuterine Insufflation of Gas

ONE OF THE greatest contributions to gynecology is the Rubin test, by means of which the patency or nonpatency of the fallopian tubes can be determined with certainty without opening the abdomen. The test consists of transuterine insufflation of gas under pressure. If the tubes are patent, the gas will escape into the peritoneal cavity and can be detected, not only by auscultation with a stethoscope and by roentgenograms which will demonstrate a pneumoperitoneum (especially under the right diaphragm), but also by clinical symptoms such as pain in the shoulders and neck after sitting up or walking around. Of course, if both tubes are closed, no gas will escape into the peritoneal cavity.

The Rubin test is indispensable in the study of sterility. Rubin listed the following 12 indications for the test:

1. Primary sterility in which contributing causes, including those for which the husband might be responsible, have been eliminated and some operative procedure is contemplated. Here it has both prognostic and diagnostic value (and sometimes therapeutic value).

2. Primary sterility in which the patient is known to have passed through a gonorrheal pelvic infection soon after marriage and at the time of inquiry has no pelvic symptoms.

3. Sterility following a pelvic exudate or abscess complicating a puerperium or abortion, with or without an operation, when resolution has taken place.

4. Primary sterility in which the patient had peritonitis of appendicular origin in the pre- or postmarital state, to exclude tubal occlusion by peritoneal adhesions.

5. One-child sterility without definite history of pelvic infection.

6. After one whole tube and part of another have been removed for hydrosalpinx or pyosalpinx.

7. After unilateral ectopic pregnancy to determine the patency of the remaining tube.

8. After salpingostomy to determine the success of the operation which was calculated to effect an opening of occluded tubes.

9. After sterilization by tube ligation to test the patency of the tied or severed tubes.

10. After multiple myomectomy in a nullipara to make certain that at least one uterine ostium of the tube has been left intact.

11. Sterility of long standing when pelvic masses are palpable and the clinical diagnosis is leiomyomas or "chronic disease of the adnexa." The test shows whether or not the tubes are open.

12. As a therapeutic measure to eliminate the tubal factor in sterility. The Rubin test is contraindicated in the following conditions.

1. Acute and subacute pelvic infection, because of the danger of spreading the infection.

2. During menstruation or any type of uterine or cervical bleeding.

3. Immediately after a curettage. This and the preceding are contraindications because insufflation may disseminate blood and endometrium into the peritoneal cavity with subsequent formation of endometriosis. Furthermore there is the rare possibility of embolism due to forcing of gas into open blood spaces.

4. Suspicion of pregnancy, either intrauterine or ectopic. (However, the test has been inadvertently performed a number of times during early pregnancy without interrupting the gestation.)

5. Serious cardiac and pulmonary diseases, which are themselves contraindications to pregnancy.

6. Pelvic tenderness, inflammatory and noninflammatory tumors, or purulent vaginal discharge.

7. Fever from any cause.

There are no real dangers associated with the Rubin test if it is properly performed. If too much pressure is used, that is, over 200 mm. Hg, there is a remote possibility of rupturing an occluded tube. Rarely, a woman faints after the test, but this reaction is transitory and harmless. There is some pain associated with the test, but it is slight. When the tubes are patent and the patient gets up and walks around immediately after the test is completed, she will have pain in one or both shoulders or neck if a sufficient amount of gas was used. To obtain immediate relief, all the patient needs to do is lie down, particularly with the head lower than the feet. In this posture the gas gravitates away from the diaphragm to the pelvis. The pain experienced on getting up and walking around is due to subphrenic irritation by the gas used.

Apparatus

The safest medium to use for the Rubin test is carbon dioxide, and the best kind of apparatus is that devised by Rubin, Kidde, and others. Simple apparatus necessitating only air may lead to embolism and death and so should never be used. Besides the gas apparatus itself, the following paraphernalia is necessary: a uterine cannula of the Keyes-Ultzmann type with an adjustable

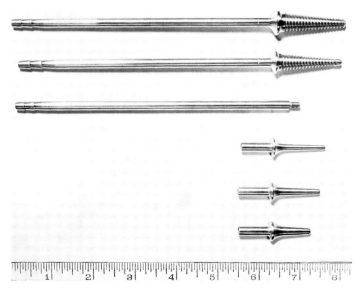

FIG. 56.—Colvin uterine cannula and tips of various sizes. (Manufactured by Thos. L. Keith Co., Atlanta, Ga.)

FIG. 57.—Light-weight apparatus for kymographic uterotubal insufflation.

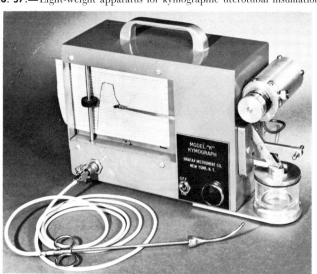

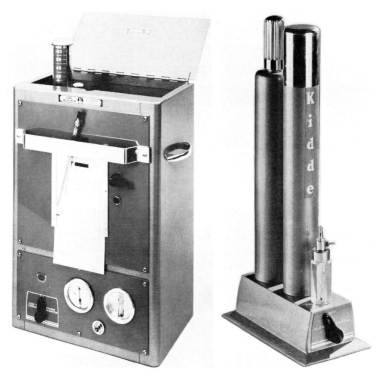

FIG. 58 (left).—Kidde kymograph insufflator.
FIG. 59 (right).—Kidde office model insufflator.

rubber acorn or the Colvin cannula (Fig. 56) with a fixed screw-shaped metal plug, a speculum, a uterine probe, a dressing forceps, and a tenaculum.

One Rubin apparatus is an automatically acting siphon volumeter to which has been added a manometer. It is not cumbersome, and, except for refilling, the gas tank needs a negligible amount of handling. Carbon dioxide is delivered commercially in tanks of large quantities under great pressure that require a reduction valve to regulate the flow. The gas from a large tank may be transferred to a smaller one without a reduction valve. The small tank is easily fastened to an examining table or placed on a small table or chair near the examining table. It may be refilled as often as necessary.

Rubin reported on the use of a simplified light-weight apparatus for kymographic uterotubal insufflation (Fig. 57). It has all the essentials of the old competent apparatus, with the advantages of smaller size and weight due to the use of an effervescent tablet having a known potential quantity of carbon dioxide for each test. The effervescent tablet, containing sodium bicarbonate, citric acid, and tartaric acid in suitable proportions as the source of carbon dioxide supply, has made possible the elimination of gas tanks, heavy pressure-reducing valves, and reserve chambers.

The smaller Grafax kymograph (Fig. 57) has been adapted to the use of the effervescent tablet. The apparatus consists of the effervescent tablet, carbon dioxide chamber, closure cap, pressure-limiting bellows, flow control valve, pressure-recording manometer, kymograph, and outlet to uterine cannula.

The oscillations resulting from carbon dioxide insufflated through the uterus and tubes as generated by the tablet are the same as those obtained when carbon dioxide flows from a compressed tank. The patient's pelvic sensations, tubographs, auscultatory findings, subjective sense of percolation, and presence of a subphrenic pneumoperitoneum are also just as characteristic when the tubes are patent as with the older types of insufflation apparatus. Shoulder pains are less intense, possibly because of humidification of the effervescent carbon dioxide bubbles, which are probably more rapidly resorbed. Figure 58 shows the regular Kidde kymograph insufflator and Figure 59, the office model designed to be used with the physician's own blood pressure manometer.

Technic

It is best to carry out the test on day 9 of a 28-day cycle. On this day and the days just before and afterward, there is a low type of endometrium which is intact, and the chances of a pregnancy being present are slight. There is no need to give preliminary medication.

The patient is placed in the lithotomy position, and a careful bimanual examination is made to rule out any infection or pregnancy and to determine the position of the uterus. The apparatus should be tested to be certain that there are no leaks and that the cannula is not plugged. A speculum is inserted into the vagina, and the external os is cleansed with cotton on a dressing forceps and painted with half-strength tincture of iodine or other antiseptic. The anterior lip is grasped with a single-toothed volsella as the patient is being told that this will hurt for a second. A uterine probe is inserted past the internal os to determine the exact direction and length of the uterine cavity. This also usually hurts a little. The cannula is then inserted into the cervical canal. If an ordinary cannula with a rubber tip is used, it should be inserted past the external os. If the Colvin cannula is used, there is no need to attach a tenaculum to steady the cervix. The cannula is simply screwed into the cervix in a clockwise direction until it feels snug. If bleeding occurs, it is best to desist and repeat the test at another time. In most cases the physician can hold both tenaculum and cannula with one hand while he uses the other to regulate the flow of gas. The tenaculum and cannula used with the Rubin or similar apparatus are self-retaining, so both hands are free after the flow of gas is started.

Nearly always, if the tubes are open the pressure rises to 80 or 100 mm. Hg, then drops suddenly to 40–50 mm., where it remains fairly steady. If this occurs it is not necessary to inject much gas. If an assistant listens with a stethoscope at either side of the abdomen while gas is being injected, sounds of intermittent bubbling can be heard. The cannula is then removed from the cervix. It is not necessary to take a roentgenogram to prove that gas has escaped into the peritoneal cavity. It is best to place a small tampon against the cervix to check any bleeding from the punctures made with the tenaculum. The tampon should be removed by the patient when she arrives at home.

If the tubes are closed, the pressure continues to rise, and the patient complains of pain in the middle of the lower part of the abdomen. Nothing will be heard with the stethoscope on the sides. The patient will not have shoulder pain, nor will roentgenograms reveal any subdiaphragmatic pneumoperitoneum. If the pressure goes up to 200, the cannula should be removed, tested for its patency, and the test repeated. If the second test shows tubal blockade, the test should be repeated the following month. If the tubes are again found to be impermeable to gas, a radiopaque preparation should be injected into the uterus (as described in Chapter 18, "Hysterosalpingography") to determine patency or the site of obstruction in the tubes.

Occasionally a woman becomes pregnant after a Rubin test, even if the test apparently showed that the tubes did not permit gas to go through.

18

Hysterosalpingography

THE INJECTION of radiopaque substances into the uterus and fallopian tubes for diagnostic purposes is an office procedure for physicians who have roentgen equipment in their offices or can perform the procedure in the office of a roentgenologist. Even when carried out in a hospital, it is equivalent to an office procedure because the patient is ambulatory and need not remain in the hospital for more than a few hours. The injection is easy to carry out but is safe only when properly performed. In sterility cases I generally do not use hysterosalpingography if the tubes are found to be patent by the Rubin test. If two Rubin tests fail to show tubal patency, I resort to the injection of a radiopaque substance.

The indications for hysterosalpingography are:

1. To detect the patency or nonpatency of the fallopian tubes (most common indication).

2. To determine the location of obstructions in the fallopian tubes, especially if an operation is contemplated to overcome tubal occlusion. The roentgenograms can be shown to the patient and her husband to demonstrate graphically just what the trouble is and what the operation is intended to accomplish.

3. To follow up patients who have had plastic operations on the fallopian tubes to see if the repaired tube or tubes remain patent after the operation.

4. To visualize the uterine cavity, especially if submucous leiomyomas, polyps, or carcinoma of the body of the uterus is suspected.

5. To determine the size and shape of the uterus in extremely obese women or when bimanual examination is unsatisfactory.

6. To determine malformations and malpositions of the body of the uterus.

7. To diagnose an abdominal pregnancy. In such cases a hysterosalpingogram will clearly reveal a normal-sized, non-gravid uterus and a fetus lying completely outside the uterus.

8. In the presence of indefinite pelvic masses, to determine the location and size of the uterus and tubes.

9. To determine the size and shape of the uterus in some cases of dysmenorrhea.

10. In all cases of habitual abortion to detect a uterine malformation, a submucous leiomyoma, or polyps.

The contraindications to hysterosalpingography are:
1. A normal intrauterine pregnancy.
2. Acute or subacute infection in any of the pelvic organs.
3. Normal or abnormal uterine bleeding.
4. Recent curettage, because the injection of radiopaque medium in the presence of open sinuses may lead to embolism.
5. Purulent discharge from the vagina or cervix.
6. Heart trouble or serious systemic disease.
7. Fever from any cause.

If hysterosalpingography is not properly carried out, there is danger of serious complications. Even if these do not occur, the roentgenograms may be unsatisfactory and hence useless. Proper interpretation of the films is of great importance in all hysterosalpingographies.

The equipment necessary for hysterosalpingography includes a bivalve speculum, one or preferably two single-toothed volsella, a 10 ml. syringe, and an intrauterine cannula that has near its tip a movable rubber or metal acorn with which to plug the cervix. Numerous simple and complicated combinations of instruments have been designed that are useful to the physician who frequently resorts to hysterosalpingography. A self-retaining cannula-tenaculum combination is most helpful.

It is best to carry out the procedure on day 9 of a 28-day cycle. Preferably, the patient should have taken an enema a few hours before the test. When the physician is ready to begin, the cannula is attached to the syringe, and both are filled with the opaque substance. If a heavy oil such as Lipiodol is used, it should be prewarmed. Aqueous contrast mediums are much safer than oil preparations because they do not cause any inflammation or remain unabsorbed. A scout film is mandatory.

Technic

Strict asepsis and antisepsis must be observed at all times during the procedure. Furthermore, every movement should be made with as much gentleness as possible to avoid hurting the patient. The patient is placed in the lithotomy position on a Bucky diaphragm at the end of an x-ray table with leg holders. A vaginal speculum is inserted and all discharge is removed from the vagina and cervix. A light is placed so as to expose the cervix clearly. Half-strength tincture of iodine or other antiseptic is applied to the entire cervix and external os. The anterior lip of the cervix is grasped transversely with a single-toothed volsella, but the patient is first warned that this will hurt for a second. It is assumed that a bimanual examination was made before the procedure was begun and that the position of the uterus is known. If the examination failed to reveal the exact position of the uterus, it is advisable to insert gently a sterile uterine probe to determine this point before inserting the cannula. Again the patient should be told that this will hurt slightly. If the Colvin cannula is used, there is no need to know the position of the uterus because the tip of the cannula does not extend beyond the internal os. If the Keyes-Ultzmann cannula is inserted in the cervical canal, the acorn is pressed firmly against the external os. This insertion also will hurt a little. At this point a second volsella may be placed on the posterior lip and both volsella held tightly to make certain that the acorn fills the cervix. The second volsella, however, is not necessary. As soon as the acorn properly fills the cervix, an assistant is asked to hold the volsella firmly. The operator then holds the cannula with the attached syringe in his left hand (if he is right-handed), and with his right hand slowly and evenly forces the radiopaque substance from the syringe into the uterine cavity through the cannula.

The patient should again be warned that this will hurt slightly. The contrast medium will first fill the uterine cavity and then the fallopian tubes. At this point the patient usually complains of uterine cramps; contrast medium may escape from the cervical canal. For the normal-sized uterus, between 5 and 8 ml. of the medium is used. As soon as the injection is completed, the speculum (modified Graves) is removed and a roentgenogram is taken with the cannula still in place. After this the cannula is removed; of course, some substance runs back from the uterus into the vagina. This should be removed and the patient given a pad to wear. If iodized oil is used, a second roentgenogram should be taken from 1 to 24 hours later to show the condition of the fallopian tubes. Lateral roentgenograms often give additional information. After 24 hours the uterus and tubes will be free from oil if the tubes are patent, and some oil will be seen in the pelvic cavity. If the tubes are closed, oil will be seen proceeding up to the point of obstruction, whether it is at the uterine end of the tube, the middle portion, or the fimbriated end.

In the last few years new contrast mediums have been prepared. Nearly all are aqueous solutions, and they have distinct advantages over oil contrast mediums. If an aqueous solution is used, the substance escapes so rapidly that there is no need to take another film the next day.

Interpretation of Results

Normally the uterine canal is sharply defined and triangular (Fig. 60). The tubes are thin and tortuous for the proximal two-thirds and dilated at the distal third. In many films, when sufficient radiopaque substance has been injected, there is visible a spill of it from the dilated distal ends. When an oily substance is used, the diagnosis of patent tubes is made from the roentgenograms taken from 1 to 24 hours later. They must show a filmy deposit of oil scattered throughout the pelvis to warrant a diagnosis of patent tubes.

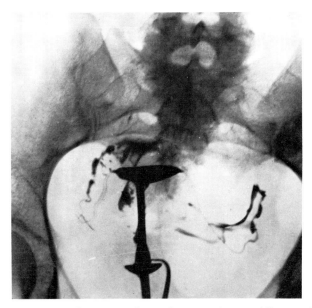

FIG. 60.—Hysterosalpingogram of normal uterus and patent fallopian tubes.

Of course, it is always possible that one tube may be open and the other one closed.

Insufficient attention is usually paid to the cervix in the roentgenograms; occasionally close observation will disclose stenoses, sacculations, and growths.

The size, shape, and position of the uterine cavity are always shown, and leiomyomas and polyps usually are obvious. However, often neoplasms are diagnosed when they are not present and, vice versa, growths are not shown. Congenital anomalies such as a double uterus are plainly shown.

The patency or nonpatency of the tubes is usually obvious at a glance. If the tubes are closed, the site of obstruction stands out prominently (Fig. 61). One may see the size of the tubal lumen and the degree of tortuosity. The lumen of a normal tube is fuzzy, while that of a chronically diseased tube is sharply outlined and wiry. When a small hydrosalpinx is present, the cornual end is frequently patent. Contrast medium then enters the distal bulbous end, which is clearly visible on the first roentgenogram as a considerably dilated distal end. No spill is visible. However, in the 24-hour exposure, the uterus and proximal two thirds of the tubes have no iodized oil, but the distal ends of the tubes contain most of the oil shown on the first plate. Roentgenograms taken a week or 2 later will reveal the same shadows in the distal ends.

The oil remains in these sacs because the musculature of this portion of the tubes is so defective that it cannot force the oil back into the uterine

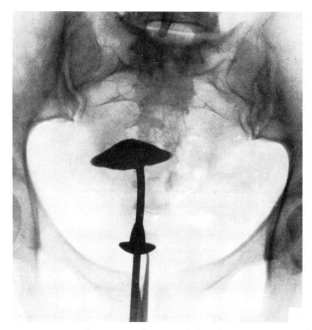

FIG. 61.—Hysterosalpingogram showing tubal occlusion at uterine ends.

FIG. 62.—Hysterosalpingogram showing hydrosalpinx characterized by globules in distal ends of tubes.

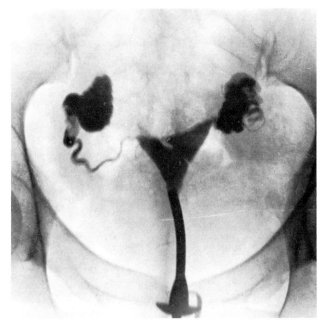

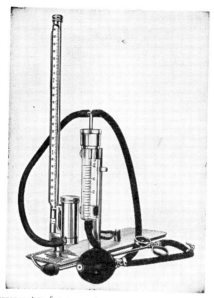

FIG. 63.—Jarcho's pressometer for accurate measurement of pressure during injection of radiopaque substance. (Apparatus manufactured by Becton-Dickinson Co., Rutherford, N.J.)

cavity. Furthermore, the oil in these cases is in the form of globules because that entering the dilated part of the tubes encounters serous fluid (Fig. 62). The findings are pathognomonic of hydrosalpinx. A rare exception occurs when oil escapes from patent tubes and drops into the free fluid in the pelvis. However, these droplets are usually in the midline instead of on either side, are very low in the pelvis, and later change their position.

Physicians who have occasion to perform many hysterosalpingographic examinations may deem it advisable to obtain a Jarcho pressometer, which was especially designed for this procedure (Fig. 63).

19

Artificial Insemination

ARTIFICIAL OR THERAPEUTIC insemination is the introduction of semen into the genital tract of the female without sexual intercourse. There are two types of artificial insemination, one in which the husband's semen is used and one in which semen obtained from a donor is used. The use of a husband's semen is a medical problem, and one need not be concerned about legal entanglements. On the other hand, many questions arise when semen from a person other than the husband is used.

Artificial insemination has been practiced for a long time, in both animals and man, and there are dangers connected with the procedure.

Artificial insemination in animals possesses a number of advantages over natural breeding. The chief advantage is that it increases the usefulness of superior sires to an extraordinary degree. For example, the semen from one bull may be used to inseminate 500 cows. The percentage of success is extremely high. In sheep, for example, 95% of pregnancies are obtained by using fresh semen at three successive heat periods. Special methods have been devised for obtaining semen and keeping it sterile and for shipping it to various parts of the world. Artificial insemination has been used not only in cattle and sheep, but also in horses, swine, birds, and fowl.

In human beings, also, artificial insemination is not new. The first to employ it was John Hunter, who was born in 1728 and died in 1793.

When to Use Artificial Insemination

In human beings there are only two indications for artificial insemination of the husband's spermatozoa: (1) inability of the husband to deposit the semen in the vagina, and (2) inability of the spermatozoa to gain access to the uterine cavity from the vagina. One reason for a husband's inability to deposit his semen in the vagina is pronounced hypospadias; another is premature ejaculation, before insertion of the penis into the vagina. Another important reason, but fortunately a rare one, is definite dyspareunia. The cause may be physical or psychic.

In nearly all cases in which coitus can take place normally but the spermatozoa do not reach the uterine cavity, the fault lies in a grossly abnormal discharge from the cervix that prevents the spermatozoa from gaining access to the uterus. In most cases the discharge can be eliminated by means of diethylstilbestrol, sulfonamides, or penicillin (see p. 139) or cauterization.

Indications for artificial insemination with a donor's semen are (1) complete absence of sperm, (2) grossly defective sperm (either decidedly diminished number, defective motility, or excessive incidence of deformed sperm) and (3) the likelihood of a child's inheriting a disease (rare).

Previous birth of babies with erythroblastosis fetalis by a woman whose husband is homozygous was formerly considered an indication for artificial insemination; but the use of gamma Rho immune globulin (human) may wipe out Rh immunization entirely and eliminate the risk of erythroblastosis.

Use of the Husband's Semen

When the husband's semen is to be used, the physician must first ascertain that the sperm are normal in number, form, motility, and endurance. Of course the wife must have no abnormalities of the internal genital organs, and the physician must also have proved that the tubes are patent and ova are present. Furthermore, he should warn both the husband and the wife that probably many attempts will have to be made over a period of a few months. Fertilization seldom follows a single insemination, any more than impregnation occurs after a single natural act of coitus.

The most favorable time for artificial insemination is at the time of ovulation. There is only one egg each month in normally menstruating women, and its life is short. Therefore it is important to know the exact time during which to perform the artificial insemination.

Unfortunately, we have no means of determining with certainty the time of ovulation in all women, though we can determine ovulation in some, especially if a combination of procedures is used. (See discussion of ovulation, p. 141.)

Despite the fact that one cannot determine exactly when a woman ovulates each month, in most women who menstruate fairly regularly, ovulation takes place 12 to 16 days after the beginning of a menstrual cycle. Mobile spermatozoa reportedly have been found in the reproductive tract up to 9 days after the last intercourse, but a conservative estimate would place the average mobile life at 48 hours. Since the life of spermatozoa is probably not more than 48 hours and the life of an ovum less than 16 hours (probably only 12 hours), insemination must take place within 2 or 3 days of ovulation. Therefore artificial insemination should be practiced between the tenth and the seventeenth day of a cycle. During these 8 days, semen should be obtained three times. The specimens of semen should be collected in a clean wide-mouthed jar (2-oz. size), not in a rubber sheath. The best way to obtain a specimen of semen for insemination is by masturbation.

Of course, not all women menstruate approximately every 28 days. We can readily determine the best days for insemination regardless of the length of the menstrual cycle, because we know that in most cases the egg ripens and therefore is ready to be fertilized about 14 days before the next menstrual period would begin. Roughly, for women with a 30-day cycle, we inseminate from day 12 to 19; for a 35-day cycle, from day 17 to 24; and so on.

It is generally useless to inseminate with defective sperm (as to number, motility, or excessive abnormalities) in cases in which normal coitus can take place. In such cases the husband's semen alone should not be used, and either a donor's semen or a combination of the husband's and a donor's semen should be tried. In some of my successful cases of insemination, I combined the husband's semen (defective in number and motility) with a donor's semen; in such cases the parents can at least hope that the offspring was really the husband's.

In cases of faulty deposition in the vagina, it is only necessary to place the semen in the vagina against the cervix. However, when the cervix is the responsible factor, as can be determined by the Sims-Huhner test (p. 147), it is essential to place a small amount of the semen inside the cervix. This procedure must be carried out with the utmost aseptic care and only after one is convinced that no infection exists in the woman's pelvis. This meticulous care is essential because, if semen (which is by no means sterile) is injected into the uterine cavity, infection of the pelvic organs may sometimes follow. Furthermore, when too much semen is injected into either the cervix or the uterine cavity, the uterus is stimulated to contract and most of the semen is expelled into the vagina.

For insemination into the cervix, it is best to use a tuberculin syringe to which is attached a uterine cannula without the rubber acorn. For insemination into the vagina, any syringe and cannula are satisfactory; even a glass pipet with a rubber bulb at the end will suffice.

With an oligospermic male, it is possible to concentrate spermatozoa by means of a split ejaculate. There should be 4 days of sexual rest before obtaining these specimens. Two sterile, wide-mouth jars are provided and the specimens obtained by self-manipulation. The first few drops of the ejaculate contain the majority of the spermatozoa. Therefore, the first few drops are collected in one container (labeled number 1) and the remainder of the ejaculate in the other container (labeled number 2). With this method a small semen volume containing a concentrate of spermatozoa is obtained in a sterile container. The "split number 1" is used for intracervical insemination at ovulation time.

Use of a Donor's Semen

Great care must be exercised in selecting candidates for artificial insemination when a donor's semen is to be used. Before undertaking it, the physician must consider the ethical, legal, emotional, and religious aspects of this procedure.

The physician should have a heart-to-heart talk with both the husband and the wife, and he should assure himself that he is morally justified in carrying out artificial insemination. From the physical standpoint, he must be sure that the husband has no sperm and that the wife has no abnormalities of the genital organs, that her tubes are patent, and that she ovulates. Furthermore, both the husband and the wife must be in excellent physical and mental condition, their Rh status must be known, and their Wassermann reactions must be negative. A written consent may act as protection for the wife, the donor, the donor's wife, and the legal status of the child.

Of great importance is the selection of a proper donor. An individual must be chosen who bears certain resemblances to the sterile husband, not only racially and physically but also emotionally and temperamentally. For example, it might be embarrassing in later life if a tall blond, placid type of donor had been selected for a short, swarthy, highly emotional couple. The donor must have no inheritable taint, such as epilepsy or diabetes; he must have a negative Wassermann or Kahn reaction; and preferably, though not necessarily, he should be married and have normal children. Of course his sperm must be normal. All donors and the women who are to be inseminated should be tested for Rh status because the woman to be inseminated and the donor must both be either Rh-positive or Rh-negative. The blood type should also be determined. Residents in hospitals are a good source of donors and most of them are happy to earn extra money. The price is $20 for each specimen. The best specimens are those obtained by self-manual manipulation. If no pregnancy occurs after a trial of 4 months with one donor, it is advisable to secure another donor.

The physician must arrange for the collection of the donor's semen and the insemination in such a way that the donor cannot possibly find out who is to receive his spermatozoa. Nor should the recipient be able to discover who the donor is. There are many valid reasons for these precautions, chiefly the possibility of blackmail on the part of the donor and the risk of transference of affection from the recipient to the donor. To eliminate all risk the donor should be asked to bring his specimen to a place other than that where the insemination is to be performed. If the specimen is to be delivered to the physician's office, it should be brought to a side door during the physician's regular office hours when there are many patients, so that the donor could not possibly identify the recipient even if he watched every woman who left the office. Of course, the physician should use his judgment in selecting a donor who would not be so low morally as to resort to dishonesty.

Technic of Insemination

The patient is placed on the examining table, a speculum is inserted, and the vagina and cervix are cleansed with cotton. There is no need to disturb the normal cervical mucus. If there is a tenacious or purulent discharge in the cervical canal, it can usually be removed by aspirating with a syringe without a needle. The semen is drawn up into the sterile syringe and the cannula attached. If the semen is to be deposited at the external os, which is the normal procedure, all the semen is used for this purpose. If the trouble lies inside the cervical canal and the secretion cannot be removed, the tip of the cannula, attached to the syringe, is carefully and slowly inserted into the cervical canal just past the external os. An antiseptic should not be used in the cervical canal, because it may kill the sperm. Nor should a tenaculum be used on the cervix. Then 2 or 3 drops of semen are gently and slowly injected into the cervical cavity. If more than this small amount is used or if the manipulations are rough, the semen will be expelled into the vagina. After the few drops of semen are inserted into the cervical canal, the cannula is withdrawn gently. A portion of the rest of the semen is gently directed at the opening of the cervical canal, and the balance is placed in the vaginal vault. The speculum is carefully removed, and the patient's legs are stretched out on the examining table, where she remains for half an hour. The speculum may be left in the vagina in such a way that the seminal fluid bathes the external os. After 20–30 minutes the excess semen is wiped away with cotton pledgets, and the patient leaves. There is no need to restrict any activities after insemination.

I usually inseminate 3 times a month. The inseminations are made at 2-day intervals during the most favorable week, namely, the fertile days selected for sexual abstinence by those who use the rhythm method of conception control (see Fig. 87, p. 209).

My incidence of success with donor inseminations is about 65% and with the husband's semen about 30%.

Guttmacher, Harman, and MacLeod were appointed a committee by the American Society for the Study of Sterility to study the question of artificial insemination. They sent questionnaires to 96 members. Of the 71 who answered, 52 registered approval of artificial insemination using a donor and 44 said they practiced donor insemination. The indications listed for donor insemination were azoospermia, 42; dyspareunia, 24; a sensitized, Rh-negative wife, 18; cacogenic factors in the husband's line, 11; increased number of abnormal forms in the husband's semen, 10; and poor sperm motility, 9. Opinion was evenly divided between 2 and 3 inseminations per month as routine practice. The total number of attempted donor inseminations by the 44 members was 568. The incidence of success varied from 0 to 100%, the most frequent incidence being 50–60%. The committee concluded that it is ethical and proper for physicians qualified in the diagnosis and treatment of infertility to perform donor artificial inseminations. The most practical method of selecting the fertile time for insemination is the temperature graph. The likelihood of pregnancy resulting from donor insemination in the ordinary case is 50–60%. The average successful case requires 3 to 6 inseminations over a period of 2 to 4 months. It is deemed proper by most physicians who carry out donor inseminations to deliver the babies themselves and to assent to the recording of the husband's name as the baby's "father" on the birth certificate.

It is unfortunate that there are no specific laws governing artificial insemination, because there are six individuals who must be protected legally: the physician, the wife, the husband, the child, the donor, and the donor's wife. All require clarifications under statutes that are yet to be enacted.

Since artificial insemination is an unsettled procedure legally, perhaps both husband and wife should sign a statement granting permission to the physician. A simple form used by Kleegman follows.

We the undersigned, request Dr. . . . .
to inseminate my wife, Mrs. . . . . with
the sperm of a donor for the purpose of making her pregnant.

The choice of the donor is to be left entirely to the discretion of
Dr. . . . . and shall be unknown to us.
We shall not hold Dr. . . . . responsible
for any untoward results as a result of this procedure.

. . . .
         Husband   Wife

Date . . . .

Witness . . . . (usually office nurse or
                                 secretary)

Witness . . . . (physician performing
                                 the insemination)

The Roman Catholic church is opposed to donor artificial insemination; therefore, this procedure should not be suggested to persons of the Catholic faith.

Vaginal Pessaries

I SHALL RESTRICT the word "pessary" to its old usage, namely, for the maintenance of the uterus in an anteflexed position or to splint the vaginal walls to prevent prolapse of the uterus.

Most gynecologists correctly believe that retroflexion and retroversion of the uterus usually produce no symptoms and require no treatment. Approximately 20% of all women have a retroflexed uterus, and most women, if not told about it, are not aware of any untoward symptoms.

When should a vaginal pessary be used? At the outset the physician must realize that the pessary is only a temporary device in nearly all instances. It is helpful but rarely curative, except in case of retroflexion in a large, soft subinvoluted uterus after labor.

The commonest indication for use of a pessary is retrodisplacement associated with relaxation of the anterior or posterior vaginal wall or both. Most women who have this condition complain of backache and a dragging sensation in the pelvis. In such women, after the uterus is elevated and a pessary inserted, definite relief from the disagreeable symptoms is obtained in some cases. However, in some women the distressing symptoms persist in spite of the pessary in the vagina. It is in women with retroflexion of the uterus associated with relaxation of the vagina that most operations for retrodeviation are performed; but only a small proportion of women who undergo suspension operations are permanently relieved of their symptoms.

Another indication for a pessary is a large, soft, boggy, subinvoluted uterus that is retrodisplaced after labor. In such cases there is usually bleeding from the uterus for several weeks after delivery. To relieve this condition, it is essential to elevate the uterus before inserting a pessary in the vagina.

Elevation of the body of the uterus from retroflexion to anteflexion is demonstrated in Figures 64–67.

First a bimanual examination must be made to be certain that the uterus is retroflexed and the adnexa are normal. In most cases the cervix will be found high up under the anterior vaginal wall. Where the body of the uterus should normally be, nothing but the abdominal and vaginal walls is felt between the fingers in the vagina and the hand on the abdomen. However, posterior to the cervix in the culdesac of Douglas and separated from the cervix by a groove is a round mass, the body of the uterus. In cases of subinvolution, this mass

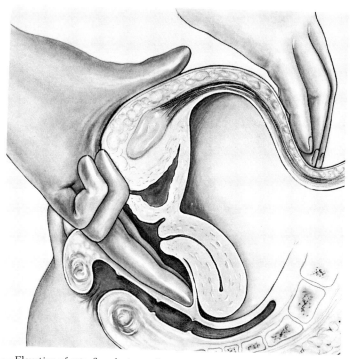

Fig. 64.—Elevation of retroflexed uterus; first step. Corpus is gently pushed out of culdesac.

Fig. 65.—Elevation of uterus; second step. Corpus is straightened out.

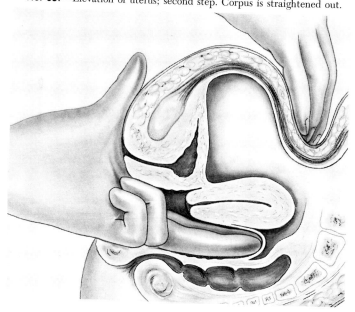

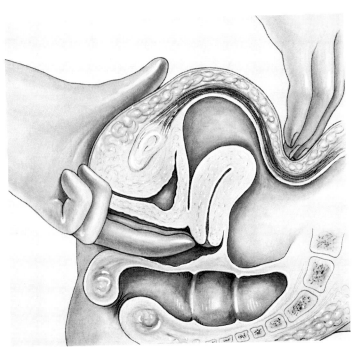

FIG. 66.—Elevation of uterus; third step. Corpus is brought up.

FIG. 67.—Elevation of uterus; fourth step. Corpus is sharply anteflexed and maintained in this position with the hand outside.

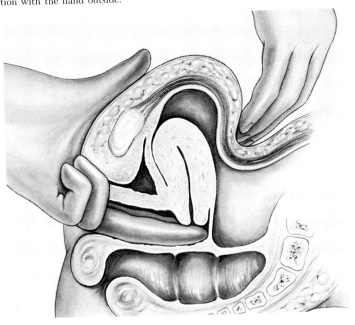

172

is soft, but, in cases of retroflexion in which there has not been a recent pregnancy, the mass is usually hard. When the cervix is moved with one finger in the vagina, the other finger will feel that the mass in the culdesac also moves.

Before the uterus is elevated, the patient should be asked to empty her bladder. The rectum also should be empty. With the two fingers in the vagina, particularly the longer one, the corpus is gently but firmly pushed back out of the culdesac and up toward the abdominal wall. Soon the hand on the abdomen feels the corpus. Pressure on the corpus with the fingers in the vagina is continued until the hand on the abdomen can grasp the corpus through the abdominal wall and hold it in place for a minute or 2. Then a pessary is inserted in the vagina.

A few weeks after a subinvoluted retroflexed uterus is elevated and a pessary is placed in the vagina, the uterus regains its tonicity, decreases in size, and the bleeding ceases. Then the pessary is removed.

In many cases of prolapse of the uterus, a pessary is useful if placed in the vagina for a few weeks before operation. It helps restore some tonicity to the pelvic tissues and permits the vaginal mucosa to regain its normal consistency.

The common belief is that, for a pessary to be beneficial, the position of the uterus must first be changed from posterior to anterior. However, Howard A. Kelly, who had more experience with pessaries than any other gynecologist, maintained that the only function of a pessary is to take up the slack and splint the vaginal walls and, in this way, limit prolapse of the uterus. The purpose is not to correct a retrodisplacement or to place the uterus in any conceivably ideal position. Therefore, in applying a pessary, there is no need to pay attention to the position of the uterus before or afterward. With these ideas I fully agree, except in rare instances of pregnancy in a retroflexed uterus and of a large subinvoluted uterus after labor. In nearly every instance in which pregnancy occurs in a retrodisplaced uterus, nothing need be done, because as the uterus grows it gradually rises out of the pelvic cavity spontaneously. After 10–12 weeks the uterus is so large that it cannot fall back into the pelvis.

The kind and size of pessary to be used depend on the amount of slack in the vaginal walls and the amount of uterine prolapse, the extent of the cystocele, and the competence of the outlet to retain a pessary.

The pessary generally used formerly was a hard rubber one of the Albert Smith type or one of its modifications. Those commonly used are shown in Figure 68. They are made in various sizes so that they properly fit vaginas of different sizes. To change the shape of a Smith type of pessary, it must be softened by heating in boiling water. Then it should be quickly pressed to the desired shape in a towel.

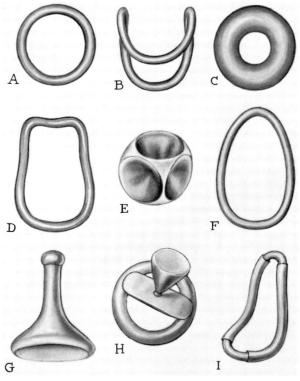

FIG. 68.—Types of pessaries. **A,** hard rubber ring pessary; **B,** Gehrung pessary, valuable in prolapse; **C,** inflated ring pessary; **D,** Thomas-Smith pessary; **E,** bee cell pessary; **F,** Smith pessary; **G,** Gellhorn pessary; **H,** Menge pessary with stem; **I,** Findley and Gynefold type pessary.

Experience is required to judge quickly which type of pessary and what size are to be used for each patient. A pessary is properly sized and placed if it is so situated in the vagina that the cervix lies in its center and it fits the vagina so loosely that a finger can be slipped between it and the vaginal wall on all sides. It must not press against any part of the vagina. On the other hand, it must not be too loose or it will be forced out when the patient has a bowel movement or urinates or even when she gets up from the examining table and begins to walk. A physician must keep a variety of pessaries on hand at all times to have the proper one when it is needed.

Technic of Inserting a Vaginal Pessary

The technic of inserting a vaginal pessary is simple. The pessary should be scrubbed with soap and water, dried, and lubricated with a lubricant or liquid green soap. The patient is placed in the lithotomy position and a bimanual examination made to be certain that there is no abnormality such as a pelvic inflammation or neoplasm. If the Smith pessary is used, one edge of it is held in the fingers of the right hand, with the large concavity toward the patient's head. The lubricated index finger of the left hand is placed in the vagina to press down on the perineum. The lubricated pessary is turned sideways and gently pushed into the vagina in such a way that it hugs the posterior vaginal wall and avoids the pubic bone, urethra, and other sensitive structures in and above the anterior portion of the vagina (Fig. 69). After the pessary is in the vagina, it is turned on the flat with the large concavity pointing up toward the patient's abdominal wall (Fig. 70). The index finger or two fingers of the left hand are then inserted deep into the vagina to depress the topmost (posterior) bar of the pessary down and behind the cervix (Fig. 71). The cervix spontaneously falls into the opening of the pessary (Fig. 72). The same fingers then sweep around the entire pessary to be certain that there is sufficient but not too much space between the pessary and the vaginal wall. If the pessary appears to fit properly, the patient is asked to strain hard to be sure that it cannot be expelled by such action. If there is too much or

FIG. 69.—Insertion of vaginal pessary; first step.

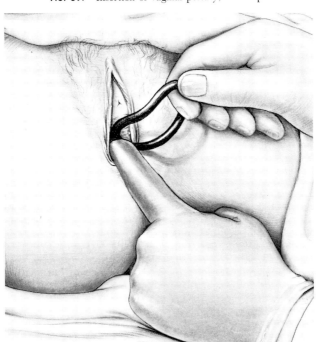

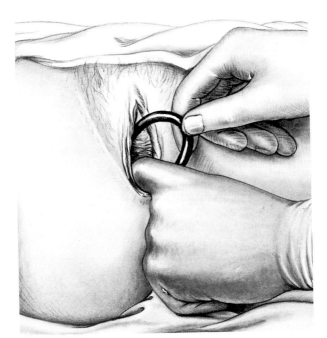

FIG. 70.—Insertion of vaginal pessary; second step.

FIG. 71.—Insertion of vaginal pessary; third step.

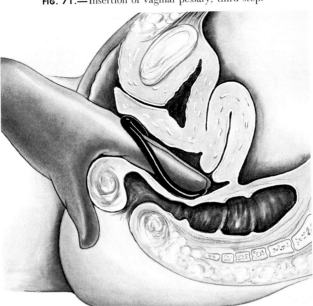

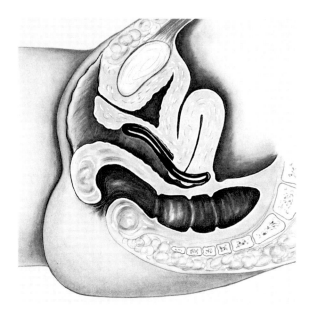

FIG. 72.—Pessary in place.

too little space between the pessary and the vagina, the pessary must be removed and another one inserted. When a pessary is removed, the steps of insertion are reversed. The Findley and Gynefold pessaries are easier to insert because they are folded in two before being inserted. The bee cell pessary is small and offers support from the suction action of its six concave surfaces. The moist vaginal mucosa invaginates into the cavities and is held there by negative pressure. However, it is necessary to remove and replace bee cell pessaries every month to make sure that the suction does not lead to ulcerations in the vaginal mucosa.

In case a heavy uterus falls back before a pessary can be properly placed, Javert's recommendation may be followed. With the patient in the lithotomy position, the uterus is properly elevated and the pessary inserted into the vagina. The patient is then placed in the knee-chest position (Fig. 73). Anteflexion of the uterus is completed, and the pessary is properly placed.

It is best to have the patient return in a week or 10 days after a pessary has been inserted to determine if it has remained in position and if the patient is comfortable. If the patient has no complaints and the pessary is in good position, she is advised to return every 2 months. At these visits, after an examination, the pessary is removed, cleaned, and reinserted. However, before the pessary is replaced a bimanual examination should be made and the vaginal and cervical mucosa inspected. If congested or otherwise abnormal areas of mucosa are seen, the pessary should not be replaced for at least 3 or 4 weeks.

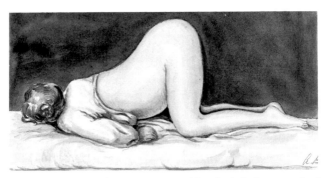

FIG. 73.—Knee-chest position. Chest must rest on table or bed, thighs perpendicular to surface of table or bed, and back depressed. In this position the body of the uterus is anteflexed by gravity.

Patients who wear pessaries should take a lactic acid or vinegar douche every day. It is advisable to remove a pessary after 6 months and ask the patient to go without one for at least a few weeks. If symptoms return, an operation is advisable.

In elderly women with prolapse of the uterus who cannot be operated on, a variety of pessaries may be used. In some, a large ball pessary will give relief; in others, a soft rubber doughnut pessary and, in still others, a cup pessary may be used with success. The need for pessaries today is far less than it was formerly, because, in spite of a woman's age, operation is now readily carried out with practically no risk, especially if local infiltration anesthesia is employed.

A great boon to women with prolapse of the uterus and those with a large cystocele and/or rectocele who are not operated upon is the daily use of estrogens, with double the dose prescribed for menopausal symptoms. The estrogens usually and remarkably restore the tonicity of the vaginal tissues and reduce the extent and symptomatology of the prolapse, cystocele and rectocele.

21

Pelvic Tuberculosis

PELVIC TUBERCULOSIS is uncommon in the United States but is a frequent disease in several foreign countries. In nearly all cases, the fallopian tubes are involved. The uterus also is tuberculous in about 70% and the ovaries in approximately 30%. The cervix is seldom implicated. Since endometrial biopsies have become almost routine in the study of sterile couples, endometrial tuberculosis has been found in some cases in which it was not suspected. In practically every case in which there is endometrial tuberculosis, both tubes are also tuberculous, and this is most likely the cause of the sterility.

A preoperative diagnosis of pelvic tuberculosis can generally be based on one or more of the following observations: (1) history of a chronic illness; (2) palpation of masses in the pelvis; (3) slight fever; (4) low white-blood-cell count; (5) no benefit from antibiotics other than streptomycin; (6) improvement with isoniazid, especially when combined with para-aminosalicylic acid (PAS) or streptomycin; (7) positive endometrial biopsy; (8) positive smears; (9) positive cultures of menstrual blood; (10) sometimes, hysterosalpingography, and (11) guinea pig inoculation.

In most cases of pelvic tuberculosis with palpable masses, a laparotomy must be done. Although streptomycin, PAS, and isoniazid may cure endometrial tuberculosis, they do not as often cure tubal lesions. Therefore, even though repeated endometrial biopsies or repeated inoculations of menstrual blood fail to reveal tubercle bacilli after streptomycin-PAS-isoniazid treatment, this does not mean that the tubes are free from disease and that the patient can conceive.

Sutherland, who has observed 511 women with a confirmed diagnosis of genital tuberculosis, now treats his patients as follows: Daily administration of 1 Gm. streptomycin sulfate (reduced to 0.75 Gm. in patients over age 40 and to 0.5 Gm. in those over age 60) and several tablets of 15 Gm. para-aminosalicylic acid (PAS) and 300 mg. isoniazid. After 120 days the streptomycin is discontinued; PAS and isoniazid are continued for up to 18 months. At this point positive bacteriologic findings or persisting symptoms require PAS and isoniazid therapy for another 6 months. Pregnancy occurring during the period of treatment indicates immediate discontinuance of streptomycin.

If a tubo-ovarian abscess is present after 3 or 4 months of antimicrobial therapy, laparatomy must be performed. In women past 40, the operation should consist of total hysterectomy and bilateral salpingo-oophorectomy. Great care must be exercised during the operation to avoid damaging the bowel and bladder, else fistulas may result. All drugs must be given again after the operation, but isoniazid must be continued indefinitely.

Intrauterine pregnancy following healed pelvic tuberculosis is rare. Schaefer reviewed 7,000 reported cases of genital tuberculosis in which there were 155 full-term pregnancies, 125 ectopic gestations, and 67 abortions. Women with advanced disease are permanently infertile.

Schaefer, Marcus and Kramer, who reported six cases of postmenopausal endometrial tuberculosis, say that it is probably safer to avoid streptomycin because elderly patients usually cannot compensate as can younger patients if the vestibular function of the eighth nerve is destroyed. With the recent development of ethambutal as an effective antituberculosis agent, Schaefer *et al.* are now prescribing this drug with isoniazid in doses of 15 mg. per kilogram or about 1000 mg. per day. Treatment with isoniazid and ethambutal is continued for two years.

Vaginal Douches

THERE IS NO unity of opinion among either physicians or women concerning the value of vaginal douches. At one extreme one finds women who take a douche every day except during menstruation, in the belief that it is a cleansing process equivalent to brushing the teeth. At the other extreme are women who never take a douche. In between are women who take douches after coitus, after the menstrual flow is over, and on special occasions. *A pregnant woman should never take a douche.* Those who douche use a variety of substances in the douche water, and physicians prescribe various douche preparations.

Are douches essential, and are there any types of douche medication that may be harmful?

I believe that women who have a normal vaginal secretion should not take douches except perhaps the morning or a few hours after intercourse and only to accomplish mechanical cleansing of the vagina. For this purpose an acid or alkaline douche may be used. The cheapest is vinegar (5% U.S.P. acetic acid), of which 4 tablespoonfuls should be added to 2 qt. of warm water (a full douche bag). A preferable preparation for douches is one of lactic acid (see p. 184).

On the other hand, douches often help women who have abnormal vaginal discharges.

Technic of Taking a Douche

The best time for taking a douche is just before a woman goes to bed. She should always lie down in a bathtub when she takes a douche, not sit on a toilet bowl. The bathroom should be warm. A bath towel placed under the torso adds to comfort and prevents chilling from the tub. A fountain type of syringe is far better than a bulb type (whirling spray form). Before getting into the bathtub, the woman should fill the rubber bag or can with 2 qt. of very warm water, around 110°F., and add the necessary amount of vinegar, lactic acid, or other substance recommended by her physician. In many cases plain water is as effective as a medicated douche. The water should be tested with the back of the hand to be sure it is not too hot. The patient should be told, or she will quickly learn, that the vulva and perineum are much more sensitive to heat than the vagina. Therefore it may sometimes be advisable for her to apply petrolatum to the labia and perineum before taking a douche. Before the water is placed in the douche container, the metal stop on the rubber tubing should be inspected to be sure it is clamped. The bag or can should be hung in a suitable place near the bathtub between 1 and 2 ft. above the pelvis (not above the top of the bathtub). If a hook is not available, the simplest way of suspending the bag or can is from the back of a chair placed next to the tub. Most douche bags and cans have a hard rubber or a glass nozzle attached to the rubber tubing. A soft rubber catheter is preferable, and this can easily be attached to the rubber tubing by means of a glass connector. Regardless of what material the tip is made of, it should be gently inserted into the vagina for about $1\frac{1}{2}$ in. after the patient lies down. Then the metal stop on the rubber tubing is slowly released so that the douche water runs into the vagina slowly.

Backache

THE WORD "BACKACHE" includes pain due to arthritis of the spine, myositis or inflammation of the muscles of the back, relaxation of the pelvic joints during or shortly after pregnancy, pain in the coccyx from injury during labor or at some other time, soreness from improper posture, and sciatica. In addition, pain in the back may be due to abnormalities in the internal genital organs. Therefore whenever pain in the back is severe enough to cause complaint, a careful physical examination must be made. One or more likely causes of the pain may be found, and if more than one etiologic factor seems to be present, these must be properly evaluated. In many instances roentgenograms must be taken before a definite diagnosis can be made. Consultation with an orthopedist is necessary in some cases.

Just as in an abdominal or a bimanual examination, a routine should be followed in examining a patient who has backache. First the patient should be carefully observed as she walks toward and away from the examiner. As few clothes as is consistent with modesty should be worn. Then the patient's back should be examined while she is standing. During the examination it is essential to have a female attendant or female relative in the room. It is important to examine the entire back from the shoulders down to the coccyx. The thighs and legs must also be surveyed. The physician should observe any difference in the height of the shoulders, the curvature of the back, any lordosis or scoliosis, asymmetry of the iliac crests and difference in length of the lower extremities. Then the patient is asked to bend forward, backward, sideward, and in a rotary manner and to tell whether any of these movements cause pain and where the pain is located.

After the back is inspected and its mobility observed, it is palpated. This procedure may elicit tender areas, spasticity of certain muscles, lipomas, or other conditions. After this, the patient lies supine on the examining table with her legs extended. One leg at a time is elevated and abducted. Each thigh is next flexed sharply on the abdomen in an attempt to reproduce the pain. The tendon reflexes are tested, along with muscle power and a sensory examination to pin prick. A bimanual examination follows.

In most cases of severe low backache, it is advisable to have roentgenograms taken not only of the sacral but of the thoracic and lumbar areas, with lateral as well as anteroposterior views. The lateral views are particularly useful for revealing abnormalities in the vertebrae and intervertebral disks. In some cases oblique films are helpful. Treat pregnant patients symptomatically without taking roentgenograms during the first trimester and, if possible, delay the examination until after birth of the baby.

Gynecologic Causes of Backache

In a certain proportion of women with backache, disturbances or diseases of the pelvic organs are responsible for the pain. The most commonly accepted gynecologic cause is retroflexion of the uterus. In fact, many physicians who find a retroflexed uterus conclude that the displacement is the cause of the backache without even trying to find another cause. However, uncomplicated retroflexion and retroversion of the uterus produce no symptoms. Other causes should be looked for by both physical and roentgen examination, and if the physician cannot find the reason for the backache, he should refer the patient to an orthopedist.

In cases of retroflexion complicated by other abnormalities, such as cystocele, rectocele, prolapse of the uterus, pelvic inflammation, and tumors, the pain in the back may be, and usually is, due to associated conditions rather than to the retroflexion itself. Correction or removal of the associated conditions nearly always relieves all or most of the backache, even if the procedure performed does not directly involve the uterus.

A second gynecologic disturbance that may be regarded as a cause of backache is that which results from injuries during labor. Such injuries include damage to the soft parts resulting in cystocele, rectocele, and prolapse and damage to the pelvic joints that brings about separation and abnormal mobility of the sacroiliac joints. Coccygodynia may also result from injury during labor.

The pain from cystocele, rectocele, and prolapse is nearly always situated in the sacral and lower lumbar areas. Backache is more often associated with cystocele and rectocele than with complete prolapse. Sometimes a vaginal pessary will prove whether or not a cystocele or rectocele is responsible for the backache, but frequently only a repair of the pelvic structures will give this information. A physician should not promise that repair of a cystocele or rectocele will cure backache.

The uterosacral ligaments are frequently damaged in childbirth and are common sources of low backache. When these ligaments are injured or inflamed, they are exceedingly sensitive to touch. This sensitivity may be elicited on bimanual vaginoabdominal examination either by palpating the ligaments themselves or by moving the cervix from side to side. However, a far better way is to make a rectoabdominal examination, by which the sensitive ligaments are easily detected.

Other sources of backache resulting from childbirth injuries are varicose veins and stasis of veins in the broad ligaments. These are difficult to diagnose clinically, but rectal examination may reveal sensitive veins in the broad ligaments. Usually, abnormal veins are detected only at operation.

Injuries to the pelvic joints and coccyx are orthopedic conditions and are discussed in the following section.

A common cause of pain in the back is inflammation of the fallopian tubes, ovaries, and pelvic peritoneum. In most cases there is not only backache but also pain in the pelvis and lower part of the abdomen. Treatment must be directed to the inflammatory condition regardless of whether or not backache is present. Sometimes conservative treatment, such as application of heat, relieves the backache, but in most instances an operation has to be performed.

Another source of backache is an infected cervix. In some cases eradication of infection in the cervix by an electric apparatus, by amputation, or by hysterectomy has relieved backache.

Neoplasms in the pelvis may cause backache, but only when they are large enough or so situated that they produce circulatory congestion or pressure on nerves or neighboring structures. Malignant growths not only produce pain in this way but may invade and destroy soft tissue and bone. Size alone is of no importance in producing pain, because large cysts of the ovary and even large leiomyomas seldom cause pain. Therefore when a mass, even a large one, is found in a woman who complains of backache, one should not conclude that the tumor is the cause of the backache but must look for other sources of the pain. Frequently other causes for the pain will be found.

Still other gynecologic causes of backache are endometriosis, dysmenorrhea, and carcinoma of the pelvic organs. For discussions of these conditions, see the respective chapters.

Backache is often associated with pregnancy. One cause is lordosis from the disturbed posture due to the large anterior protrusion of the uterus during the latter half of pregnancy.

Orthopedic Causes of Backache

In well over 50% of women with backache, an orthopedic, not a gynecologic, disorder is the cause. The usual orthopedic lesion is arthritis of the spine, but other changes may be present in the bones, joints, intervertebral disks, ligaments, muscles, or nerves in the back.

The joints of the back are subjected to great strain during the latter part of pregnancy and during labor because of the physiologic relaxation of all the pelvic ligaments. There is also much relaxation during menstruation. Strains may be acute or chronic. In acute cases there is a history of a sudden, severe "catch" in the back while lifting or bending over. The pain is most commonly unilateral but may be bilateral in some cases. There is often, however, pain down the leg along the course of the sciatic nerve, along the lateral aspect of the thigh, or in the gluteal region. Examination of the patient's back while she is standing reveals definite deviation of the spine to the opposite side, shifting of the weight to the opposite foot, exquisite sensitivity over the joint, and decided limitation of motion and spasm of the muscles of the back. Pronounced pain is elicited when the iliac crests are approximated or when the extended legs are raised while the patient is in the dorsal recumbent position. The foregoing signs and symptoms as well as those in chronic cases may be due to the herniated disk syndrome.

In chronic cases of strain the patient complains of pain in the low back region but there may be pain in the leg. Examination reveals tenderness in the involved joint, muscle spasm and pain when the extended leg is elevated. Most women maintain that the pain began after a childbirth. Some patients have difficulty in getting up from a chair; in others, the pain is aggravated after walking, and some cannot stoop without pain to put on their shoes or pick up objects. Many have more pain at night; this can be relieved by a pillow placed in the hollow of the back. When the pain is in front, it is often mistaken for tubo-ovarian disease or ureteral pathology. Relief may be obtained in chronic cases by a properly fitted surgical corset.

Incorrect posture due to poor muscular development, unfavorable occupation, flatfoot, or other disturbance is sometimes the cause of backache. Treatment depends on the cause and usually requires a long time.

Other orthopedic causes of backache are abnormal conditions in the bones and joints, such as fractures, tuberculosis, arthritis, local malignancy, and metastases from malignant growths elsewhere, and spinal anomalies, such as occult spina bifida, scoliosis, and sacralization of the first sacral vertebra.

Other Causes of Backache

There are also neurologic causes of backache, including tumors of the spinal cord or meninges.

In some women there is a psychoneurotic basis for backache, but all other possible sources must be ruled out before such a diagnosis can be made.

There is some controversy as to the importance of coccygodynia, or pain in the coccyx, as a source of backache. Some orthopedists dismiss it as being inconsequential, while others regard it as of some importance. In most cases pain in the coccyx follows an injury during labor, but it may be due to falls, blows, or kicks. Pain in the coccyx is felt while the patient sits or when she arises after having been seated for awhile. Patients with this condition usually sit on one buttock at a time in order to relieve pressure on the coccyx.

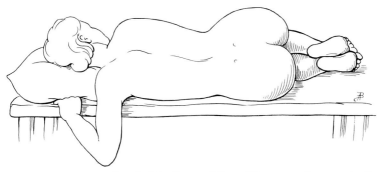

FIG. 74.—Sims's position, described by Sims as follows: "For a speculum examination, the patient is to lie on the left side. The thighs are to be flexed at about right angles with the pelvis, the right being drawn up a little more than the left. The left arm is thrown behind the back, and the chest rotated forward, bringing the sternum very nearly in contact with the table, while the spine is fully extended with the head resting on the left parietal bone. The head must not be flexed on the sternum, nor the right shoulder elevated. Indeed the position must simulate that on the knees as much as possible, and for this reason the patient is rolled over on the front, making it a left lateral semi-prone position."

Coccygodynia is easily diagnosed. The patient is placed either on her left side in the Sims position (Fig. 74) or on her back in the lithotomy position with the buttocks well over the edge of the examining table. With the index finger in the rectum and the thumb over the coccyx on the outside, the coccyx is compressed and gently moved. If the coccyx has been injured this manipulation will cause severe pain. It is best to treat coccygodynia conservatively with heat and sedatives. Removal of the coccyx is sometimes necessary if conservative measures fail to give relief.

Exercise in the Treatment of Genital Relaxation, Urinary Stress Incontinence, and Sexual Dysfunction

BY ARNOLD H. KEGEL, M.D.

THE MUSCLES of the pelvic diaphragm—particularly the pubococcygeus—are largely responsible for the quality of the tissues in this area and the satisfactory performance of the sphincters. Exercise of any muscle group promotes tissue tone and facilitates the function of adjacent structures. The support provided by the pelvic diaphragm is its unique feature. Flaccidity of these muscles can have serious consequences on the circulation and on the anatomical relationships of other pelvic organs as well as on their functioning.

Urinary stress incontinence, genital relaxation, sexual problems, rectal stasis, and other pelvic complaints are often related to dysfunction of the neuromuscular structures. Exercise of the pubococcygeus muscle, although a simple procedure, will many times completely relieve the patient's complaints.

Functional disturbance in the pelvic region is best illustrated by urinary stress incontinence. The success of any treatment, including the many surgical procedures that have been developed, is determined by a single criterion: when control is established, the woman becomes dry. This objective can usually be achieved by the physiologic approach of strengthening the pelvic muscles and re-educating their functional pattern.

Even if an operation could remove the cause of urinary stress incontinence, it cannot restore good function to muscles that have lost body, tone, and contractility. On the other hand, active exercise of the pubococcygeus, a voluntary muscle in the levator ani group, can reverse deficiencies brought about by lack of activity. In promoting healthier tissues, exercise therapy can also be a valuable adjunct to any other form of treatment.

The physiologic approach of pelvic exercise has been used to treat thousands of women with urinary stress incontinence, both in private practice and at the Research Clinic of the University of Southern California Medical School (Los Angeles County General Hospital). In patients without surgical or obstetric injuries and without neurogenic or other systemic disease, the success rate was better than 86%. Few recurrences were seen, because a good functional pattern brings comfort to the patient and, once established, tends to become habitual.

Pelvic Examination

History.—In addition to a conventional history, the patient is asked particularly about earlier genitourinary problems, since these probably have a bearing on diagnosis and prognosis. As a child, the woman may have been slow to learn control, with enuresis persisting until 9 or 10 years. It is well worth some effort to jog the patient's memory about these details as evidence of such early weakness is an important indication of a correctable physiologic disturbance. In adolescence, the patient may have had vague feelings of pelvic fatigue or discomfort; during early married life, there may have been nonspecific bladder disorders and difficulties in sexual adjustment; deliveries may have been difficult, with consequent injury; in later years she may have had other functional problems, often attributed to childbearing.

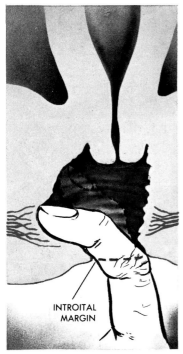

Fig. 75.—Weak or atrophic pubococcygeus muscle offers little resistance to pressure. Palpation shows a thin, fibrous muscle along a narrow area of the vaginal wall. Contractile ability is limited.

INTROITAL
MARGIN

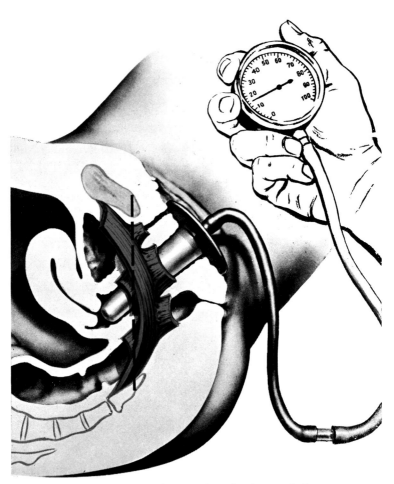

Fig. 76.—Perineometer, consisting of a vaginal air chamber attached to a manometer calibrated from 0 to 100 mm. Hg. Contractions over a wide area, as produced by a well-developed pubococcygeus muscle, register 30 mm. Hg or more. A poorly developed muscle contracts over a narrow area, registering 10–15 mm. Hg.

Abdominal palpation.—Diastasis of the rectus abdominis is often associated with diastasis of the pubococcygeus through which herniation of the bladder or rectum may occur. With disturbed reflexes, any downward strain, such as produced by coughing, causes the abdomen and the perineum to bulge and may be accompanied by involuntary expulsion of urine.

Examination of the perineum.—In the presence of weak musculature, the perineum is prolapsed, a condition usually described as lax or parous outlet. As a rule, contractions of weakened muscles are inadequate to lift the perineum more than slightly. The orifices of the urethra, vagina, and rectum lie in a descended position as if ready to empty.

DIGITAL EXAMINATION OF THE VAGINA.—Only one finger is used for palpation. Two-finger palpation spreads the vaginal canal and thus does not permit accurate identification of the structures. Gentle palpation with the tip of the index finger is required when looking for evidence of motor function and sensory perception. Bimanual examination is useful in the general survey of the pelvis but contributes little in determining the performance of neuromuscular structures or the presence of any old obstetrical or surgical injuries. The speculum conceals significant details in the middle third of the vagina.

In patients with weak or atrophic pelvic muscles, the vagina is short and shaped like a wide-mouthed funnel. The pubococcygeus muscle can be palpated only over a narrow area, probably no more than one fingerbreadth along the lower wall of the vagina on each side. A weak muscle offers little resistance to pressure (Fig. 75); even if the patient succeeds in tightening it, the contractions, confined to a narrow area, are weak. Measured with the perineometer (Fig. 76), they rarely exceed 10 mm. Hg.

Patient Education and Exercise Program

RE-TRAINING OF MUSCLES.—Many patients will not be able at first to contract the pubococcygeus muscle, but will notice a tightening when an attempt is made to draw up the perineum. Some can be made aware of the correct muscle contractions while pretending to stop the flow of urine or to check a bowel movement. Such marginal contractions indicate a degree of residual function that can be improved through voluntary effort and with practice. When the patient succeeds in activating the pubococcygeus muscle, the contractions must be identified for her as the correct way of performing the exercises. In our clinic, the perineometer is introduced so that the patient may observe on the manometer the results of correct effort. A few minutes' use of the instrument to visualize her contractile ability is a distinct aid in instruction.

While the patient is learning to recognize the voluntary contractions of the pubococcygeus, her early attempts may involve extraneous muscles, such as those in the gluteal and thigh areas as well as in the abdominal wall. Such mistakes as holding the breath, squeezing the thighs together, or bearing down must be corrected at once so that the proper pattern is learned before the wrong contractions become habitual.

MOTIVATION.—Every effort must be made to motivate the patient to learn the exercise routine correctly and to practice it conscientiously. Any woman who already understands the value of exercise on fitness and health will not need further convincing. In patients with urinary stress incontinence, the goal of being dry is the strongest motive. Incentive may also be fostered by pointing out the advantages of avoiding an operation—in saving expense, discomfort, and time, as well as the possible aftermath of surgical scarring.

EXERCISE PROGRAM.—As soon as the patient is able to discern the correct contractions of the pubococcygeus muscle and to repeat them unerringly, she must also be made to understand that the more frequent the practice, the more rapid will be the improvement in muscle function. A program of several hundred contractions throughout the day, broken into sessions of 5 to 10 contractions every half hour, is recommended. Each contraction should be held at least 3 seconds, relaxed for an equal period, and the next contraction then attempted. The patient must be warned *never* to bear down. After 2 weeks, a follow-up examination should be made to confirm the patient's proficiency in following the routine.

The first series of contractions should be practiced in the morning before the woman gets out of bed. At this time, the pubococcygeus, which has been relieved of supportive functions during the night, lies in a relatively high position, leaving less slack to be taken up. When pointed out to her, nearly every woman with genital relaxation can distinguish between the feeling of comfort in the pelvic region with the muscles contracted and the heavy, dragging sensation experienced when the muscles sag on arising.

As part of the regular exercise routine, the patient should interrupt the flow of urine several times while holding the thighs apart. In this position, the muscles at the level of the bladder outlet are being used rather than the external muscles.

FOLLOW-UP EXAMINATIONS.—Follow-up examinations are essential to assure success in physiologic treatment. Patients who have been using the pelvic musculature incorrectly all their lives find it difficult to learn to use a new group of muscles. Instructions must be carefully repeated whenever the patient is found to be using muscles other than the pubococcygeus. Many such repetitions may be required before the woman has mastered the technique. The perineometer is helpful in such difficult cases by making it possible for the woman to visualize the effect of her efforts. The instrument can be used at home for a 20-minute session 3 times daily in addition to the regular routine. The patient should be cautioned that a high reading on the manometer is meaningless if extraneous muscles are being used.

In uncomplicated urinary stress incontinence, consistent exercise will usually bring symptomatic improvement within 6 weeks. This is the time to impress upon the patient the necessity of keeping to the exercise routine as initiated. Progress will probably be faster from this point on, although several months more will be required to bring all supportive and sphincteric structures to optimal capacity. Every patient should be followed for a full year, giving encouragement and careful supervision of her performance. Only then can one be sure that pelvic exercise has been given a fair chance to overcome the patient's disability.

Tissue Response to Pelvic Exercises

Exercise of the pelvic muscles correctly performed for a sufficient length of time will produce many changes throughout the pelvis. Improved tone and color indicate a healthier state of the tissues. The pelvic floor is raised to a position that affords more normal functioning of all the pelvic viscera, and the orifices of the urethra, vagina, and rectum remain closed without conscious effort. The most noticeable changes occur in the vagina. The middle third of the organ, formerly short and funnel shaped, becomes long, snug, and cylindrical. This transformation is evident upon digital palpation and may also be visualized in three dimensions with moulages (Figs. 77 and 78). An alginate colloid that gels in about 1 minute is used to obtain such impressions of perivaginal structures.

Continued exercise not only strengthens the pubococcygeus muscle but increases its bulk. When functioning efficiently, it can be palpated along the lateral walls of the vagina for a distance of about three fingerbreadths (Fig.

FIG. 77 (left).—Moulage, anterior view, disturbed muscular function. Weak pubococcygeus muscle (*area 2*) gives the vaginal canal a short, wide, funnel shape, resulting in poor supportive, sphincteric, and sexual functions. (*Arrow* indicates urethral meatus.)

FIG. 78 (right).—Moulage, anterior view, good muscular function. The pubococcygeus muscle (*area 2*), with a normal width of about three fingers, gives the middle third of the vaginal canal a firmly supported, long, cylindrical shape. (*Upper arrow* indicates the sulcus between the urogenital diaphragm and the pubococcygeus muscle.)

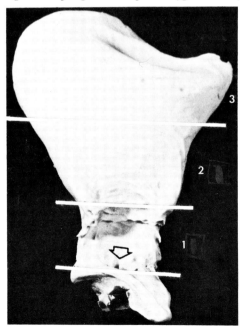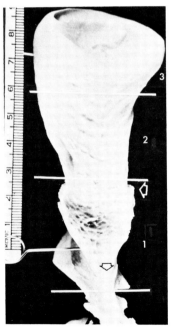

79). Contractions can be felt along the entire width. Clinical improvement of urinary stress incontinence can be expected with better tone and hypertrophy of the pubococcygeus, since these qualities enable the muscle to give adequate support to the proximal urethra and bladder neck, with reinforcement of the sphincters. Bulging of the anterior vaginal wall due to muscle weakness (often referred to as cystocele and urethrocele) will diminish. However, herniation of the bladder through a hiatus of the pubococcygeus muscle will not be corrected by exercise.

In response to active exercise of the pubococcygeus, all muscles of the pelvic diaphragm are benefited. As a consequence, malposition of the uterus frequently improves. Circulation, particularly venous flow, is increased throughout the pelvic area, leading to relief of pelvic vascular congestion and fibrosis. Similarly, infertility as well as functional bleeding associated with genital relaxation can be favorably affected. While on exercise therapy, patients have also reported relief of rectal stasis and hemorrhoids. Because a physiologic treatment such as exercise has so pervasive an influence, it is indicated for almost any functional disorder of the pelvic organs before more radical approaches are used.

For many women, pelvic exercises have enhanced sexual sensory perception. Guided by the responses of these patients, we were able to identify two centers

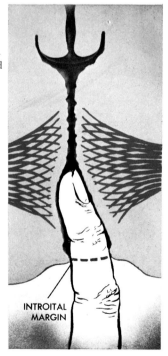

Fig. 79.—Pubococcygeus muscle with good tone and efficient pattern of contractions extends along the entire middle third of the vagina, keeping the organ snug and elongated.

INTROITAL
MARGIN

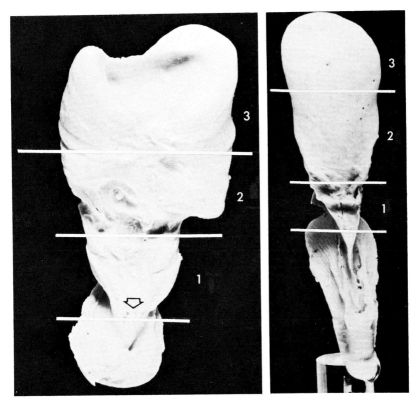

FIG. 80 (left).—Moulage, anterior view. Surgical injury of left pubococcygeus muscle (*area 2*), opposite bladder sphincter, caused severe urinary incontinence. Deeply placed, excessively tight sutures strangulate tissues and result in atrophy.

FIG. 81 (right).—Moulage, anterior view. Evidence of neurologic disease, characterized by loss of tone and contractility of pubococcygeus muscle as well as lack of rugae in the walls of the middle third of the vagina (*area 2*).

of acute sexual perception in the posterolateral quadrants of the vagina at the sulcus between the upper and middle third of the pubococcygeus. Women who claim to have lost the enjoyment of sex after childbirth have found that exercise therapy helped them to regain their former sexual response.

Injuries from childbirth or surgical intervention may play a part in dysfunction of the pubococcygeus muscle. Although such injury is usually confined to one side, atrophy from disuse of the muscle occurs on both sides. After exercise therapy, it can be observed that the injured side has only partially responded. The injured area can be palpated as a gap in the musculature (Fig. 80). Discovery of an injury involving the area of sexual perception has explained certain cases of sexual maladjustment and relieved these women of the psychological burden of so-called frigidity.

The pubococcygeus muscle can also be incapacitated by loss of nerve function due to spinal injury, congenital anomalies, and neurologic or metabolic disease (Fig. 81). In these categories the most common disorders are diabetes, lower neuron lesions, nerve compression by an intervertebral disk, spina bifida, and Parkinson's disease. However, any evidence of residual function calls for pelvic exercises as a means of preserving or improving the remaining traces of neuromuscular performance.

Additional Indications for Pelvic Muscle Exercise

Pelvic muscle exercises are a great aid before and after childbirth. If the pubococcygeus muscle is supple and strong, with unimpaired contractility and in its normal high location, it retracts during the second stage of labor to a position behind the rami of the os pubis; here it is protected from injury. On the other hand, a prolapsed, fibrotic pubococcygeus may be pushed forward with the fetal head and may be torn or involved in a mediolateral episiotomy. Exercises of the pelvic muscles should be taught routinely to every pregnant woman. Only if she has become aware of the correct muscle contractions before labor will it be possible to resume the exercise routine immediately after childbirth. Such exercise aids in prompt closure of the birth canal and facilitates return of pelvic organs to normal position and function.

The preventive use of pelvic muscle exercises is recommended during each of the developmental phases of a woman's life. In pre-adolescence they are effective in correcting imperfect urinary control and should be taught during the teens as an essential part of sex education. They should certainly be included in the premarital examination. These technics are already being applied in the field of marriage counseling. At the American Institute of Family Relations, they have been used successfully since 1954. When necessary, women are referred to a physician for more explicit instruction and for treatment of specific disorders.

Pelvic muscle exercise is indicated before and immediately after any operation involving the neuromuscular tissues of the pelvis. The longer the course of preoperative exercises, the more will tissue quality be improved. Postoperatively, the exercises promote recovery and help to restore supportive, sphincteric, and sexual functions.

ENURESIS IN CHILDREN.—Prolonged bed wetting or diurnal enuresis in children can be treated by the same principles that apply to urinary stress incontinence. Young children can be taught to interrupt the flow of urine several times while voiding. Older children can advance from this procedure to pretending to stop urinary flow and can then practice the exercise at frequent intervals during the day, as recommended for adults.

Functional Anatomy

Although the response to pelvic muscle exercise can be clearly demonstrated, the nature of this phenomenon will be fully appreciated only when the functional anatomy of the pelvis is understood. The pubococcygeous muscle is the central structure of the pelvic diaphragm (levator ani group) which attaches anteriorly to the os pubis and the obturator fascia and extends posteriorly to the coccyx. With normal, healthy tone and contractility, the pubococcygeus stretches between the two bony points of attachment in an almost straight line (Fig. 82). In this state, the muscle helps to support the pelvic structures in the proper position to perform their various physiologic functions efficiently. It is able to adapt to the numerous demands put upon it, adjusting to a full or empty bladder and rectal pouch and enabling the vagina to accommodate itself to intercourse as well as to the passage of the fetus.

FIG. 82.—With a normal, efficient pattern of contractions, the pubococcygeus muscle lies high in relation to a line drawn between the os pubis and the coccyx.

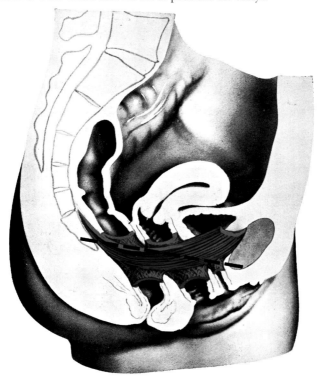

The pubococcygeus contracts the middle third of the vagina, with tiny fibers actually inserted into the muscular tunic of the organ. Through this intimate connection, muscular contractions influence not only the function of the vagina but its very configuration. Normally, the pubococcygeus extends along both sides of the vaginal wall for a distance of approximately 6 cm. This portion of the organ consequently presents a long, cylindrical shape (Figs. 78 and 79).

When any muscle is in poor condition due to non-use, it loses tone and body. The pubococcygeus, too, suffers in the same way from lack of adequate activity. Without proper tone it cannot maintain its high position but sags like a hammock between the two fixed points, and the soft tissues of the pelvic area descend with it (Fig. 83). With a flaccid pubococcygeus the area of insertion into the vaginal wall may be reduced to as little as 2 cm.; this portion of the organ then becomes shortened and widens into a funnel shape. Loss of tension in the pubococcygeus also affects sphincteric action of the bladder neck and rectum.

The relationship between function and structure of the pelvic tissues can be observed in young children. The infant is born with all pelvic organs in

FIG. 83.—An atrophic pubococcygeus muscle sags below the normal line of the taut muscle, allowing other pelvic organs to prolapse.

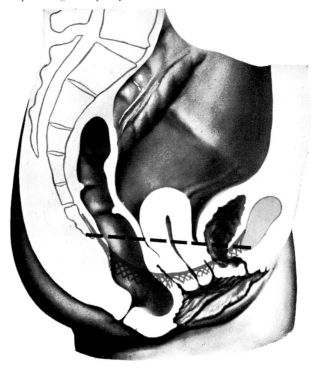

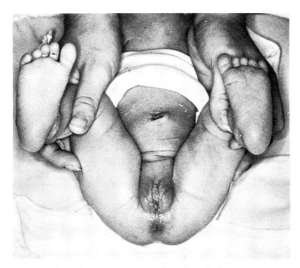

Fig. 84.—Newborn infant. Lax perineum and orifices before supportive and sphincteric functions have developed.

the emptying position (Fig. 84). Voluntary control of urine and feces is not yet possible. The supportive capacity of the pelvic diaphragm is not called upon, since the infant is always recumbent. Anatomical studies of the newborn show only rudimentary development of the levator ani.

As the child assumes an upright posture and achieves control of urination and defecation, the configuration of the pelvic structures changes (Fig. 85).

Fig. 85.—Five-year-old child, normal development of supportive and sphincteric functions. Perineum retracted and orifices closed.

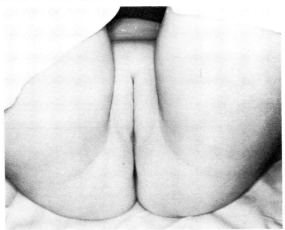

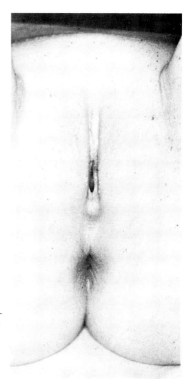

Fig. 86.—Five-year-old child, poor development of supportive and sphincteric functions. Perineum prolapsed, orifices gaping. Early correction with exercise therapy will prevent later problems.

The downward pressure engendered by the erect position evokes resistance in the pelvic diaphragm, with consequent increase in tension. The action of the sphincters is thereby facilitated, and reflex control is made possible.

Individuals, however, differ in the development of pelvic support and in their ability to learn sphincteric control. A surprising number of women seem unable from childhood to achieve a correct pattern of pelvic muscular contractions (Fig. 86). Inadequate muscular activity can develop from a variety of causes: congenital factors, childhood training, poor nutrition, lack of motivation, or other reasons.

Fortunately, the faulty pattern of contractions that leads to muscular deterioration can be corrected by exercise. The pubococcygeus as a voluntary muscle can be re-educated at any time, and the entire muscle group tends to respond. Since the neuromuscular structures of the pelvis serve as a functional unit, all organs affected by them will benefit.

Control of Conception:
Oral Contraceptives

Hormonal Inhibition of Ovulation

THE FIRST 19-norprogestational steroids studied proved to be the most consistent suppressors of ovulation. Two of them are remarkable also in their control of menstrual flow, cycle length, and dysmenorrhea. The three earliest-studied, effective inhibitors of ovulation were: 17-α-ethyl-19-nortestosterone (norethandrolone; Nilevar, Searle); 17-α-ethinyl-19-nortestosterone (norethindrone; Norlutin, Parke, Davis; also a major component of Ortho-Novum, Ortho), and 17-α-ethinyl-5, 10-estraenolone (norethynodrel; major component of Enovid, Searle). Norethynodrel not only is the most active oral ovulation inhibitor among the three initial compounds but is neither androgenic nor antiestrogenic. Norethynodrel and norethindrone are equally effective in regulating cycle length.

In recent years lower doses of progestin have become available, such as ethynodiol diacetate 1.0 mg. (Ovulen) and 1.0 mg. (Demulen), norethindrone acetate 1.0 mg. (Norlestrin), norethindrone 1.0 mg. (Ortho-Novum, Ortho, and Norinyl, Syntex), and norgestrel 0.5 mg. (Ovral). The estrogen component is either ethinyl estradiol 50 μg. or mestranol in a dose of 50, 80, or 100 μg. Many compounds with a progestin as the major ingredient in combination with an estrogen are now being used with equal success (see Table 2).

It is important that the user of the oral contraceptive method be taught to maintain *strict adherence to the regimen*. The effectiveness of the method can be assured only if the medication is started before follicular development is under way. Therefore it is essential that medication be started early in the cycle; beginning on day 5 of the first pill-taking cycle will assure this effectiveness. Moreover, skipping or forgetting to take the medication at any time during the 20 or 21 days of the regimen will predispose to escape or "breakthrough" bleeding and may even allow release of an ovum.

When the oral contraceptive is taken faithfully, cycle lengths average 28 days and pregnancy is prevented in practically 100% of cases.

By resumption of medication on the seventh or eighth day following the last pill and indefinite repetition of the prescribed course, a continued state of nonfertility can be established. If, however, after the recommended 20-

TABLE 2.—ORAL CONTRACEPTIVES AVAILABLE IN THE U.S.A., JUNE 1970

AGENT	ESTROGEN	PROGESTIN	MANUFACTURER	°ESTROGENIC POTENCY Fluid Retention	°PROGESTATIONAL POTENCY Effect on Menses	RATIO Estrogen:Progestin
Enovid-E (Conovid-E)	Mestranol 0.10 mg.	Norethynodrel 2.5 mg.	Searle	++ INTERMEDIATE	+ LOW	1:25
Enovid-5 (Conovid, Enadrel)	Mestranol 0.075 mg.	Norethynodrel 5.0 mg.	Searle			1:67
Enovid-10	Mestranol 0.15 mg.	Norethynodrel 10.0 mg.	Searle			1:66
Norlestrin-1 Norlestrin-(21) Norlestrin-(28) (21 + 7 placebo) Norlestrin-(Fe) (21 + 7 Fe)	Ethinyl estradiol 0.05 mg.	Norethindrone acetate 1.0 mg.	Parke-Davis	++ INTERMEDIATE	INTERMEDIATE	1:20
Norlestrin 2.5 (Etalontin, Orlestrin, Prolestrin)	Ethinyl estradiol 0.05 mg.	Norethindrone acetate 2.5 mg.	Parke-Davis	+++ HIGH	+++ HIGH	1:50
Ortho-Novum-1-20 Ortho-Novum 1/50-21's	Mestranol 0.05 mg.	Norethindrone 1 mg.	Ortho	± VERY LOW	+ LOW	1:20
Norinyl-1 20's 21's Noriday (21 + 7 placebo)	Mestranol 0.05 mg.	Norethindrone 1 mg.	Syntex	± VERY LOW	+ LOW	1:20
Ortho-Novum 1/80 -20 and -21	Mestranol 0.08 mg.	Norethindrone 1 mg.	Ortho			1:12.5
Ortho-Novum-2 (Ortho-Novin, Novulon)	Mestranol 0.10 mg.	Norethindrone 2 mg.	Ortho	+ LOW	+++ HIGH	1:20
Norinyl-2	Mestranol 0.10 mg.	Norethindrone 2 mg.	Syntex	+ LOW	+++ HIGH	1:20
Ortho-Novum-10	Mestranol 0.06 mg.	Norethindrone 10 mg.	Ortho			1:167
Ovral	Ethinyl estradiol 0.05 mg.	Norgestrel 0.5 mg.	Wyeth			°°1:5
Ovulen (Metrulen-M) Ovulen 21	Mestranol 0.10 mg.	Ethynodiol diacetate 1.0 mg.	Searle	+ LOW	++ INTERMEDIATE	1:10

COMBINED

Product	Estrogen	Progestin	Manufacturer	Estrogen activity	Progestin activity	Ratio
Provest† (Provestral)	Ethinyl estradiol 0.05 mg.	Medroxyprogesterone acetate 10 mg.	Upjohn	VERY LOW	± VERY LOW	1:200
C-Quens† (Estirona, Sequens)	15: Mestranol 0.08 / 5: Mestranol 0.08	Chlormadinone acetate 2 mg.	Lilly	+++ HIGH	± VERY LOW	
Oracon (Ovin)	16: Ethinyl estradiol 0.10 mg. / 5: Ethinyl estradiol 0.10 mg.	Dimethisterone 25 mg.	Mead-Johnson	+++ HIGH	± VERY LOW	
Ortho-Novum Sq (Ortho-Novin Sq, Novulon S)	14: Mestranol 0.08 mg. / 6: Mestranol 0.08	Norethindrone 2 mg.	Ortho	+++ HIGH	± VERY LOW	
Norquen		Norethindrone 2 mg.	Syntex			
Demulen	Ethinyl estradiol 0.05 mg.	Ethynodiol diacetate 1.0 mg.	Searle			

SEQUENTIAL (C-Quens, Oracon, Ortho-Novum Sq, Norquen)

°ESTROGEN EXCESS
Nausea
Edema & leg cramps
Vertigo
Leukorrhea
Increase in leiomyoma size
Chloasma
Uterine cramps

°ESTROGEN DEFICIENCY
Irritability, nervousness
Hot flushes
Uterine prolapse
Monilia Vaginitis
Early and midcycle bleeding
Decreased amount of menstrual flow

°PROGESTIN EXCESS
Increased appetite and weight gain
Tiredness & fatigue
Depression, change in libido
Oily scalp, acne
Loss of hair
Cholestatic jaundice
Decreased length of menstrual flow

°PROGESTIN DEFICIENCY
Late breakthrough bleeding & spotting
Heavy menstrual flow and clots
Delayed onset of menses

°SYMPTOMS WITH MULTIPLE CAUSES

Headache:
During medication cycle: estrogen excess
Between medication cycles: progestin excess
Migraine and visual disturbances: unknown

Mastalgia:
With fluid retention: same as headache
Without fluid retention: progestin excess

Spotting and breakthrough bleeding:
Early and midcycle: estrogen deficiency
Late cycle: progestin deficiency

° Dickey, R. P., & Dorr, C. H. II: Oral Contraceptives: Selection of the Proper Pill, Obst. Gynec. 33:273, 1969.

°° Ratio is 1:10, but since only 50% of this isomer is active, it is rated 1:5.

† Withdrawn by manufacturer October, 1970.

(Courtesy, Family Planning Division, NYU School of Medicine.)

or 21-day interval of tablet taking, the medication is suspended, ovulation usually, but by no means always, occurs in the ensuing cycle.

The incidence of break-through bleeding (usually as intermenstrual spotting) is highest in the earliest cycles and at the lower dosages. As the individual becomes more faithful in adhering to the regimen, and perhaps as the endometrium readjusts to the new hormonal level, there seems to be a steady lowering of the occurrence of this phenomenon.

When break-through bleeding occurs as a stain or spotting, the patient can be reassured as to the continued effectiveness of the pill and that the bleeding will usually disappear. If it persists, a higher dose may be prescribed or another compound with different estrogen-progestin ratios can be substituted, depending upon the time of the cycle in which the bleeding occurs.

If, however, break-through bleeding is an actual flow, it should be treated as such: medication should be terminated and the individual instructed to resume medication 5 days later.

The exact time to initiate therapy in the postpartum period for the non-lactating mother depends on the urgency of its effectiveness. It seems likely that the suppression of ovulation consequent to the recently terminated pregnancy may be extended if the oral contraceptive regimen is started by at least 3 weeks, and certainly not later than 4 weeks, post partum. In fact it appears to be safe to start therapy in non-lactating women as early as 3 or 4 days post partum. In instances of less urgency, one may elect to wait for the resumption of catamenia and initiate therapy on day 5, as in the case in nonpregnant, regularly ovulating women.

All of the orally administered progestins have similar physiologic effects. There is a rapid sequence of progestational changes in the endometrium through which the endometrial glandular elements pass, ending in an inactive type of structure. The stroma of the endometrium, and even that of the cervix, undergoes predecidual transformation very early in therapy. Effect on cervical mucus seems to be variable. There generally is an increase in the 24-hour production, but the appearance is usually consistent with effects of progestational therapy on the progestational phase. In those instances in which inspection of ovaries has been possible after one or more cycles of norethindrone or norethynodrel, a gross picture of ovarian inactivity has been noted.

Suppression of ovulation by this method does not reduce the ovarian potential for producing normal ova.

There is great concern regarding the potential predisposition of the oral contraceptives to lead to complications, especially thrombophlebitis and pulmonary embolism.

The Commissioner of the Food and Drug Administration of the Department of Health, Education, and Welfare sent a letter to all physicians on January 12, 1970. Enclosed was the revised labeling for oral contraceptives, as reported by the Obstetrics and Gynecology Advisory Committee in August, 1969. The

Commissioner said an American study confirms previously reported studies in Great Britain that show a relationship between the use of oral contraceptives and the occurrence of certain thromboembolic diseases. These retrospective studies show that users of oral contraceptives are more likely to have thrombophlebitis and pulmonary embolism than non-users. Studies in Great Britain also show increased risk of cerebral thrombosis and embolism in users of oral contraceptives. The American study also suggests there may be an increased risk of thromboembolic disease in users of sequential products. The British Committee on Safety of Drugs recently advised practitioners in that country that only products containing 0.05 mg. or less of estrogen should normally be prescribed because reports of suspected adverse reactions indicated there is a higher incidence of thromboembolic disorders with products containing 0.075 mg. or more of estrogen than with products containing the smaller dose. This finding has not been confirmed by other studies.

The "Oral Contraceptive Labeling" is extensive. Following are a few items:

ACTIONS

Combination oral contraceptives: The mechanism of action is inhibition of ovulation resulting from gonadotrophin suppression. Changes in cervical mucus and endometrium may be contributory mechanisms.

Sequential oral contraceptives: The mechanism of action is inhibition of ovulation resulting from gonadotrophin suppression.

SPECIAL NOTE

The effectiveness of the sequential products appears to be somewhat lower than that of the combination products. Both types provide almost completely effective contraception. The possible carcinogenicity due to the estrogens can neither be affirmed nor refuted at this time.

INDICATIONS

The Obstetrics and Gynecology Advisory Committee considered the following indications acceptable: contraception, endometriosis, and hypermenorrhea.

CONTRAINDICATIONS

(1) Thrombophlebitis, thromboembolic disorders, cerebral apoplexy, or a past history of these conditions. (2) Markedly impaired liver function. (3) Known or suspected carcinoma of the breast. (4) Known or suspected estrogen dependent neoplasia. (5) Undiagnosed abnormal genital bleeding.

Warning.—Since the safety of the pills in pregnancy has not been demonstrated, it is recommended that for any patient who has missed two consecutive periods, pregnancy should be ruled out before continuing the contraceptive regimen.

PRECAUTIONS

(1) The pretreatment and periodic physical examinations should include special reference to breasts and pelvic organs, including Papanicolaou smear, since estrogens have been known to produce tumors, some of them malignant,

in five species of subprimate animals. (2) Endocrine and possibly liver function tests may be affected. Therefore, if such tests are abnormal in a patient taking the pills, the tests should be repeated after the drug has been withdrawn for 2 months. (3) Under the influence of estrogen-progestogen preparations, pre-existing uterine leiomyomas may increase in size. (4) Because these agents may cause some fluid retention, conditions that might be influenced by this factor, such as epilepsy, migraine, asthma, cardiac or renal dysfunction, require careful observation. (5) In break-through bleeding, and in all cases of irregular bleeding per vaginam, nonfunctional causes should be borne in mind. In undiagnosed bleeding per vaginam, adequate diagnostic measures are indicated. (6) Patients with a history of psychic depression should be carefully observed and the drug discontinued if the depression recurs to a serious degree. (7) A decrease in glucose tolerance has been observed in a significant percentage of patients on oral contraceptives. For this reason, diabetic patients should be carefully observed. (8) The age of the patient constitutes no absolute limiting factor. (9) The pathologist should be advised when relevant specimens are submitted. (10) Susceptible women may experience an increase in blood pressure following administration of contraceptive steroids.

ADVERSE REACTIONS OBSERVED IN PATIENTS RECEIVING
ORAL CONTRACEPTIVES

A statistically significant association has been demonstrated between use of oral contraceptives and the following serious adverse reactions: thrombophlebitis, pulmonary embolism, and cerebral thrombosis.

Although available evidence is suggestive of an association, such a relationship has been neither confirmed nor refuted for the following serious adverse reactions: neuro-ocular lesions, e.g., retinal thrombosis and optic neuritis.

The following adverse reactions are known to occur in patients receiving oral contraceptives: nausea, vomiting, gastrointestinal symptoms (such as abdominal cramps and bloating), break-through bleeding, spotting, change in menstrual flow, amenorrhea during and after treatment, edema, chloasma or melasma, breast changes (tenderness, enlargement and secretion), change in weight (increase or decrease), changes in cervical erosion and cervical secretions, suppression of lactation when given immediately post partum, cholestatic jaundice, migraine, rash (allergic), rise in blood pressure in susceptible individuals, and mental depression.

The following laboratory results may be altered by the use of oral contraceptives: hepatic function: increased sulfobromophthalein retention and other tests; coagulation tests: increase in prothrombin, factors VII, VIII, IX, and X; thyroid function: increase in PBI and butanol extractable protein-bound iodine and decrease in T^3 uptake values; Metyrapone test; and pregnanediol determination.

Control of Conception:
The Rhythm Method

THE MOST NATURAL and the least harmful method of birth control is that commonly known as "the rhythm" or the "Ogino-Knaus" method. This is based on animal physiology. Thus it is known with certainty that in most animals and almost surely in human beings, the gametes are capable of fertilization for only a short time. It is generally assumed that ova are incapable of fertilization after 24 hours and spermatozoa are not fertile ordinarily after 48 hours, even though they may be motile for much longer periods. Therefore, unless an ovum and a spermatozoon meet within a very short time, conception cannot occur. An ovum is extruded from the ovary at the time of ovulation, and in women with a 26–30-day menstrual cycle, ovulation usually takes place sometime between the tenth and the seventeenth day after onset of the menses. Theoretically, therefore, conception should be possible only during this time, that is, during the time an ovum can be present. Ogino and Knaus assume that ovulation recurs in each menstrual cycle with almost mathematical precision as regards the subsequent menstruation. Both agree that because of this it is possible to calculate the fertile and sterile days every month for most women.

Ogino maintains that ovulation occurs between the twelfth and the sixteenth day before onset of the next menstruation regardless of the cycle, allowing 5 days for minor variations in any given number of regular cycles. Knaus believes that ovulation takes place only on the fifteenth day before the beginning of the next menstrual period. Basing their conclusions on these assumptions, Ogino and Knaus specify certain days in each menstrual cycle as days of absolute sterility and others as days of fertility. The greatest exponents of the Ogino-Knaus theory in the United States have been Latz and Reiner, who formulated the following rules to be observed in determining the safe period.

1. A written record is made of the dates menstrual periods begin for a period of at least 8 months to 1 year before the method is practiced. This is necessary to determine the variation between the shortest and the longest cycle. Patients should also be instructed to record disturbing factors that may upset the regularity of menstruation such as sickness (even colds), mental

shock or upset, physical strains, and even great changes in climate or altitude. This will enable the physician to make an intelligent interpretation of the data, which are of no value when furnished from memory.

2. There must be no sexual intercourse during the time of possible conception.

3. A regularity in menstruation must prevail. The menstrual cycle may be either long or short, but the variation should not be more than 10 days; a longer variation would make use of the method impractical. However, according to Latz and Reiner, 90% of women have variations of from 2 to 8 days regardless of whether their cycles are short or long, and therefore they maintain that most women menstruate regularly enough to make use of this method of natural conception control.

4. After these three rules have been satisfied, the woman is told that her fertile period extends from the twelfth to the nineteenth day before her expected menstruation (the expected first day of menstruation being calculated from the longest cycle in the last 8 months) plus the days of variation between the longest and the shortest cycle in the last 8 months added to the beginning of the fertile period. For example: suppose a woman has varied between a 26- and a 30-day cycle in the last 8 months. Then her first 7 days, counting from the first day of menstruation, are sterile. The next 12 days (8 days of regular fertility plus the 4 days of variation) are fertile, and the remaining days until menstruation are sterile. The patient is then asked to record conscientiously on a calendar the day of each intercourse as well as the first day of each menstrual period.

This method of birth control should not be used: (1) After labor or abortion until the regularity of the cycle is re-established (usually in 3 to 6 months). About 50% of women menstruate irregularly for a short time after childbirth. (2) After febrile or debilitating diseases or severe physical injuries. (3) After severe psychic or emotional upsets. (4) After any drastic alteration in the ordinary routine of life such as prolonged travel in a different climate and strenuous exercise. During and after these unusual occurrences, the method should not be used until regular menses have been definitely established.

Figure 87 is a chart published by Latz and Reiner to show at a glance the fertile days for menstrual cycles varying from 21 to 38 days. Latz and Reiner added 3 days to the fertile days laid down by Knaus, 1 day before and 2 days after the fertile period, to allow for possible errors in computation. This gives 8 days of abstinence for those who want to avoid conception.

Unfortunately the rhythm method of conception control cannot be applied as universally as its proponents believe. In the first place, only 80% of women, at most, menstruate with a degree of regularity that will permit accurate calculation of a fertile period. Certainly not more than 60% of all women menstruate approximately every 28 days. Second, a large proportion of women

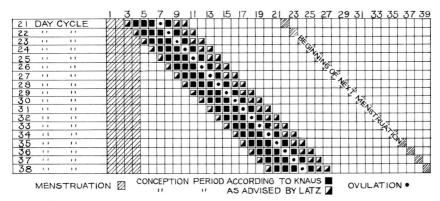

FIG. 87.—Latz-Reiner chart for determining fertile days each month for women with menstrual cycles varying from 21 to 38 days.

at more or less periodic intervals encounter the contraindications enumerated by Latz and Reiner. Thus, most women at various times have full-term pregnancies or abortions, minor or major illnesses, and psychic or emotional upsets or they take trips to other climates. Third, certainly not all, or even the majority, of women ovulate on the fifteenth day before every menstrual period. Many women ovulate a few days before or after this date.

An objection to the Ogino-Knaus method raised by many couples, particularly recently married ones, is that there is an excessive number of days each month when coitus cannot be indulged in. In some cases less than half of each month is safe or convenient for coitus because to the 8-day period of possible conception must be added the number of days the woman menstruates.

Despite all these arguments against the Ogino-Knaus theory, there is no doubt that the rhythm method of controlling conception can be followed successfully by a large number of women. Certainly women who have a fairly regular 26–30-day menstrual cycle are candidates for this method of birth control. (See p. 141 for discussion of ovulation.)

Control of Conception: Mechanical Devices

Physiology

As HAS BEEN stated many times in this book, the reaction in the normal vagina is acid and that in the normal cervix is alkaline. Since the reaction of semen is alkaline, the ideal arrangement, and the one that usually obtains during coitus in normal women, is for the semen to be deposited on the cervix and in the posterior vaginal vault. In some animals, the semen is sucked into the uterine cavity almost immediately after it is ejaculated into the vagina. Perhaps there is a somewhat similar action in women. Even if this does not occur after ejaculation, the spermatozoa, of which there are normally between 200 and 500 million in each ejaculation, remain in an alkaline medium long enough so that some of them gain access to the depths of the cervical canal and from there to the uterus and fallopian tubes. It is in the tubes that fertilization takes place. The speed with which spermatozoa travel is great, for they usually cover 2.5 cm. (1 in.) in about 8 minutes, so it does not take long for spermatozoa to reach the fallopian tubes. Spermatozoa have a remarkable way of overcoming obstacles, as proved by the pregnancies that have occurred in girls with intact hymen after semen had been deposited only on the vulva. In such cases the spermatozoa not only must travel over a physical barrier, the hymen, but must overcome a chemical medium in the vagina, which has an acid reaction.

Ordinarily spermatozoa are destroyed by acids, weak antiseptics, and heat. The ideal contraceptive device is one that acts both mechanically and spermicidally. Therefore, not only must it prevent the spermatozoa from gaining access to the external os, but it must destroy them.

No mechanical contraceptive is completely satisfactory. First, most mechanical devices are unesthetic, many interfere to some degree with the emotions of the female or male or both, and in some instances they produce an undesirable psychologic reaction.

Devices Used by the Male

Practically the only device used by men is the *condom*, or *sheath*, which may be made of rubber, latex compounds, or "fishskin." The last mentioned are made from the peritoneal covering of the cecum of animals. Condoms are used more often than any other mechanical contraceptive device. The rubber and latex sheaths are much cheaper than the "skins," are more readily applied and are elastic. Before a condom is applied it must be rolled, and the distal half-inch should be pinched off to permit a free portion to remain and also to prevent the accumulation of air during application of the sheath. After use and before it is discarded, the sheath should be tested by filling it with water, pinching off and twisting the open end, and compressing the distended sac. Escape of water from the distended portion, of course, indicates a defect in the sheath.

"Fishskin" condoms are more expensive than rubber or latex ones, and they are not elastic. They are more difficult to put on and are best tested by filling with water. The small amount of water that remains in the sheath after emptying helps in drawing on the sheath, or the sheath may be drawn on like a glove and then moistened. A major defect in "fishskin" sheaths is the looseness at the top. A rubber condom fits snugly at the top and prevents any leakage of semen during an ejaculation and shortly afterward. Regardless of whether the rubber, latex, or skin sheath is used, the penis should be withdrawn shortly after ejaculation. During withdrawal, care must be exercised to see that the sheath does not slip off.

Although condoms are the most convenient mechanical devices in use and are highly dependable in preventing unwanted pregnancies, they are by no means the most satisfactory. Some men cannot use them because they interfere with complete sensation, and some women object to their use for the same reason. Couples should not rely on condoms alone but should use a contraceptive jelly or cream in addition. The condom may prove helpful for some men in whom the orgasm occurs too quickly; a condom will often dull sensation sufficiently to permit prolongation of coitus to a satisfactory conclusion.

For protection against venereal disease, nothing is more ideal than a condom except antibiotics. Men who have a venereal infection and insist on having intercourse must be instructed to use condoms, and women who are infected should be warned about the danger to which they expose male partners who do not use a sheath.

The chief reason for the failures that occur when condoms are used is that many men engage in the preliminary acts of coitus, including penetration of the penis into the vagina, before they use a condom, not putting it on until just before the orgasm. Under such conditions conception may follow because during the preparatory acts some spermatozoa escape into the vagina.

Another method of contraception that the male partner can use is *coitus interruptus*, known more popularly as "withdrawal." This is one of the oldest methods of birth control known and requires the man to withdraw his penis when he feels that ejaculation is imminent and to ejaculate the semen between the female's thighs. Coitus interruptus is effective for those couples who have used it consistently for a long time with success.

Devices Used by the Female

The devices that may be used by women for the prevention of conception are numerous. They consist chiefly of douches (plain water or medicated), spermicides (jellies, creams, foam, suppositories, or tablets) and mechanical devices (diaphragms, cervical caps, and intrauterine devices). (See Table 3.)

Douches are unsatisfactory as a means of contraception, regardless of whether plain water is used or drugs are added to the douche water. The chief reason is that no matter how quickly after coitus a douche is taken, it will do little good, because during ejaculation some spermatozoa are deposited at the external os of the cervix. These immediately find their way into the cervical canal and the uterus, out of reach of a douche. (Douche water does not extend much beyond the external os.) Another undesirable factor with douches is that many women object to getting out of bed immediately after coitus. Third, douche bags or cans are not always available, and, fourth, in many instances there are no facilities for the privacy of a douche.

Spermicides may be applied in the form of jelly, foam, or suppository. Their primary purpose is to destroy the spermatozoa, but the vehicles for the drugs also act as mechanical barriers. This is an ideal combination and a simple one, but unfortunately there is no completely satisfactory spermicide. Because of this, it is wise for the physician to prescribe both a spermicide and a mechanical barrier such as a diaphragm.

TABLE 3.—Pregnancy Rates Based on
Use Efficacy°

Pregnancy Rate—100 Women Using Technic for One Year

Less than 1	Orals (Combinations)
Less than 2	Orals (Sequentials)
2–5	Intra-Uterine Devices
10–15	{ Diaphragm & Jelly or Cream { Condom (Rubber)
15–20	Aerosol Vaginal Foam
20–30	Jelly or Cream Alone
35	{ Rhythm { Withdrawal
35–40	{ Suppositories { Vaginal Tablets
More than 40	Douche
80	Nothing

° Use efficacy: A combination of both method failure and patient failure.

An effective spermicide must kill spermatozoa in a minute or two, it must be fluid enough to cover the entire vaginal wall and portio of the cervix, it must be acid in reaction, it must not be injurious to the vaginal mucosa, it must not burn or produce any annoyances to either the male or the female, it must not have a bad odor, it must not contain any substance that may be absorbed and produce toxic symptoms, and it should be stable, cheap, easy to apply, and simple to remove from the vagina if all of it is not absorbed.

A *jelly* is a frequently used spermicide in the vagina and on the cervix. Most of the jellies sold commercially are acid in reaction and contain a water-soluble base such as gum tragacanth or glycerite of starch. Many spermicides are used, chief among them being lactic acid, quinine or quinoline salts, boric acid, and acetic acid. Jellies are fairly stable, they are easily spread all over the vagina during coitus, they remain effective in the vagina for many hours, and they are easily removed by douching if desired. Nearly all jellies are put up in collapsible tubes from which the jelly is squeezed into the vagina through a specially prepared nonbreakable nozzle. In nearly all instances, women should be advised to apply jelly on the diaphragm before the latter is inserted into the vagina. If a special diaphragm inserter is used, there is no need to place additional jelly in the vagina after the diaphragm has been inserted. In other instances, jelly should be placed in the vagina in front of the pessary. To accomplish this, the nozzle attached to the collapsible tube is inserted deep into the vagina and the key on the base of the tube turned halfway. A half-turn usually deposits about 1 teaspoonful of jelly, which is sufficient. It is best to use a measured amount of jelly. This may readily be done with any one of a number of measuring tubes that may be purchased with or without the commercial tubes of jelly.

If coitus is to take place a second time shortly after the first, additional jelly should be placed in the vagina with the use of an applicator before the second act. Whenever jelly is used, either alone or with a diaphragm, it should be left in the vagina for at least 6 hours after coitus. If women desire to take a douche after coitus, they should wait at least this length of time. There is, however, no absolute necessity to take a douche after the use of a jelly, because the latter is usually entirely absorbed. Women who experience some irritation from retained jelly should take a douche in order to remove all the jelly.

Vaginal foam tablets.—Only one vaginal foam tablet is approved by the United States Food and Drug Administration for contraceptive use (Durafoam Vaginal Tablet, Durex Products, Inc.). The foam spreads throughout the vagina and acts as a chemical and mechanical barrier to immobilize spermatozoa and prevent their entrance into the cervix. The tablets can be purchased without a prescription and should not be kept for more than 6 months.

Immediately before coitus, and lying on the back, the woman inserts a slightly moistened tablet high up in the vagina. At least 5 minutes should elapse after insertion, and not more than 1 hour should elapse before having intercourse.

An additional moistened tablet should be inserted at least 5 minutes before each time that intercourse is repeated.

This simple method is as effective as jelly alone but not as safe as the diaphragm plus jelly.

Aerosol foams.—An aerosol foam acts like a jelly or cream alone, but the foam is in a container under pressure and is extruded into an applicator when the container is manipulated. Because only a small amount of foam is necessary, it is not messy and there is little postcoital leakage. If a douche is taken after use, at least 6 hours should elapse.

Suppositories.—The suppository is a small solid cone which usually melts at slightly below body temperature and contains either cocoa butter or glycerogelatin. It should be inserted not less than 15 nor more than 60 minutes before intercourse. As with tablets, a second suppository should be inserted before each ejaculation, and a douche should not be taken until 6 hours after the last ejaculation.

Vaginal Diaphragms

The most satisfactory mechanical measure for contraception is a combination of a vaginal diaphragm (or "pessary") and a jelly. When used intelligently, this method may be 95% reliable, but it depends on the sustained motivation of the couple and consistent use. The failure rate varies from 10 to 30%. There are various types of diaphragms, but the following ones are in general use. (1) A rubber dome and a base containing a flat steel watch spring. This diaphragm is flexible in only one plane; that is, it can be compressed laterally only. (2) A rubber dome with a base containing a coiled steel spring. This spiral type of diaphragm is flexible in two planes, laterally to form an oval and also at an angle to the plane of the rim. Diaphragms vary in diameter from 50 to 105 mm. and are sold in sizes varying 5 mm. The sizes generally used are from 65 to 85 mm. Diaphragms can be fitted to almost all women except those with complete prolapse, extensive cystocele and rectocele, and girls with an intact hymen.

Before a diaphragm is inserted, a careful bimanual examination should be made not only to rule out any abnormalities, including an early pregnancy, but also to decide on the size of diaphragm to be fitted. Generally, in women who have not had children, a 65- or 70-mm. diaphragm is the proper size, whereas in women who have had one or more children, the size will depend on the degree of pelvic relaxation and will usually be a 70-, 75-, or 80-mm. diaphragm. Most manufacturers of diaphragms supply a series of rings of varying sizes for the purpose of determining the proper size of diaphragm to use. After a little experience, these trial rings can be dispensed with.

A properly fitting diaphragm is one that, after insertion, extends from behind the symphysis to the posterior vaginal vault and covers the entire cervix. It must cause no discomfort and must remain in place even after straining. The entire rim of the diaphragm is kept in close contact with the vaginal wall all around by the steel spring in the base. The diaphragm therefore acts as a mechanical barrier. Furthermore, as will be explained later, there is jelly on the rim of the diaphragm which helps further to seal off any possible space between the diaphragm and the vaginal wall. During coitus, the penis comes in contact only with the anterior surface of the diaphragm, not with the cervix or the vaginal fornix.

A diaphragm has both a concave and a convex side. Some physicians advise women to place the diaphragm in the vagina in such a way that the cervix fits into the concave side or hollow of the diaphragm. It really makes no difference into which side the cervix fits. However, it is much easier to remove the diaphragm when the cervix is against the convex surface, that is, the outside of the dome. It is easy to insert the diaphragm this way if a special inserter is used. To simplify the instructions, the woman may be told to consider the vagina and the diaphragm as cups. Then if she will visualize the insertion of one cup inside another, she will grasp the idea of inserting the diaphragm with the outside of the dome toward the cervix.

Before having a woman insert a diaphragm, it is best to show her illustrations and a model of the external and internal genitals. (These can be purchased.) After this, the patient should insert an index finger into the vagina to feel the lower surface of the symphysis, the direction of the vaginal canal, and particularly the cervix. She should learn to recognize the position of the cervix to be sure that it will be covered by the diaphragm after it is inserted.

It is well to demonstrate the insertion of a diaphragm on the model. The patient's attention should be directed to the fact that when a diaphragm is in place, it lies obliquely and not vertically and extends from the base of the symphysis, past the cervix to the posterior fornix. When the penis is inserted, it passes under that part of the rim of the diaphragm that is behind the symphysis.

In most women, the spiral spring diaphragm may be used. However, in women with a short anterior vaginal wall and therefore an indefinite posterior pubic space and in women with a cystocele and rectocele and a long cervix, it is best to use the flat spring type of diaphragm because it is much more rigid and is flexible in only one plane.

After the insertion of a diaphragm is demonstrated on the model or explained, the patient should insert the diaphragm in her vagina and the physician should check it to see that it has been placed properly. The patient should

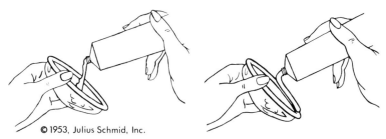

© 1953, Julius Schmid, Inc.

FIG. 88.—Application of jelly to diaphragm **(left)**, and around rim **(right)**. (Figs. 88–91, courtesy of Julius Schmid, Inc., New York, manufacturers of Ramses Gynecological Products.)

then remove the diaphragm and should replace it and remove it at least twice more. She should return with the diaphragm a week or two later to show that she has been using it properly.

There are various ways of inserting a diaphragm. If the fingers alone are to be used and no special inserter, about 1 teaspoonful of jelly (a half-turn of the key on the tube) is placed on the inside of the dome and a small amount of it is spread all around the rim (Fig. 88). Then the patient compresses the rim of the diaphragm between the thumb and the first two fingers of the right hand in such a way that the diaphragm is held at an angle of 45 degrees. With the index finger and thumb or the index and middle fingers of the left hand, the labia are spread apart and the diaphragm is gently inserted in the vagina, first in a horizontal direction and then down toward the rectum. After the diaphragm is in the vagina, the right index finger is inserted into the vagina and the upper rim of the diaphragm (the last portion to enter the vagina) is pushed behind the symphysis to be sure that the cervix is covered. The woman can be taught to detect the cervix through the diaphragm. After the diaphragm is in place, the nozzle of the tube of jelly is inserted in the vagina for 2.5–3.5 cm. (1–1½ in.) and an additional teaspoonful of jelly is squeezed into it.

Whether the diaphragm is inserted with the fingers or with a special inserter, the woman may assume a reclining (gynecologic) position or an upright position. Figure 89 illustrates the correct position and the method of insertion

→

FIG. 89.—Inserting diaphragm in reclining position. After assuming gynecologic position **(top left)**, patient locates cervix **(top right)**. **Center left,** she holds diaphragm between thumb and fingers and compresses it until inner edges are about ½ in. apart. **Center right,** holding diaphragm in this position, she inserts it high in vagina, so that it passes cervix and catches in hollow behind it; using first finger, she pushes last portion of diaphragm rim forward and upward in vagina until it hooks behind bony projection at top front of vagina. Inserting diaphragm at an angle pointing downward will help make certain that it is correctly placed. **Bottom left,** patient tests for proper placement by inserting forefinger and making sure that cervix can be felt through pliant rubber dome of diaphragm. **Bottom right,** care must be taken to prevent entering rim of diaphragm from catching in front of cervix, leaving it unprotected.

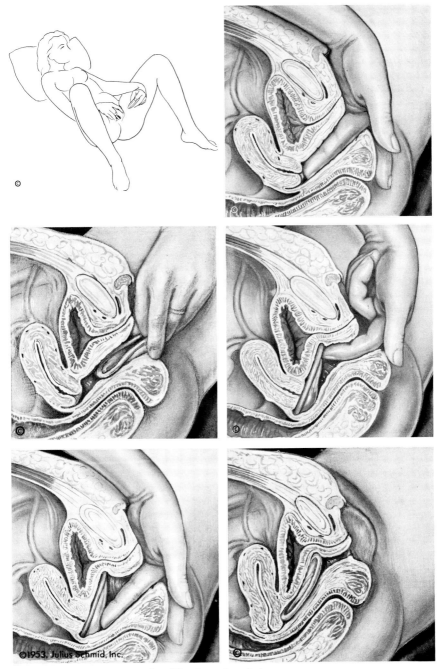

©1953, Julius Schmid, Inc.

FIG. 89.—Legend on facing page.

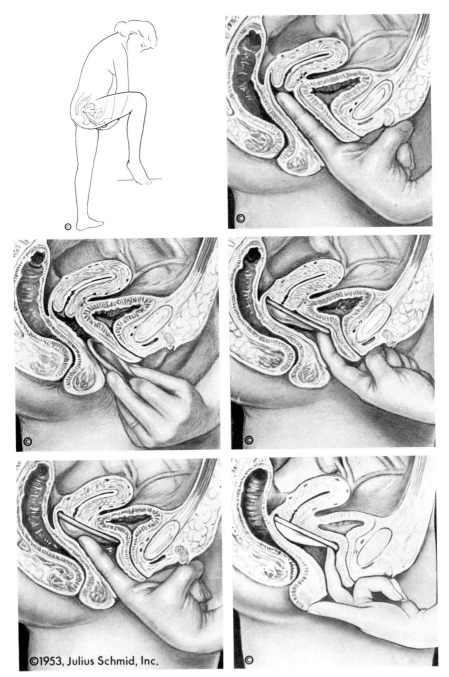

©1953, Julius Schmid, Inc.

FIG. 90.—Legend on facing page.

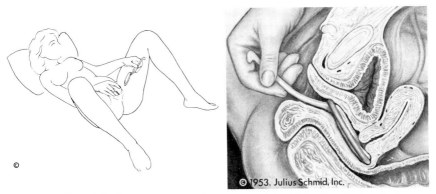

FIG. 91.—Use of diaphragm inserter. **Left,** correct position. **Right,** introducing diaphragm. Inserter should be introduced with diaphragm on top, then passed down and slowly forward along floor of vagina until forward rim of diaphragm passes cervix and lodges in posterior fornix. A simple twist or turn of handle disengages diaphragm from inserter, after which instrument is gently withdrawn.

in the gynecologic position; Figure 90, the correct posture and the method for the upright position; and Figure 91, the use of an inserter. A number of different types of inserters can be purchased. All are devised to hold the diaphragm in an elongated and therefore narrowed shape. After the diaphragm is placed on the inserter, jelly is spread on both the outside and the inside of the dome and all around the rim. Nearly all inserters have a curve to correspond to the posterior vaginal wall, and when the inserter with the attached diaphragm is directed into the vagina, the diaphragm readily slides beyond the cervix and covers it. To free the inserter from the diaphragm, it is turned to the right or left, after which it is easily withdrawn from the vagina. There is no need to add jelly after the diaphragm is in the vagina, because jelly was placed on both sides of the diaphragm before insertion.

Coitus may be indulged in immediately after insertion of the diaphragm. The following morning the diaphragm is easily removed by inserting the index or middle finger high up into the vagina, flexing this finger sharply against the rim of the diaphragm, and pulling it down and out of the vagina. The diaphragm can also easily be removed with the inserter. A plain warm water douche may then be taken if desired to remove the material in the vagina. The diaphragm is washed with soap and water, dried, covered with talcum powder, and replaced in its container. A woman may also use a small amount of the douche water before she removes the diaphragm if she so desires. As

←**FIG. 90.**—Insertion and removal of diaphragm in upright position. **Top left** shows correct position. **Top right to bottom left** represents same steps as those in Figure 89, but with patient in upright position. **Bottom right,** removal of diaphragm. Index finger is inserted behind diaphragm rim and gently pulls out diaphragm, following direction of vaginal floor.

mentioned previously, it is not necessary to use a douche either before or after removal of the diaphragm, but most women feel cleaner if a douche is taken after a diaphragm is removed.

A diaphragm may be used for a year or two, but the user should test it from time to time by stretching the dome away from the rim all around. Also, every few weeks water should be placed inside the dome to see whether any holes have appeared. Petroleum jelly and cold cream should not be placed on a diaphragm, because they lead to deterioration. Furthermore, they are messy.

Intrauterine Contraceptive Devices

In 1928 Graefenberg was the first to popularize an intrauterine device for the purpose of contraception. He employed a ring design made of silk and later evolved a spiral design made of silver or gold. His results were excellent, but in the hands of less-expert physicians, who did not adhere to the strict requirements of Graefenberg, the ring met with disfavor and its use was discontinued. It was not until 1959 that a second look was taken at intrauterine contraception by Oppenheimer, who reported the use of the Graefenberg ring in 1,000 cases in Israel.

Several factors were responsible for the reappraisal of intrauterine devices but most important was the use of biologically inactive materials such as plastic and stainless steel. The stretching and recoiling properties of plastic materials enable insertion into the uterus and removal without having to dilate the nulliparous cervical canal. The presence of a transcervical appendage of nylon strings makes for ease of identification and removal. The Population Council and the International Planned Parenthood Federation have spent considerable time and money on research and clinical trials of various designs. (See Table 4.)

More clinical data have been accumulated on the loop design of Lippes than on any other modern device and it appears to be the most popular choice. There is a 2.5% failure rate in the first year's use, a 1.5% failure rate in the second year, and a 0.5% failure rate in its third year—the same effectiveness as the oral combination pill. It has about a 6–7% expulsion rate, and in the first year of use about 15% of the devices must be removed because of pain, bleeding, and annoying vaginal discharge. Thus in the first year of use, about 25% of the patients are no longer wearing the device, in the second year another 10% have stopped wearing it, and in the third year only about 60% of the patients still wear the device. The most important cause of discontinuation is the necessity for removal because of bleeding or pain or both.

Numerous changes in design and material are being studied in an effort to reduce the expulsion rate, pain, and bleeding and to facilitate introduction

TABLE 4.—Intrauterine Devices Available in U.S.A.†
(August 1969)

Device	Size	Type	Material	Manufacturer or Distributor	Pregnancy Rate	Expulsion Rate*	Removal Rate**	Continuation Rate	Perforation Rate
Birnberg Bow	Small	Closed with tail	Polyethylene Ba impreg. Nylon tail	I.C.D. Corp.	8.8/100	0.9/100	7.9/100	78.5/100[1]	50/10,000
	Large				3.9	0.6	12.5	80.7[1]	89[2]
Gynekoil (Margulies Spiral)	Small	Open with tail	Polyethylene Ba impreg. Beaded tail	Ortho	2.9	8.6	9.7	67.4[1]	3/10,000 (Cervical 1/10,000)
	Large				1.3	6.1	13.8	73.0[1]	
Hall-Stone Ring	—	Closed No tail	Stainless Steel	Goshen Instr. Corp.	6.2	4.6	8.6	76.3[1]	10[2]
Lippes Loop	A (small)	Open with tail	Polyethylene Ba impreg. Nylon tail	Ortho	4.9	5.7	7.7	74.9[1]	4.3[5]
	B				2.8	4.3	13.7	75.1[1]	
	C				2.4	4.2	12.0	77.1[1]	
	D (large)				2.4	2.9	12.8	77.5[1]	
Majzlin Spring	—	Closed with tail	Stainless Steel Silk tail	Anka	1.4	0.5	14.0[4]	—	—
Saf-T-Coil	—	Open with tail	Polyethylene Ba impreg. Nylon tail	Julius Schmid	2.2	7.8	15.7	72.7[1]	—

Ref: (1) Tietze, C., Eighth Progress Report, Cooperative Statistical Program for the Evaluation of IUD, 1967.
(2) Tietze, C., Am. J. Obst. & Gynec. 96:1043, 1966.
(3) Hill, A. M., Am. J. Obst. & Gynec. 103:200, 1969.
(4) Kings County Report (unpublished data).
(5) Liao, S. C., et al., Am. J. Obst. & Gynec. 103:224, 1969.
* First insertion only
** Medical reason only
† Family Planning Division, Dept. of Obs/Gyn, NYU School of Medicine.

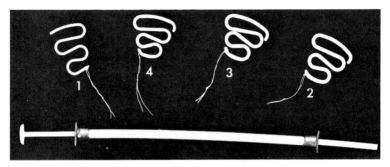

Fɪɢ. **92.**—Intrauterine contraceptive devices. **1,** 25 mm.; **2,** 31 mm.; **3,** 30 mm.; **4,** 27.5 mm. (Courtesy of Dr. Jack Lippes.)

of intrauterine devices through the nulliparous cervical canal. Individual, packaged, sterile disposable units with directions for use are now sold (Lippes Loop, Ortho Products Co. [Fig. 92] and Saf-T-Coil, Julius Schmid, Inc. [Fig. 93]) and have advantages but the cost is prohibitive for use on a mass scale in underdeveloped countries. The only serious side effect of intrauterine devices is uterine perforation, which occurs once in about 1,500 insertions.

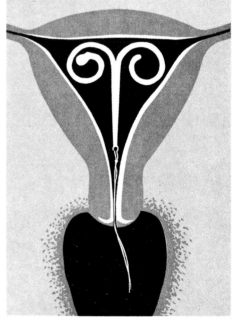

Fɪɢ. **93.**—Saf-T-Coil, an intra-
uterine contraceptive device.
(Courtesy of Julius Schmid, Inc.,
New York, N.Y.)

This complication usually requires a laparotomy for removal of the device.

There are three categories of contraindications. (1) Pre-existing conditions that may be exacerbated, disseminated, or masked by the added presence of any device; these are acute or subacute pelvic inflammatory disease, carcinoma, unexplained menorrhagia or metrorrhagia, abnormal Papanicolaou smear, and history of infected abortion or postpartum endometritis within the first 6 weeks. (2) The possibility of a pregnancy. The introduction of such a device into a uterus containing an undetected pregnancy is fraught with the immediate danger of perforation and hemorrhage and the less immediate but equally serious risk of sepsis and septic abortion. Therefore an intrauterine device should never be introduced until pelvic examination has ruled out a diagnosable pregnancy. Because it is difficult to detect an early pregnancy, the introduction of the intrauterine device should be deferred until the end stages of menstruation, when in any case the isthmic-cervical segment is most patulous and accommodating. (3) A pre-existing condition that would diminish contraceptive effectiveness of the intrauterine device. These include (a) septate or double uterus, (b) any condition in which there is coexisting enlargement of the cavity, such as that due to leiomyomas or the early postpartum period, and (c) cervical incompetence, because such will tend repeatedly to eject the device.

The method's potential popular appeal is believed to rest on the facts that the couple is subjectively unaware of the presence of the device, they need never intrude a repetitive contraceptive action into their sexual life, and they need not remember to keep contraceptive supplies on hand. It cannot be forgotten at the critical moment, it is inexpensive, and it can be used by breast-feeding mothers without fear of suppression of lactation. These advantages are especially appreciated in economically underdeveloped countries. The disadvantage is that it is not as effective as the pill, it requires trained personnel, preferably a physician, to insert it, and it does have a fairly high non-acceptability rate due to disagreeable side effects.

Gynecologic and
Obstetric Endocrinology

by Robert B. Greenblatt, M.D.

Hypothalamus.—The pituitary gland, long considered the master gland of the body, often was referred to as the leader of the endocrine orchestra. With newer knowledge of the role of the hypothalamus in controlling the secretions of the hypophysis, the master gland has been relegated to a secondary role. Neurohumoral substances are secreted by the ganglionic cells in the hypothalamus, and these exert profound influences by stimulating the release of the follicle-stimulating hormone (FSH), luteinizing hormone (LH), adrenocorticotrophic hormone (ACTH), and thyroid-stimulating hormone (TSH) and by inhibiting the release of lactogenic hormone. There is now strong support for the concept proposed by Harris and others that the hypothalamus exerts its effect on the anterior pituitary not through purely nervous pathways but through secretion of neurohumoral substances, which are transmitted to the hypophyseal cells by means of the hypophyseal portal circulation.

The hypothalamus should be considered the master ganglion of the autonomic nervous system, motivating, associating, and transmitting impulses along the sympathetic and parasympathetic nerves to the soma. The hypothalamus is also influenced by impulses from the other elements of the brain, including the cerebral cortex, and much of this is reflected in unconscious behavior, as demonstrated by psychosomatic, glandular, and sexual dysfunctions. Conversely, the endocrines temper and influence the hypothalamus, as can be noted in the irritability of this organ during the menopause, giving rise to vasomotor disturbances.

Pituitary gland.—A functioning pituitary gland is of prime importance to growth and adequate thyroid, gonadal, and adrenal activity. All the glands of internal secretion, however, are mutually interdependent, and a disturbance in one may upset the others.

From a clinical point of view, only the anterior and posterior lobes of the pituitary gland need be considered. The *posterior lobe* contains two hormones.

1. One, the *vasopressor factor*, or vasopressin, has a stimulating effect on the vascular and intestinal muscles; it brings about an elevation in blood pressure and an increase in peristalsis. Vasopressin is believed to be the

hormone that inhibits diuresis, and in its absence diabetes insipidus ensues.

2. The second hormone, the *oxytocic factor*, or oxytocin, controls uterine contractions and is therefore used clinically to initiate or increase labor pains and to control uterine bleeding by stimulating uterine contractions. It also has an effect on lactation as the milk "let-down" factor. By this term is meant the flow of milk from one nipple when the baby nurses from the other. This reflex is a sign of successful nursing rather than of an abnormality and is not present in a mother who is worried or upset.

It has been shown that the posterior lobe of the pituitary is not the center of manufacture of vasopressin and oxytocin but is only the repository of these neurohormones, which originate in the supraoptic and paraventricular nuclei.

The *anterior lobe* of the pituitary gland has multifold and important functions. The chief hormones produced in the anterior lobe are the following.

1. *Thyroid-stimulating hormone* (TSH). This pituitary hormone is responsible for normal function of the thyroid gland. If the pituitary gland is removed, the thyroid partially atrophies. On the other hand, thyroidectomy and the ingestion of thyroid substance produce changes in the hypophysis; hence there is a reciprocal action between the thyroid and the pituitary gland.

Administration of pituitary extract containing TSH induces hypertrophy and hyperplasia of the thyroid gland and increases the basal metabolic rate.

The most active factor isolated from the thyroid is thyroxin, which has been obtained in pure form. Iodides, an essential element of the diet, are necessary for the formation of thyroxin. Iodine deficiency and faulty or incomplete synthesis of thyroxin are the commonest causes of colloid goiter.

2. *Lactogenic hormone.* The pituitary gland affects the breast in two ways, directly and through the ovaries. The breasts enlarge during pregnancy as a result of the action of one or both ovarian hormones. With the withdrawal of these hormones after parturition, the lactogenic hormone stimulates the production of milk. The flow of milk is maintained reflexly by the repeated emptying of the breasts by the baby's nursing.

3. *Adrenocorticotrophic hormone* (ACTH). The cortex of the adrenal glands is dependent on the pituitary gland for much of its activity. Removal of the pituitary gland results in atrophy of the zona fasciculata and zona reticularis but not the zona glomerulosa. Conversely, removal of the adrenal glands results in certain changes in the anterior pituitary lobe. The adrenal cortex aids in the maintenance of optimal concentrations of sodium and potassium in the blood and of normal blood volume. The cortex also is concerned with conversion of protein to glucose and the storage of glucose as glycogen in the liver. The adrenal cortex is the major contributor to the defenses of the body and, under the stimulation by stress or the alarm reaction, secretes additional corticosteroids to meet the demands of the stressful situation.

The adrenal cortex also elaborates androgens, an excess of which may produce masculinization. This is reflected in an increased output of 17-ketosteroids in the urine. The growth of sexual hair in the normal female is dependent on adrenal cortical androgens.

The adrenal medulla may or may not be dependent on the anterior pituitary lobe, but it definitely is associated with the involuntary nervous system. Epinephrine and nor-epinephrine are the hormones of the medulla. Epinephrine participates in the acute emergency mechanism and emotional response of the body; it increases oxygen metabolism and glycolysis, decreases dextrose combustion in muscles, and affects the circulatory, respiratory, digestive, and other systems. Nor-epinephrine is concerned with the maintenance of blood pressure levels and vascular tone.

4. *Gonadotrophic hormones.* The anterior lobe of the pituitary is essential to the development and continued activity of the ovaries and testes. There are at least two distinct anterior pituitary gonadotrophic hormones, one that stimulates follicles (FSH) and another that induces ovulation, the luteinizing hormone (LH). There is a definite reciprocal action between the pituitary and the ovaries, because removal of the gonads results in changes in the pituitary and removal of the pituitary induces atrophy of the gonads.

These two gonadotrophic hormones work in sequence. First, the follicle-stimulating hormone stimulates the primordial follicle to grow and, with the addition of LH, causes maturation of several graafian follicles. One of the follicles will take pre-eminence over the others, and when the minor FSH and major LH surge occurs (usually at midcycle), the chosen follicle ruptures and the ovum is extruded—thus ovulation (Fig. 94). A corpus luteum develops from the ruptured follicle. The corpus luteum blooms for a while, then atrophies, and a new cycle begins. The graafian follicle with its garland of theca cells produces estrogen, whereas the luteinized granulosa cells of the corpus luteum are thought to produce progesterone, while the luteinized paralutein or theca cells continue to produce estrogens. Rising titers of estrogen have an inhibitory action on the anterior pituitary, suppressing follicle-stimulating hormone secretion. Estrogen levels as a consequence fall and the pituitary gland becomes active again, and the cycle repeats. Thus the ovarian-pituitary cycle is a self-regulating system.

Animal experiments suggest that there is a third gonadotrophic anterior pituitary hormone, luteotrophin, which is thought to maintain the corpus luteum. Luteotrophin is probably identical with the lactogenic hormone from the anterior pituitary lobe, but there is no proof that it is necessary for the maintenance of the human corpus luteum.

The ovarian cycle in human beings and in the rodent can be followed by examination of smears from the vaginal canal. In most women the desquamated vaginal epithelial cells are large and clear with pyknotic nuclei as a result of estrogen stimulation which reaches its zenith at about the time of ovulation.

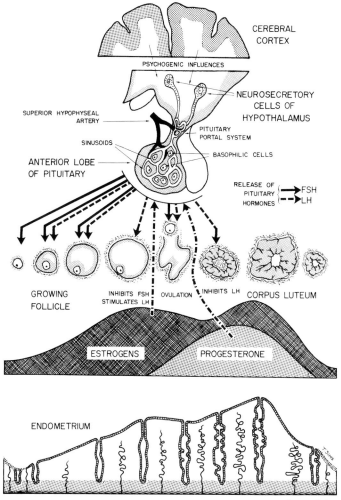

FIG. 94.—Cerebral, hypothalamic, pituitary, and ovarian interrelationships of the menstrual cycle.

After ovulation, progesterone prevents complete maturation of the vaginal epithelium, and desquamation of intermediate cells in large numbers becomes apparent in the vaginal smears. These phenomena are clear cut in the rodent but may be difficult to follow in human beings. In the menopause, if the estrogen deficiency is severe, the vaginal smears are composed of cells that are prepuberal, arising from the basal layers of the mucosa. Estrogen administration induces vaginal maturation. Frequently, however, the deficiency is only relative, and both intermediate and superficial cells are also found in menopausal women.

Normal menstruation is usually held to be dependent on the consecutive action of estrogen and progesterone on the uterus. However, pseudorhythmic bleeding, clinically indistinguishable from the normal menses, may occur in the absence of a corpus luteum. In other words, menstruation may occur in the absence of an ovum (anovular menstruation). In such cases, throughout the entire interval between the bleeding periods, only the follicular phase of the endometrium (or, in pathologic cases, hyperplasia), but not the progestational or luteal phase, is seen on microscopic study.

Uterine bleeding can be induced in castrated primates by the injection of estrogen alone. Seven to 10 days after cessation of injections, bleeding may occur, indicating that progesterone is not necessary for the induction of uterine bleeding. However, bleeding may be induced with greater regularity by the administration of both estrogen and progesterone.

The foregoing information is graphically presented in Figure 94.

5. *Growth hormone.* The pituitary elaborates a growth hormone that has its greatest effect during the pubescent period. Its many functions are not yet fully appreciated. No satisfactory commercial preparations are available for therapeutic use.

Clinical Endocrinology

From a clinical point of view the following hormones are useful in gynecology and obstetrics.

1. The two hormones from the posterior lobe of the pituitary: (*a*) the *oxytocic factor,* or oxytocin (Pitocin), which is used chiefly in obstetrics as an oxytocic and occasionally by some gynecologists during vaginal hysterectomy and myomectomy to maintain uterine tonus and lessen bleeding during operations, and (*b*) *vasopressor factor,* or vasopressin (Pitressin), to stimulate peristalsis or inhibit diuresis in diabetes insipidus. DuVigneaud and his associates were responsible for synthesizing oxytocin, the first synthetic polypeptide hormone. The synthetic hormone is practically identical to natural oxytocin in regard to its biologic activity and chemical and physical properties.

2. The *gonadotrophic hormones* from the anterior lobe of the pituitary (FSH and LH). Preparations of these hormones are available only for experimental purposes. Only preparations made from human pituitaries or menopausal urine are of any value because of species specificity. Such preparations contain mostly the follicle-stimulating and variable amounts of the luteinizing factor. Pituitary gonadotrophic hormones of animal origin are not recommended for clinical use.

3. *Prolactin.* Excellent results have been obtained with prolactin in certain animals, but its use in human beings is still in the experimental stage.

4. The *chorionic hormones*. Human chorionic gonadotrophin, a pituitary-like hormone with LH- and LTH (luteotrophin hormone)-like properties is produced by the chorionic epithelium of the placenta. Though it is capable of stimulating the growth of follicles and corpora lutea in rodents and other laboratory animals, it has little effect on human ovaries. Chorionic gonadotrophin in the urine of pregnant women is responsible for positive results of the Aschheim-Zondek, Friedman, and other biologic tests for pregnancy. It may be detected in the urine 4 to 10 days after the first missed menses. At this early stage there may be insufficient gonadotrophin to cause a response in test animals, but after the second week the concentration is great enough to yield uniformly positive results in tests for pregnancy.

During pregnancy the amount of gonadotrophin in the urine increases rapidly to a sharp peak about 70 days after the last menstrual period. At this time the amount of hormone may be tremendous, excretion reaching several hundred thousand rat units in 24 hours. For this reason bioassays of urine for the diagnosis of hydatidiform mole should not be attempted at this time—a most important fact to remember. However, before and after this period of abnormally high excretion, markedly elevated titers are suggestive of hydatidiform mole. In normal pregnancy the concentration of gonadotrophic hormone decreases rapidly after the 12th week, and, from then on, the 24-hour level is maintained at 1,000–5,000 rat units until term. A week after delivery there is little evidence of this substance in the urine.

A rich source of gonadotrophic hormone (follicle-stimulating type) was found by Cole and Hart in the blood serum of pregnant mares. In animals this hormone produces effects similar to those achieved by extracts of the anterior pituitary gland. Thus it is capable of stimulating the germinative epithelium of the ovaries and testes in laboratory animals; it can induce ovarian growth in primates and produce fertile ovulation in rats, cows, sows, and other animals. It is mentioned here solely to discourage its use for the induction of ovulation in human subjects. It is excellent for horses, as its name, equine gonadotrophin, implies.

5. *Ovarian steroids*. Knauer, in 1900, demonstrated the role of the ovary as an endocrine organ when ovarian transplants prevented atrophy of the uterus in ovariectomized rabbits. Allen and Doisy observed, in 1923, that injections of follicular fluid of hog ovaries induced full estrus in bilaterally oophorectomized mice and rats, while Courrier was making more or less similar observations in France in other experimental animals. In 1927, Aschheim and Zondek found that pregnancy urine was rich in estrogenic substances, and, within the next 2 years, Doisy in the United States and Butenandt in Germany announced the isolation of estrone from urine. Subsequently, estrone and estradiol were isolated from the ovary. At about the same time, Corner and Allen isolated a hormone from sow ovaries which they named progestin. Although a wide variety of clinical and animal studies have provided much

information on the biosynthesis and secretion of steroids from the ovary, there is much work to be done before we achieve full understanding of the various pathways involved.

The isolation of hormones from ovarian tissue and the demonstration of pituitary dependency constitute classic chapters in the literature of reproductive physiology and will not be elaborated on here. Attention will be directed to some of the advances made in our knowledge of the biosynthesis, physiology, and pharmacology of ovarian hormones.

BIOSYNTHESIS, PHYSIOLOGY, AND METABOLISM OF PROGESTERONE.—Progesterone is a steroid hormone with 21 carbon atoms and is related structurally to the adrenocortical hormones. Although it is an intermediate in the biosynthesis of most steroid hormones in the body, it is secreted in significant quantities only by the corpus luteum and the placenta. It is thought that cholesterol is an essential precursor in the major pathway of the biosynthesis of progesterone. The various steps in its biosynthesis are shown in Figure 95.

In the menstrual cycle, progesterone is secreted only after ovulation has taken place. This is indicated by a rise in basal body temperature and urinary pregnanediol. Pregnanediol is the major metabolite of progesterone and occurs in the urine in the water-soluble conjugated form. The liver and kidneys are considered to be chiefly responsible for the metabolism of progesterone.

The physiologic functions of progesterone have been adequately recognized

FIG. 95.—Biosynthesis of progesterone in the ovary.

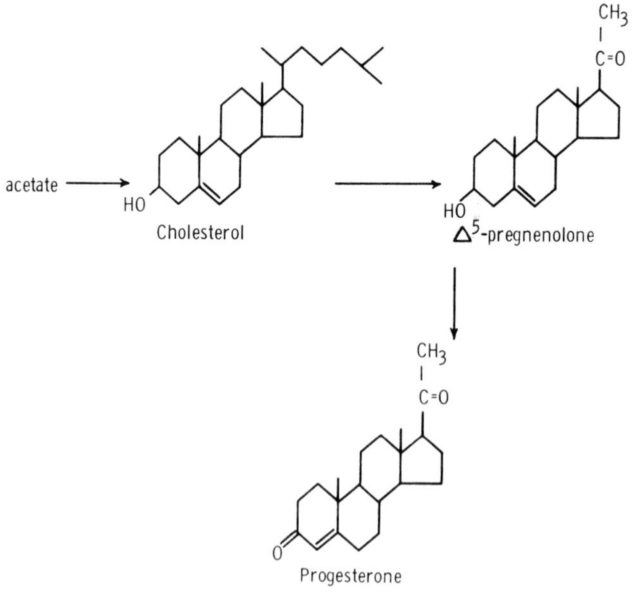

and warrant brief summarization. It induces a secretory endometrium which is believed to be indispensable for nidation of the fertilized ovum. It also causes an increase in mucin and glycogen in the lining epithelial cells of the endometrium in association with diminished activity of alkaline phosphatase. Progesterone modifies the vaginal epithelium, causing desquamation. It develops the alveolar system of the breasts in conjunction with estrogen. It is believed to maintain the uterus in a quiescent state during pregnancy.

Progesterone exerts a significant thermogenic effect. It is said to be a saluretic and mildly catabolic. Selye has shown that it decreases pulmonary alveolar tension of carbon dioxide and has anesthetic properties.

PROGESTERONE PREPARATIONS AND ROUTES OF ADMINISTRATION.—The progestational agents are administered by several means: intramuscular injection, vaginal suppository, and orally. Progesterone is rapidly metabolized in the body and therefore should be administered at least at 8- to 12-hour intervals. The esters of progesterone, such as Delalutin and Depo-Provera, are long lasting; only one injection every 10–30 days is necessary. The testosterone analogues with progestational activity are potent progestational agents but may have mild androgenic properties. Progesterone and its analogues are of value in functional uterine bleeding, endometriosis, dysmenorrhea, amenorrhea, mazoplasia, premenstrual tension, habitual and threatened abortion, and dermatoses associated with menstrual molimen, and in pregnancy. The dosages and routes of administration of the more commonly used progesterone preparations and progestational agents are listed in Table 5.

TABLE 5.—DOSES AND ROUTES OF ADMINISTRATION OF
PROGESTERONE AND PROGESTATIONAL AGENTS

Progesterone
  Parenteral—short-acting
    1. Lutocylin (Ciba), 25 mg./ml.
    2. Proluton (Schering), 25 mg./ml.
  Parenteral—long-acting progestational agents
    1. Delalutin (Squibb), 125 and 250 mg./cc. (17α-hydroxyprogesterone caproate)
    2. Depo-Provera (Upjohn), 50 mg./cc. (17α-hydroxy-6β-methyl progesterone acetate)
  Oral—progesterone derivatives
    1. Provera (Upjohn), 2.5 and 10 mg.
    2. Duphaston (Philips-Roxanne), 5 and 10 mg. (6-dehydro-retroprogesterone)
    3. Gynorest (Mead Johnson), 5 and 10 mg. (6-dehydro-retroprogesterone)
Testosterone analogues with progestational activity
  Oral
    1. Lutocylol (Ciba), 10 and 25 mg. (ethisterone)
    2. Pranone (Schering), 10 and 25 mg. (ethisterone)
    3. Progesterol (Organon), 10 and 25 mg. (ethisterone)
    4. Norlutin (Parke, Davis), 10 mg. (norethindrone)
    5. Norlutate (Parke, Davis), 2.5 and 5 mg. (norethindrone acetate)
Suppository
  Colprosterone (Ayerst), 25 and 50 mg.

BIOSYNTHESIS, PHYSIOLOGY, AND METABOLISM OF ESTROGENS.—Although the presence of an ovarian hormone that had estrogenic properties was discovered as early as 1923 by Allen and Doisy, the exact nature of the secretion of estrogens by the ovary has only recently been elucidated. In a careful study carried out by Brown in 1957, it was concluded indirectly from experimental evidence that the ovaries secrete estrone and estradiol but not estriol. Estradiol was isolated from ovarian vein blood by Mahesh *et al.;* estrone and estriol were not detectable in these specimens.

Estrone and estradiol are synthesized in the ovary from acetate and cholesterol. The various pathways of the synthesis of estrogens in the ovary are shown in Figure 96. Among these, conversion of cholesterol to estrone and estradiol via Δ^5-pregnenolone to progesterone to 17α-hydroxyprogesterone and Δ^4-androstenedione is considered to be the major pathway.

FIG. 96.—Biosynthesis of estrogens in the ovary.

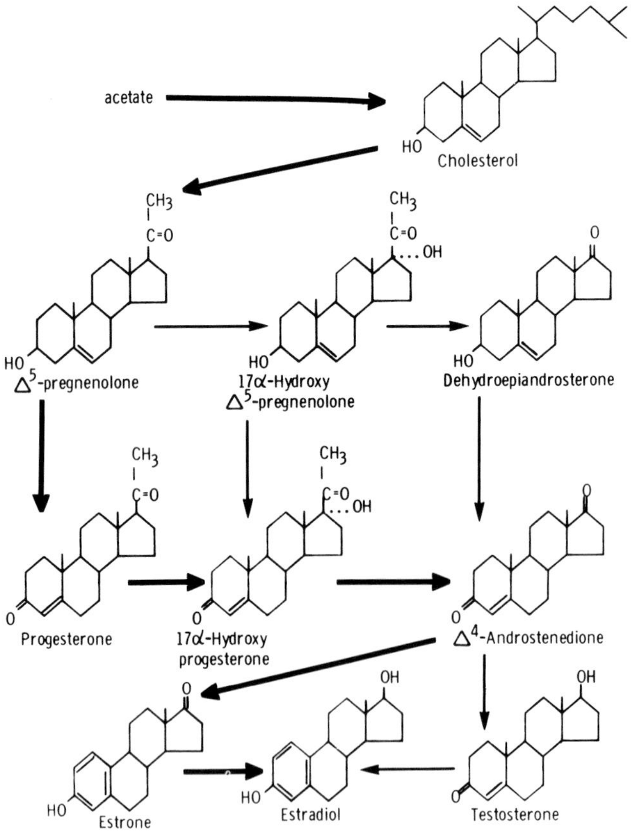

Estrogens are present in the blood plasma, partly in the free form and partly conjugated as estrone sulfate and estradiol sulfate. The hormone production at various periods of life ranges from the minimal values found between ages 5 and 10 to the maximal values attained during pregnancy. The highest estrogen secretion in the normal nonpregnant adult occurs about the time of ovulation and is generally referred to as the ovulation peak. Another, but lesser peak, occurs at about day 21 of the cycle and is known as the luteal peak. After the menopause, production of estrogens decreases rapidly in many, slowly in others.

The placenta is believed to play a significant part in the conversion of dehydroepiandrosterone sulfate to estriol sulfate and estriol, in addition to the production of estrone and estradiol through the biosynthetic progesterone pathway. The levels of urinary estrogens in the normal menstrual cycle, in pregnancy, in postmenopausal women, and in normal males, based on the results of Brown, are shown in Table 6.

Among the natural estrogens available for clinical use, the most widely used are conjugated estrogens of equine origin (Premarin). Other natural estrogens available are simple estrone, estradiol, and estriol. Synthetic estrogen derivatives for parenteral use such as estradiol benzoate, estradiol valerate, and estradiol cyclopentyl propionate have particular value because of their prolonged activity. Among the synthetic estrogens, ethinyl estradiol is worthy of mention because it is many times more potent than estradiol. Several synthetic nonsteroid compounds possess estrogenic activity; among them are stilbestrol and chlorotrianisene (TACE). The structural formulas of several estrogens and synthetic compounds are shown in Figure 97.

The doses of some of the commonly used estrogen preparations are given in Table 7. The advantages of oral therapy are that the dosages can be manipulated readily and that medication can be terminated at any time. Pellets are exceedingly useful when oral medication is not tolerated well and when

TABLE 6.—Average Amounts of Urinary Estrogens Excreted in
Normal Conditions (μG./24 Hr.)

	Estriol	Estrone	Estradiol-17-β
Menstrual cycle			
Onset of period	6 (0–15)°	5 (4–7)	2 (0–3)
Ovulation peak	27 (13–54)	20 (11–31)	9 (4–14)
Luteal maximum	22 (8–72)	14 (10–23)	7 (4–10)
Full-term pregnancy	30,000	2,000	750
Postmenopause	3.3 (0.6–8.6)	2.5 (0.8–7.1)	0.6 (0–3.9)
Normal men	3.5 (0.8–11)	5.4 (3–8.2)	1.5 (0–6.3)

° Figures in parentheses represent range.

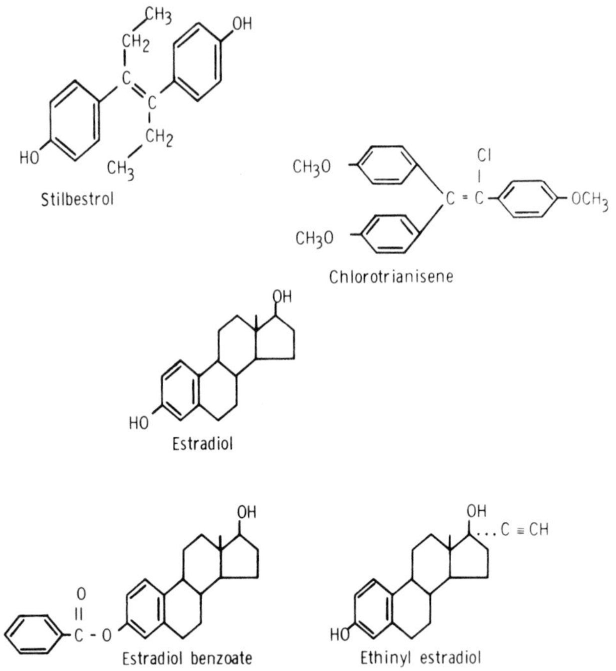

Fig. 97.—Comparison of structures of synthetic and natural estrogens.

a constant dosage is desirable. Injectable estrogens have more precise systemic effects, but their use is inconvenient if frequent injections and office visits are thereby necessary.

As to the various estrogens given orally, it is of value to know that ethinyl estradiol is approximately five times more potent than stilbestrol, and stilbestrol is five times more potent than conjugated equine estrogens on a milligram basis; i.e., 0.05 mg. ethinyl estradiol = 0.25 mg. of stilbestrol = 1.25 mg. of conjugated estrogens. This comparative potency holds for certain conditions such as the management of menopausal symptoms. The values, however, differ considerably when inhibition of ovulation is attempted; for instance, 0.1 mg. of ethinyl estradiol from day 5 to day 25 of the cycle is adequate to inhibit ovulation in almost all instances, whereas 2–3 mg. of stilbestrol or 3.25–5 mg. of conjugated equine estrogens are necessary.

EFFECT OF ESTROGENS.—Estrogens, in general, may be categorized as a proliferative hormone with selective affinity for tissues of Müllerian origin. At puberty they are responsible, in a large part, for transformation of the female body contours and maturation of the genitalia, vaginal mucosa, and duct system of the breasts and nipples. The corpus-to-cervix ratio converts

TABLE 7.—Doses and Routes of Administration of Some
Commonly Used Estrogen Preparations

Parenteral use
  Short-acting
    1. Theelin (Parke, Davis), 1 mg.
    2. Estrone (Lilly), 1 mg.
  Long-acting
    1. Progynon B (Schering), 1 and 1.66 mg. (estradiol benzoate); 7–10 days
    2. Delestrogen (Squibb), 10 mg. (estradiol valerate); 10–14 days
    3. Depo-estradiol (Upjohn), 1 and 5 mg./ml. (estradiol cyclopentyl propionate); 14–21 days
Pellet implantation
  Progynon pellet (Schering), 25 mg. (estradiol); 6 months
Oral ingestion
    1. Premarin (Ayerst), 0.3, 0.625, 1.25, and 2.5 mg. (conjugated equine estrogen; natural
       estrogen)
    2. Diethylstilbestrol (Lilly), 0.1, 0.2, 0.5, 1 and 5 mg. (synthetic nonsteroid)
    3. TACE (Merrell), 12 mg. (chlorotrianisene; synthetic nonsteroid)
    4. Estinyl (Schering), 0.02 and 0.05 mg. (ethinyl estradiol; synthetic estrogen)
    5. Eticylol (Ciba), 0.02 and 0.05 mg. (ethinyl estradiol; synthetic estrogen)
Suppository
  Diethylstilbestrol (Lilly), 0.1 and 0.5 mg.
Topical application
    1. Dienestrol (Ortho), 0.1 and 0.5 mg./Gm. (diethylidineethylene; synthetic nonsteroid
       estrogen)
    2. Premarin cream (Ayerst), 0.625 and 1 mg./Gm. (conjugated equine estrogens)

epithelium is modified in such a manner that the mucus increases in quantity
and transmigration of spermatozoa is enhanced. Cervical mucus under the
influence of estrogens crystallizes into a fern pattern when allowed to dry.
Progestins inhibit this property.

Estrogens, through a feedback mechanism, suppress FSH and LH. They
facilitate the maturation of the primordial follicle of the ovary to the antrum
stage and the migration of the prime follicle toward the surface. Estrogens
effectively revert abnormal serum lipids associated with atherosclerosis and
therefore, it is believed, may curb atherosclerosis during the premenopausal
years. Estrogens favor epiphyseal closure in the pubescent individual. In
postmenopausal women, the prevalence of osteoporosis has led many investigators to consider estrogen deficiency one of the most common contributory
factors in this bone disease. Postmenopausal patients with incontinence and/or
vaginal prolapse due to a weak bladder sphincter tone have exhibited improvement subsequent to estrogen therapy. Often estrogens (cream or oral)
make repair operations unnecessary. In the postmenopausal individual, episodes of psychic depression are common. The administration of estrogen
frequently imparts a sense of well-being and helps to overcome this depressive
state.

The influence of estrogens on sexual hair growth in the female (pubic and axillary) is secondary, not primary. In hypo-ovarianism due to primary hypo-pituitarism, sexual hair growth is as a rule absent. The administration of estrogens induces, in such cases, breast development and maturation of the internal and external genitalia but does not cause sexual hair growth. If androgens are added to the estrogens, sexual hair growth occurs. On termination of androgen therapy while estrogens are continued, loss of sexual hair usually ensues.

During aging there is epithelial regression; the skin, in losing its soft pliant character, becomes abnormally dry, scaly, and inelastic. It is surmised that estrogens cause hydration of the skin, but this refers to hydration of the dermis, not of the stratum corneum. The integrity of nasal, buccal, gingival, and vaginal mucosa is also largely dependent on estrogens. Spider telangiectases of the skin are most commonly associated with cirrhosis of the liver and with pregnancy. It has been theorized that accumulation of estrogenic substances is responsible for vascular spiders.

Estrogen preparations may be used for the following conditions: amenorrhea, dysfunctional uterine bleeding, dysmenorrhea, sexual infantilism, postpartum breast engorgement, abnormal lactation, atrophic vaginitis, kraurosis vulvae, and for the many conditions in which inhibition of ovulation is advantageous, as in the treatment of cyclic acne. For cyclic acne of young women, sequential estrogen-progestin therapy may be employed. Ethinyl estradiol, 0.1 mg., may be administered from day 5 to day 25 of the cycle; during the last 5 days, a progestin is added. The estrogen is sufficient to inhibit ovulation and the progestin to give constancy to the withdrawal uterine bleeding. For many years we, among others, have advocated the use of estrogens for the treatment of acne and as early as 1952 (*Office Endocrinology* [4th ed.; Springfield, Ill.: Charles C Thomas, Publisher]), I proposed the inhibition of ovulation for severe cyclic acne. Considerable lessening of the acneform eruptions has been noted in patients so treated. Sequential therapy is preferable to combined estrogen-progestin preparations, although Strauss and his colleagues have found the latter quite useful in their patients with acne. Therapy, if need be, may be continued for several years. Furthermore, there is some experimental evidence that (corticoid) suppression of adrenal steroids with dexamethasone and estrogen suppression of ovarian steroids may lessen severe acne and modify the rate of facial and sexual hair growth.

6. *Male sex hormones.* Testosterone is the most potent and perhaps the only true androgen produced by the body. Androgen therapy (Table 8) may be administered in three different ways:

A-*1*, Intramuscular injection: For this purpose, testosterone propionate in oil or in an aqueous suspension is used.

A-2, Repository intramuscular injections: There are now available long-acting testosterone preparations whose effects may last 2 to 4 weeks.

TABLE 8.—DOSES AND ROUTES OF ADMINISTRATION OF ANDROGENIC AND
ANABOLIC AGENTS

ANDROGENIC AGENTS

Oral (tablets)
  Fluoxymesterone
   1. Halotestin (Upjohn), 2, 5, and 10 mg.
   2. Ora-testryl (Squibb), 2, 5, and 10 mg.
  Methyltestosterone
   1. Metandren (Ciba), 10 mg.
   2. Methyl-Testosterone (Lilly), 10 and 25 mg.
   3. Neo-Hombreol(M) (Organon), 10 and 25 mg.
   4. Oreton-M (Schering), 10 and 25 mg.
Parenteral
  Testosterone:
   1. Oreton (Schering), 25 and 50 mg./ml., in aqueous suspension
   2. Mertestate (Breon), 25 mg./ml. in aqueous suspension
  Testosterone cyclopentylpropionate: Depo-testosterone cyclopentylpropionate (Upjohn), 50,
    100, and 200 mg./ml.
  Testosterone enanthane: Delatestryl (Squibb), 200 mg./ml. in aqueous solution
  Testosterone propionate:
   1. Neo-Hombreol (Organon), 50 mg./ml. in oil
   2. Oreton Propionate (Schering), 25 mg./ml. in oil
   3. Perandren (Ciba), 25, 50 and 100 mg./ml. in oil
Buccal and sublingual
  Methyltestosterone
   1. Metandren (Ciba), 5 and 10 mg. Linguets
   2. Oreton-M (Schering), 10 mg. buccal tablets
  Testosterone propionate
   1. Oreton Propionate (Schering), 5 and 10 mg. buccal tablets
   2. Perandren (Ciba), 5 mg. Buccalettes
Pellet implantation
  Oreton (Schering), 75 mg. testosterone

ANABOLIC AGENTS

Oral
  Oxymetholone
   1. Adroyd (Parke, Davis), 2.5, 5, and 10 mg. tablets
   2. Anadrol (Syntex), 2.5 mg. tablets
  Stanazolol: Winstrol (Winthrop), 2 mg. tablets
  Methandrostenolone: Dianobol (Ciba), 2.5 and 5 mg. tablets
Parenteral
  Nandrolone decanoate: Deca Durabolin (Organon), 50 mg./ml.
  Nandrolone phenpropionate: Durabolin (Organon), 25 and 50 mg./ml.

B-1, Oral administration: For this route, methyltestosterone is the most effective androgen. However, 4 or 5 times the amount of androgen must be given orally as compared with a dose of testosterone propionate given intramuscularly.

B-2, Sublingual or buccal administration: With this method testosterone propionate or methyltestosterone may be used; they are about equally effective. This method yields variable results but is believed to be more effective than oral administration.

C, Pellets: An excellent method for long-term therapy is pellet implantation. Each pellet contains 75 mg. of free testosterone.

Androgen therapy is frequently employed in gynecology. It may be used for hypermenorrhea, dysmenorrhea, premenstrual tension, mittelschmerz and/or intracyclic bleeding, menopausal symptoms, endometriosis, painful breasts, suppression of lactation, loss of libido, in women with mammary metastases, and in conjunction with progesterone for dysfunctional uterine bleeding.

Caution must be exercised in the use of androgen therapy because of possible virilizing effects such as growth of hair, especially on the upper lip and chin, change of voice, and enlargement of the clitoris. In addition, there are frequently an increase in weight and development of an acneform skin eruption. Disagreeable reactions seldom appear if the amount of testosterone propionate administered intramuscularly in 1 month is less than 75 mg. Side effects may disappear if androgen treatment is promptly discontinued. One or 2 pellets of 75 mg. of testosterone implanted at 6-month intervals have proved useful in the management of frigidity, migrainoid headaches, endometriosis in some patients, and as adjunctive therapy in the menopause.

Light-skinned women tolerate androgens more readily than do dark-skinned women, especially those who already have an excess of dark hairs on the face and elsewhere on the body. Whereas in some women, androgens are given deliberately to increase libido, in others, especially older ones with cancer of the breast, testosterone can bring about undesired libido. In women with bone metastases from breast carcinoma, pellets of testosterone may be implanted under the skin to maintain a fairly constant supply of this hormone over a long period.

Satisfactory results are usually obtained in cases of premenstrual painful and swollen breasts by giving 10 mg. of methyltestosterone orally or 5 mg. of testosterone buccally every day during the last 10 days of the menstrual cycle. To control puerperal lactation, excellent results may be obtained with Deladumone, a long-acting preparation of testosterone enanthate and estradiol valerate. A single intramuscular injection of 4 ml. will often suppress the discomforts associated with postpartum lactation in a great percentage of women who are not breast-feeding their babies. This combination has a sustained effect for 2 to 4 weeks. Delatestryl, an androgen, is also often effective in suppressing lactation. A single intramuscular injection of 100–200 mg. given immediately after delivery suffices.

It may seem strange to recommend the male hormone to overcome the disagreeable symptoms of the menopause, but in some cases testosterone gives relief from hot flashes, irritability, and other disturbances in this period. The substance is to be used by women who have been treated for cancer and endometriosis and those in whom estrogens produce uterine bleeding, breast discomfort, or other untoward side effects. Five mg. of methyltestosterone may be taken orally every day. In women who bleed after the use of estrogens, a combination of estrogens and androgens could be used to advantage. A satisfactory combination is Premarin with Methyltestosterone (Ayerst), containing 0.625 mg. of the former and 5 mg. of the latter. The androgen usually prevents uterine bleeding, helps further in assuaging menopausal disturbances, and acts as a tonic.

7. *Thyroid.* Thyroid therapy is valuable in certain gynecologic disturbances. Before modern endocrine preparations were developed, it was the mainstay in treatment of various ovarian disturbances. However, its use is indicated only for conditions in which there are definite symptoms of thyroid deficiency, such as dryness of the skin and hair, constipation, and lethargy, together with laboratory evidence of hypothyroidism based on basal metabolism tests and estimations of protein-bound iodine (PBI), blood cholesterol, and I^{131} uptake. Basal metabolic studies alone are not reliable indices of low thyroid activity or the need for thyroid therapy. Determinations of serum cholesterol, PBI and I^{131} uptake, and T_4 estimations are needed for confirmation.

Thyroid medication is specific in cases of excessive bleeding when there is definite evidence of underfunction of the thyroid gland. Whereas hypothyroidism is often associated with excessive uterine bleeding, it may result in amenorrhea in a small percentage of cases. Adequate thyroid therapy alone may restore the menstrual periods. A trial of thyroid therapy is indicated in subclinical or suspected hypothyroidism. If, however, the patient fails to respond in 6 to 8 weeks, continued treatment is useless.

Thyroid treatment has also been used empirically for functional sterility. It has been stated that some patients without a clinical diagnosis of hypothyroidism respond to such therapy, but there is little controlled supporting evidence. Thyroid extract should not be given empirically to infertile women; it should be given only to those with proved hypothyroidism.

Thyroid may be prescribed as thyroid extract U.S.P. Starting with $\frac{1}{8}$–$\frac{1}{4}$ gr., the dosage may be gradually increased according to response until $1\frac{1}{2}$–3 gr. daily is administered. Rarely if ever are larger doses than these necessary. If untoward symptoms appear, the dose should be diminished.

Thyroxin and triiodothyronine are the pure forms of synthetic thyroid hormones. These, at times, are preferable to the extracts because they are well standardized. If a patient is to be followed by PBI studies, pure thyroxin is the preparation of choice because triiodothyronine suppresses PBI values and thyroid extracts yield too variable results of either increased or decreased values.

Bioassays

Bioassays are useful in selected cases. They should be considered only in conjunction with the clinical manifestations and are not to be regarded as conclusive diagnostic procedures except in the case of chorionic tissue growths.

The most popular and reliable bioassay is the test for pregnancy. It is reliable in about 95% of cases. The Aschheim-Zondek test on mice or rats requires 96–100 hours and the Frank-Berman test 24 hours. The frog test requires only 1 to 3 hours and in some hands is as reliable as the other tests, provided the test is not done during the summer months in the Southern states. Newer immunologic tests have, more or less, replaced the standard pregnancy tests now in vogue. The UCG test (Wampole) can be completed in 2 hours, and the Gravindex test in 3 minutes. The Gravindex is highly reliable if performed after the thirteenth or fourteenth day of the missed period.

In the diagnosis of hydatid mole or choriocarcinoma, a quantitative procedure is used based on the normal excretion values. The excretion of urinary chorionic gonadotrophins during pregnancy rarely exceeds 10,000 rat units except during the first trimester, when tremendous amounts, from 100,000–200,000 rat units, may be excreted per day from the eighth to twelfth week of gestation. High values found at other times, therefore, should suggest an abnormal chorionic growth—hydatid mole and choriocarcinoma. If a growth is found and removed, tests for the urinary hormone should be performed subsequently to detect the presence of retained tissue, metastases, or recurrences. These tests should be repeated every few months. It should be understood that not all chorionic tumors are associated with excessive hormone excretion. Rats are usually used for the quantitative determinations.

Assays for urinary gonadotrophic hormone of pituitary origin are of value in differentiating primary or secondary amenorrhea of ovarian or pituitary origin. In the differential diagnosis of primary and secondary amenorrhea, this test has a definite place. In ovarian failure, there are as a rule increased amounts of urinary gonadotrophic hormone. In pituitary failure, urinary gonadotrophins are not detectable on assay. Radioimmunoassays of serum FSH and LH are rapidly replacing urinary gonadotrophin estimations. Figure 98 serves as an example to show the effect of an antigonadotrophin (Danazol) in suppression of the ovulatory surge, as determined by radioimmunoassay of serum.

Estrogen assays on urine are useful in certain cases but have little value in routine gynecologic endocrinology. Vaginal cytology and endometrial biopsy frequently yield the necessary information. Increased estrogen values are found with granulosa cell tumors and thecomas and certain adrenocortical tumors; hence estrogen assays should be used when these tumors are suspected.

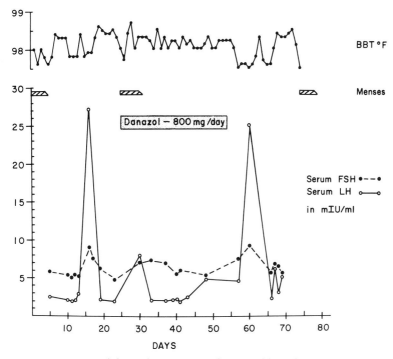

FIG. 98.—Suppression of the ovulatory surge as determined by radioimmunoassay of serum. Note the normal ovulatory surge of FSH and LH about day 14 or 15 of the first cycle, which was suppressed while on Danazol therapy during the second period; a rebound surge of FSH and LH followed discontinuation of medication. (From Greenblatt, Dmowski, Scholer, and Mahesh: Clinical Studies with an Antigonadotrophin—Danazol, Fertil. & Steril. [in press].)

Urinary 17-ketosteroid studies are frequently requested by gynecologists. Certain adrenocortical tumors with virilizing action elaborate large amounts of androgen which can be detected by 17-ketosteroid assays. Patients with virilism without demonstrable tumors may have no abnormal excretion of 17-ketosteroids, although occasionally the values are slightly above normal. Congenital adrenal hyperplasia with virilism is associated with high 17-ketosteroid values as well as markedly increased urinary pregnanetriol.

Vaginal Smears

Stockard and Papanicolaou described the technic of obtaining vaginal smears in rodents for the purpose of studying the activity of the ovaries. Allen and Doisy applied this procedure as a quantitative method of assaying estrogens and Papanicolaou introduced vaginal cytology for clinical use. He described cyclic changes in the cytology of the vaginal secretions corresponding to the follicle changes in the ovary. Papanicolaou and Shorr reported that, after the menopause and after castration, the vaginal smears revealed striking cytologic characteristics that differed from those observed in smears obtained from women with normally functioning ovaries. They also proved that by administering adequate amounts of estrogen the smears of women after the menopause could be changed to resemble those of women with normal menstrual cycles. Hence the study of vaginal smears should be a good index of the functional activity of the ovaries and also of the effect of estrogenic therapy. The study of vaginal smears is far simpler and cheaper than the quantitative method of assaying estrogen in the blood and urine and probably gives as much information.

Vaginal smears were classified many years ago by Geist and Salmon into four groups to indicate various degrees of estrogen response, and this arbitrary form of classification may be used even now.

Reaction I (advanced estrogen deficiency, Fig. 99).—The characteristic features of this type of smear are complete absence of superficial epithelial cells and presence of small, round or oval epithelial cells with rather large, darkly staining nuclei (castrate or basal cells) and presence of leukocytes. Leukocytes and erythrocytes are present in varying numbers.

Reaction II (moderate estrogen deficiency, Fig. 100).—There is a variable

FIG. 99.— Reaction I. Advanced estrogen deficiency. Vaginal smear showing typical "castrate cells" and leukocytes.

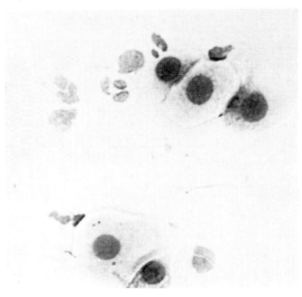

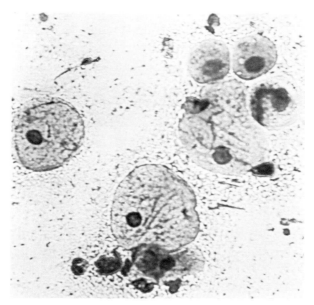

FIG. 100.—Reaction II. Moderate estrogen deficiency. Smear contains moderate-sized epithelial cells, basal cells, and occasional leukocytes.

number of larger epithelial cells. The nuclei are relatively large. Interspersed among these cells is a number of parabasal cells and leukocytes. The relative proportion of the larger epithelial cells to the basal cells is variable.

Reaction III (slight estrogen deficiency, Fig. 101).—Predominance of rather large irregular epithelial cells with vesicular nuclei is the striking feature of this smear. The cells vary in size and shape; their edges are somewhat irregular and frequently are folded. They usually occur in clumps; leukocytes may be present. The increased desquamation of cells may be due to the effect of endogenous progesterone or to moderately insufficient estrogen stimulation. This type of smear is seen in the luteal phase of the cycle.

Reaction IV (Fig. 102).—The smear consists of large, flat, clearly outlined squamous epithelial cells with small, deeply staining nuclei. These cells are larger and more clear cut, and the nuclei are relatively smaller than those in Reaction III. No parabasal cells or leukocytes are seen. Such smears are obtained from women just prior to ovulation or those on large doses of estrogen.

Mack studied certain estrogen functions by a method of staining vaginal smears that is based on the presence of glycogen in the normal vaginal epithelium and its dependence on estrogenic activity. The technic makes use of the specific color reaction resulting from the well-known affinity between

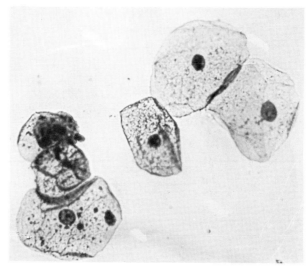

FIG. 101.—Reaction III. Slight estrogen deficiency. Smear taken in the luteal phase of cycle. Epithelial cells are larger than in Reaction II; they vary in shape, are irregular, and have a tendency to folding edges and to form in clumps.

FIG. 102.—Reaction IV. Smear taken on fourteenth day of cycle from young woman with normal regular menstrual cycle. Cells are large and flat, edges clean cut, and nuclei pyknotic. No parabasal cells are present.

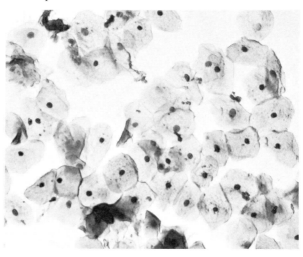

iodine and glycogen. This test is far simpler than the procedures originally described by Papanicolaou and Shorr and modified by Geist and Salmon and hence may be used more readily in office practice. The technic follows.

In the preparation of smears, a cotton applicator is inserted in the vagina and twirled lightly (one complete rotation) against the vaginal wall. The cotton end of the applicator is then rolled lengthwise over the surface of a clean glass slide. By rolling rather than rubbing, a uniformly thin film of cells with minimal clumping and cell distortion results. The film dries almost immediately and may be stained at once.

Staining is accomplished by laying the slide face down over a shallow dish containing Lugol's solution. Iodine vapors that arise insensibly from the solution suffice to stain the glycogen-containing cells in 2 or 3 minutes. Microscopic examination may be carried out immediately. Although stains made in this manner fade in 24–48 hours, restaining by the same method may be carried out repeatedly if subsequent examinations are desired.

The iodine vapor method for staining vaginal smears for glycogen provides a sensitive index of human estrogenic activity. Persistence of variable amounts of vaginal glycogen in menopausal women provides additional evidence that there is continued estrogen elaboration by the ovary or from extragonadal sources.

The vaginal smear methods (including the glycogen index) are occasionally useful in the control of estrogen therapy in atrophic vaginitis and in clinical investigations of sterility and in menopausal patients.

Suggested Laboratory Tests for Endocrine Cases

The diagnosis and treatment of endocrine disturbances frequently require the aid of the laboratory. However, before any tests are conducted or treatments are carried out, a complete history must be taken. Special emphasis should be laid on the period from birth to maturity. Then a routine physical examination should be made; this, in almost every case, will have to be supplemented by one or more special examinations. The following tests and procedures are the most often needed to obtain an accurate picture of the patient's endocrine status.

1. BMR, PBI, and I^{131} uptake for thyroid activity

2. Roentgen examination
   a) Sella turcica (for lesions of and about the pituitary gland)
   b) Vertebrae for evidence of demineralization, etc. (particularly in Cushing's syndrome, parathyroid disorders, and estrogen deficiency states)
   c) Hand and wrist for bone age (for evidence of advanced or delayed epiphyseal maturation)

    d) Chest plate (for size of heart in hypothyroidism and acromegaly and for substernal thyroid)

    e) Pyelograms (adrenal tumors may distort kidney position; presacral aerograms may be needed to outline suspected adrenal tumors)

    f) Pneumoperitoneogram (for ovarian tumors, polycystic ovaries, and gonadal dysgenesis)

3. Blood chemistry

    a) Glucose content and glucose tolerance curves (for hyperglycemia, hypoglycemia in thyroid, adrenal, pituitary, pancreatic, and liver disorders)

    b) Cholesterol (in diabetes mellitus, thyroid dysfunction, and liver disease)

    c) Sodium and potassium (in adrenocortical insufficiency and hyperactivity)

    d) Calcium and phosphorus (in parathyroid dysfunction)

    e) Chlorides (adrenocortical disturbances)

    f) Carbon dioxide-combining power (diabetic acidosis and alkalosis of primary aldosteronism, etc.)

4. Urine chemistry

    a) Chloride for conditions previously mentioned

    b) Sugar for conditions previously mentioned (glucose, lactose, pentose)

    c) Creatinine for thyroid disease and muscular dystrophies

5. Hormone assays

    a) Pregnancy test (Friedman or frog), or newer immunologic tests (UCG and Gravindex)

    b) Urinary gonadotrophins or serum FSH and LH for pituitary or ovarian failure

    c) Estrogens for adrenal and ovarian tumors

    d) Urinary 17-ketogenic steroids in Addison's disease and Cushing's syndrome

    e) Urinary 17-ketosteroids in cases of hirsutism, to rule out adrenal hyperfunction, ovarian tumors, etc.

    f) Pregnanetriol for cases of suspected congenital adrenal hyperplasia

6. Special studies

    a) Endometrial biopsy

    b) Vaginal cytology

    c) Cervical mucus

    d) Visual fields

    e) ECG for potassium deficiency, etc.

    f) Culdoscopy or laparoscopy for ovarian tumors, polycystic ovaries, gonadal dysgenesis

Intersexuality

BY ROBERT B. GREENBLATT, M.D.

IN THE HISTORY of human events there is recorded for all to read man's earliest conception of the establishment of the sexes (Genesis 1:29). The effects of castration were known to Aristotle (384–322 B.C.), and congenital eunuchoidism was mentioned in the Gospels (Matthew 19:12); nevertheless the role of the gonads in sexual development remained incomprehensible for more than 15 centuries. From the time of Galen to that of Vesalius, the ovary was called the female testis, and it was believed that the structure of the ovary and testis was identical. The discovery of the microscope and the study of cellular structure that followed gave the ovary and testis their proper distinctions. The remarkable progress in the field of endocrinology, the demonstration of specific virilizing or feminizing effects of the gonadal steroids, the induction of sex reversal in fishes, amphibia, fowl, and the opossum, the finding of sex chromatin in the nuclei of somatic cells of females, and the clarification of the embryologic development of the gonads in sexual differentiation have contributed to a profound interest in abnormalities of sexual development.

Intersexuality may be defined as the simultaneous presence of male and female somatic characteristics in the same individual. The term is generally applied to individuals with gonads of one or both sexes and some degree of ambisexual development of the accessory sexual structures. Recently the definition has been expanded to include individuals with defective gonads in whom there is a discrepancy between chromosomal sex and sexual development.

An insight into the problems of intersexuality is possible with an appreciation of the concept that competition between cortex and medulla for predominance is inherent in every embryonal gonad. Every gonad, whether destined to become a testis or an ovary, has a common anlage—cortical elements from the genital ridge and medullary elements from the mesonephros. The former are the female components; the latter, the male. Arrest of development or defective development of the gonads or exogenous and endogenous hormonal influences may alter the genetically determined balance between cortical and medullary components during the period of sexual differentiation.

TABLE 9.—INTERSEXUALITY

1. True hermaphroditism
2. Gonadal dysgenesis
3. Ovarian dysgenesis with vestigial medullary development
4. Seminiferous tubule dysgenesis
5. Pseudohermaphroditism
    Male   *a*) with ambisexual genital development
             b) women with feminizing testes
    Female *a*) congenital adrenal hyperplasia
             b) nonadrenal
6. Miscellaneous: embryonal genital malformations
    "There is a divinity that shapes our ends. . . . "

From research done on the rabbit by means of surgical castration of the intrauterine fetus, Jost concluded that the testis plays the principal part in the differentiation of the sexes. The fetal testis exerts two actions: (1) male-stimulating activity promoting masculine differentiation of the wolffian ducts, of the urogenital sinus and its derivatives, and of the genital tubercle; (2) an inhibiting activity which leads to retrogression of the müllerian ducts.

Table 9 gives an oversimplified classification of intersexuality. It serves, however, to relate those congenital intersex forms that have their basis in a disturbance of the embryonal gonad and the development of the internal and external genital structures. In our present state of incomplete knowledge, this classification helps to integrate such clinical disorders as Turner's syndrome, Klinefelter's syndrome, and male and female pseudohermaphroditism with true hermaphroditism. The diverse clinical manifestations of intersexuality may be linked to a common basic mechanism if viewed from the aspect of gonadal arrest and defective development and from the view of hormonal interference with normal fetal maturation of the accessory sexual apparatus.

1. TRUE HERMAPHRODITISM.—The classic example of true hermaphroditism is the so-called hermaphroditismus verus lateralis, i.e., the presence of a testis on one side and an ovary on the other. In true hermaphroditism, there are innumerable variations in the male and female differentiation of both the external genitalia and the genital duct structures. Ovarian and testicular elements are present in any one of many combinations. About 80 cases of true hermaphroditism have been reported. In true hermaphroditism, the sex chromatin pattern° may be either male or female; thus far there has been, according to Barr, a preponderance of the latter. In individuals with a female chromatin pattern, there is apparently a corticomedullary imbalance during the embryonic differentiation of either one or both ovaries that permits the latent medullary component to persist and subsequently to be transformed into testicular tissue (Fig. 103).

° Nuclear sex chromatin

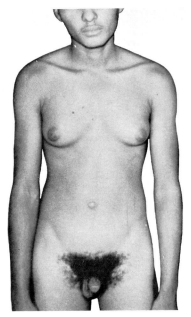 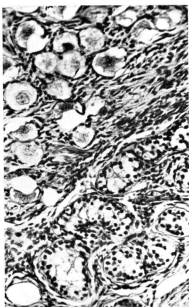

FIG. 103 (left).—True hermaphrodite with right testis in scrotum. Menses occurred at cyclic intervals through a urogenital sinus. At laparotomy a uterus unicornis with fallopian tube and ovary were found and removed. (Courtesy of Dr. J. Schutte.)

FIG. 104 (right).—Histologic section of ovotestis from a child with ambisexual genital development. (Courtesy of Dr. Henry Turner.)

The germinal elements of the ovary (ova) are usually present, but spermatogenesis in the tubules is quite rare. However, in a few instances mature ova as well as sperm were found in their respective gonads. It appeared logical to Wilkins to consider the development of ovotestes and true hermaphroditism as another form of gonadal dysgenesis in which the cortical and medullary elements develop to some degree but neither attains complete dominance over the other (Fig. 104).

2. FEMALES WITH GONADAL DYSGENESIS AND NEGATIVE SEX CHROMATIN PATTERN.—It is now generally appreciated that most cases of Turner's syndrome are examples not simply of ovarian agenesis but rather of gonadal dysgenesis. The striking application by Polani *et al.* of Barr's sex chromatin test in three cases of "ovarian agenesis" with a negative chromatin pattern proved a significant contribution to our understanding of human intersexuality.

From the experimental standpoint, Jost and Raynaud have demonstrated that early castrated fetuses of different rodents develop as females regardless of their genetic sex, provided the gonad is destroyed during the indifferent phase of its development. The similarity of these findings and the applicability in human cases was promptly recognized by Wilkins and his group and has served to explain gonadal dysgenesis.

Segal and Nelson found a negative sex chromatin pattern in 98 of 117 cases of gonadal dysgenesis and classified these cases as a subform of hermaphroditism. Many variants of Turner's syndrome have been described because of the variance in appearance of the patients, and they consequently are known under different nomenclature, but all have a common fundamental feature, i.e., rudimentary gonadal streaks. These vestigial ridges have been described in the past as aplastic ovaries, agenetic ovaries, and rudimentary ovaries. Histologic characteristics of the rudimentary gonads, whether the patient has a negative or positive sex chromatin pattern, are, in general, quite similar. The distinctive features are (1) a cortical stroma varying from scanty to a well-defined, dense, wavy connective tissue, (2) scanty to well-defined vestigial glandular structures of the rete ovarii in the hilus, and (3) Leydig cells varying from a diffuse scattering to large, well-defined clusters of cells in the medullary portion of the cortex or in the hilus, although in many instances such cells are not to be found. (See Figs. 105 and 106.)

In general, the gonadal streak is composed of stromal tissue without primordial follicles. However, in some instances there has been evidence of primordial follicles and small follicular cysts. Moreover, in the few cases reported with primordial follicles, the sex chromatin has proved to be positive. In our series of so-called Turner's syndrome with negative sex chromatin pattern in which gonadal tissues were removed at laparotomy, occasional primordial follicles were found in one case. On culture of leukocytes from this patient, an XO/XXX mosaicism was found. Ashley also found one case of gonadal dysgenesis with a negative sex chromatin pattern in which oocytes were demonstrated on histologic study of the vestigial streak removed at laparotomy. Nine cases are on record of gonadal dysgenesis in which laparotomy disclosed a testis on one side and a dysgenetic gonad on the other (Fig. 107).

3. Ovarian dysgenesis with vestigial medullary development.—Another link in the chain of gonadal arrest and defective development in relation to hermaphroditism was provided when we described a tall eunuchoid female with an enlarged phallus, rudimentary gonadal structures, and a positive sex chromatin pattern. This case differed from the cases of gonadal dysgenesis with androgenic manifestations with negative sex chromatin pattern reported by Gordan et al. as a variant of Turner's syndrome. Their patients were of short stature and had congenital anomalies, enlarged clitoris, and some hirsutism.

Our case provided a bridge between gonadal dysgenesis of the female (Turner's syndrome) and seminiferous tubule dysgenesis of the male (Kline-

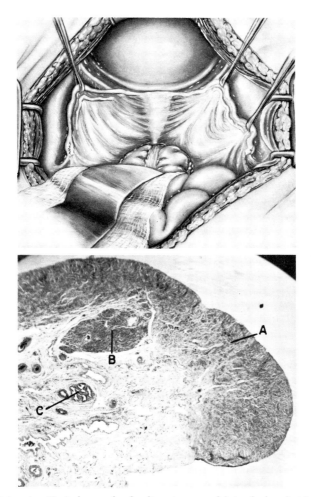

FIG. 105 (above).—Typical example of rudimentary gonadal streaks found at laparotomy in eight cases of females with gonadal dysgenesis and negative sex chromatin pattern. (From Greenblatt, R. B., Vazquez, F., and de Acosta, O. M.: Obst. & Gynec. 2:258, 1957.)

FIG. 106 (below).—Typical histologic findings: *A*, dense ovarian stroma; *B*, nest of Leydig cells; *C*, rete ovarii. (From Jungck, E. C., Greenblatt, R. B., and Martinez Manautou, J.: Pediat. Clin. North America, February, 1958, p. 127.)

felter's syndrome), because individuals belonging in the latter category also may have a positive sex chromatin pattern and are usually tall, eunuchoid, and have a phallus (Fig. 108).

This syndrome of ovarian dysgenesis with vestigial medullary development in a genetic female with eunuchoid proportions and enlarged phallus is indeed

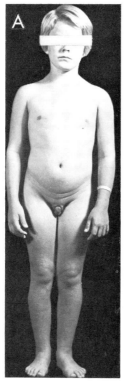
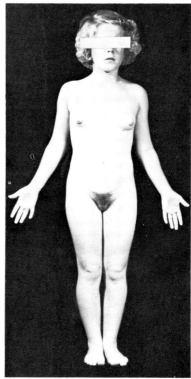

FIG. 107.—**A, left,** hermaphroditic child, 13, with female orientation and negative sex chromatin pattern in whom laparotomy revealed a uterus and fallopian tubes, a testis on one side and a dysgenetic gonad on the other. The gonads were removed. **Right,** with substitutional therapy by cyclic estrogen and progesterone, menses have been induced at regular intervals (*continued*).

a form of hermaphroditism. In fact, Robert Meyer in 1925 described a case that fits into the general category of the subject under discussion as hermaphroditismus externus asexualis.

4. SEMINIFEROUS TUBULE DYSGENESIS.—The finding of the positive type of somatic cells in males with Klinefelter's syndrome helped to complete the concept of hermaphroditism due to gonadal arrest or defective development. The breast growth, female escutcheon, and lack of beard growth are in accord with the positive sex chromatin pattern noted in these cases. Bunge and Bradbury found that the seminiferous tubule sclerosis did not completely dominate the histologic picture, for on serial sections they were able to find occasional tubules with spermatogonia, spermatocytes, spermatids, and even

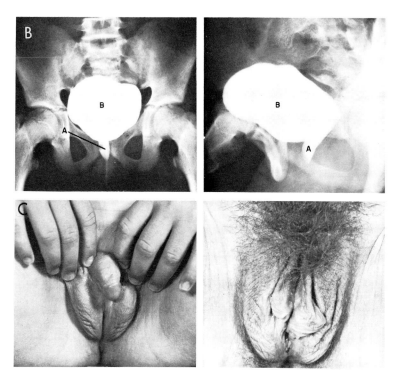

Fig. 107 (cont.).—B, anteroposterior and lateral views of A, vaginogram, and B, cystogram. **C,** before and after plastic surgery. (From Greenblatt, R. B.: Recent Prog. Hormone Res. 14:341–342, 1958.)

spermatozoa. The doubts at first expressed by Bradbury as to the validity of sexing by chromatin patterns were soon dissipated when Jost's experiments were applied to this seeming enigma. Jost's experiment showed that the medullary (testis) inductors are necessary for development of the male reproductive organs. If the cortical (ovarian) portion of the gonad of a genetic female should fail, the medullary remnant would exert its male inductor actions, the embryo would develop as a male and any remaining germ cells would be in a male environment.

The Klinefelter syndrome with a positive chromosomal pattern is Nature's experiment demonstrating in the human the bipotential of the germ cells, i.e., genetically female germ cells differentiated as spermatogonia.

5. Pseudohermaphroditism.—*Male pseudohermaphroditism.*—The testes may occupy any position, abdominal to scrotal, in any of a variety of combinations. Since the testes more or less lose their control over differentiation of the accessory sex organs early in fetal life (before the tenth week), any

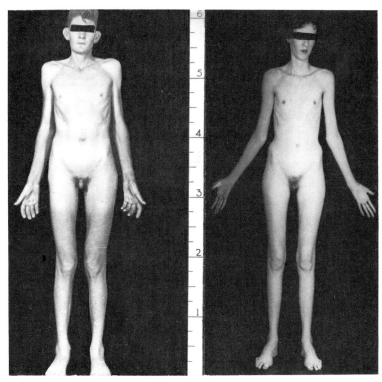

FIG. 108.—Tall eunuchoid female with markedly enlarged clitoris and ovarian dysgenesis with vestigial medullary development and a positive sex chromatin pattern shown next to a tall eunuchoid male with positive sex chromatin pattern and seminiferous tubule dysgenesis. (From Greenblatt, R. B., Carmona, N., and Higdon, L.: J. Clin. Endocrinol. 16:235, 1956.)

series of compromises between male and female differentiation may occur. The normal-appearing female with feminizing abdominal testes is at one end of the scale and, in progressively increasing phases of masculinization, the other end of the scale is reached, i.e., the hypospadic with fully descended scrotal testes who simulates most nearly the anatomically normal male. Male pseudohermaphroditism is, for practical purposes, divided into two main groups:

A. Those with ambiguous sex differentiation (Fig. 109).

    1) Hypospadic phallus with urethra or urogenital sinus but with apparent testes (inguinal or scrotal).

    2) Hypospadic phallus with urethra or urogenital sinus and abdominal testes. A vaginal dimple or abortive vaginal canal may be present. Occasionally, müllerian duct structures persist.

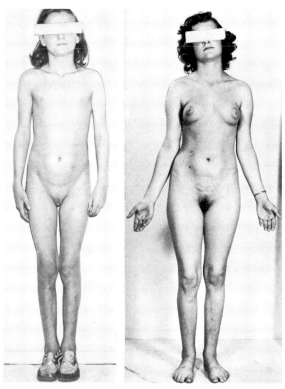

FIG. 109.—Male pseudohermaphrodite with ambisexual genital development before and after surgical removal of abdominal testes, plastic surgery of genitalia and substitutional hormonal therapy. (Courtesy of Dr. Robert B. Greenblatt.)

3) Normal penis with urethra but with empty scrotal sac (abdominal testes with persistence of wolffian and müllerian duct structures).

B. Females with feminizing abdominal testes.

    1) Vaginal canal (blind pouch) without or with scanty pubic hair and usually with excellent breast development (Fig. 110).

    2) With enlarged clitoris, vaginal canal (blind pouch), mild to moderate hypertrichosis, and breast development.

Women with feminizing abdominal testes usually have normal female genitalia at birth. In some instances, the clitoris may enlarge early in childhood, or at puberty some masculine features may develop. Wolffian duct derivatives such as vas deferens and epididymis are present. Imperfect remnants of müllerian duct structures may be found, and the vagina may be essentially normal or little more than a urogenital sinus. The inductive capacity

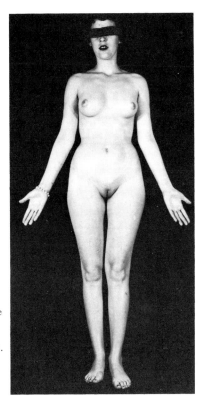

FIG. 110.—Male pseudohermaphrodite with feminizing abdominal testes. Note well-developed breasts and scantiness of pubic hair. (From Greenblatt, R. B.: Am. J. Obst. & Gynec. 70:1165, 1955.)

of the fetal gonads in these cases is lost before müllerian duct regression and wolffian duct development are completed, so that the remaining caudal region of the secondary sex apparatus including external genitalia is left to differentiate without testicular influence; thus the female condition is predominant.

Female pseudohermaphroditism.—The external appearance of the genitalia in congenital adrenal hyperplasia of the female may vary considerably and in the infant may simulate that seen in the male pseudohermaphrodite. An attempt at sexing should not be made from the appearance of the external genitalia. The clitoris may be small or phallus-like in size. A urogenital sinus is the usual defect, but in some instances the vaginal orifice is separate from the urethra. One case of female pseudohermaphroditism with a penile urethra is on record. As the child grows older, linear growth and advance in bone age are accelerated, and pubic hair usually appears by the third or fourth year.

In 1950, Wilkins and co-workers demonstrated that the administration of cortisone to children with congenital adrenal hyperplasia resulted in markedly decreased excretion of 17-ketosteroids. Furthermore, they noted that in several of their adult female pseudohermaphrodites, ovulatory menses were induced and that there was an unquestionable decrease in hirsutism. Wilkins and his group postulated that the increased output of adrenal androgens and estrogens in patients with congenital adrenal hyperplasia suppressed the formation and secretion of pituitary gonadotrophin, resulting in ovarian failure. Cortisone administration depressed adrenocorticotrophin production, which resulted in a diminution of the adrenal estrogens and androgens. The inhibition of gonadotrophin release was thus removed, and ovarian function was restored.

The electrolytic disorder resulting from abnormalities in adrenal chemistry or steroidogenesis permits the division of congenital adrenal hyperplasia into three groupings: (1) those without obvious electrolyte imbalance, (2) the salt-losing type with tendency to addisonian crisis, and (3) those with hypertension and retention of electrolytes.

Female pseudohermaphroditism without an adrenal component is the rarest form of intersex. In the few cases on record, it appears that in some instances the mother either had a virilizing tumor or received androgens or synthetic progestins in large doses during pregnancy. These cases resemble certain of the feminized cases of male pseudohermaphroditism in that hormonal values, bone age, and appearance of pubic hair are normal except that menstruation occurs at puberty.

6. EMBRYOLOGIC ERRORS.—Gross embryonic errors resulting in genital malformations appear to be far more common in genetic males than in females. In the male, failure of penile development occasionally is encountered; this results in a perineal urethra with a clitoris, without scrotum or labia. Such

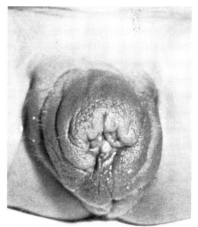

FIG. 111.—Multiple malformations resulting from error in embryologic development. Note the cloaca. The patient had imperforate anus, rotation of intestines, wolffian and müllerian remnants and ovaries, and a negative sex chromatin pattern. (From Greenblatt, R. B.: Recent Prog. Hormone Res. 14:377, 1958.)

individuals are readily mistaken for females. As they grow older the bodily contour and general make-up are similar to those of the eunuchoid male. In the female, a markedly enlarged clitoris may be found in otherwise normally developing females. Such a condition in pre-adolescent girls is distinguished from feminizing abdominal testes by the fact that the former have a female sex chromatin pattern.

Multiple malformations resulting from serious errors in embryonic development are associated with the most bizarre abnormalities of sexual development. There may be rotation of the intestines, imperforate anus, and anomalies of development of the internal and external genitalia (Fig. 111).

Diagnosis

1. HISTORY.—Particular attention to certain points in the history may prove revealing, such as (*a*) history of vomiting and rapid skeletal development in childhood or in other members of the family, (*b*) history of large doses of synthetic progestins or testosterone given the mother during pregnancy, or history of the mother harboring an arrhenoblastoma during pregnancy, and (*c*) family history of abnormalities in sexual development.

2. PHYSICAL EXAMINATION.—External appearance of the genitalia is deceiving. The diagnosis in cases of abnormalities of sexual development should be established as soon after birth as possible. This is not always possible because of indifference on the part of the obstetrician or the parents, the lack of facilities, or the seemingly minor nature of the anomaly. In gonadal dysgenesis, webbing of the neck, low posterior hairline, increased carrying angle, lymphedema, coarctation of the aorta, and other congenital anomalies may lead to an early diagnosis. However, some females do not show any of these signs, and the diagnosis may not be suspected until after pubescence. Short stature, amenorrhea, and hypoestrogenic vaginal mucosal smears then become highly significant. In congenital adrenal hyperplasia, the early appearance of pubic hair, rapid growth, and accelerated skeletal development in association with ambisexual genital development are sufficient to suggest the diagnosis.

The presence of an inguinal or labial hernia in childhood at times may furnish a clue, for a hernia may harbor a testis in a perfectly normal-appearing female child. An Addison-like syndrome in the presence of ambisexual development is not uncommon in female pseudohermaphroditism. Only in the rarest instances has there been an associated adrenal insufficiency in male pseudohermaphroditism. Absence or scantiness of pubic hair and axillary hair, primary amenorrhea, or a blind vaginal pouch in an otherwise normal-appearing female should lead to a suspicion of the syndrome resulting from feminizing abdominal testes.

3. SEX CHROMATIN PATTERNS.—The determination of chromosomal sex in patients with endocrine disorders has become an increasingly important diagnostic aid. Chromosomal sex determination in the human being dates from the work of Moore and Barr in 1953 when they demonstrated the presence of a dense pyknotic area in the nucleus of the cell that was characteristic in the female. They postulated that this was due to a fusion of the hetero-chromic portions of the XX chromosomes of the female cells. It has since been shown that each chromatin body is actually derived from a single X chromosome and that any X chromosomes in excess of one may form chromatin masses. Therefore, since the XY male with only one X chromosome does not form a chromatin mass, the presence or absence of a chromatin mass has been used to distinguish between the genetic male and the genetic female. For this reason it has been referred to as the "sex chromatin." The phenomenon has been demonstrated in human skin biopsies and in buccal and vaginal smears. A simplified staining technic that may prove useful to the gynecologist follows.

Oral mucosal and vaginal smears.—Material for the oral mucosal smear is obtained after first wiping away the saliva with a sponge and vigorously scraping the inner surface of the cheek with the edge of a tongue depressor and spreading the material so obtained on a glass slide. The vaginal smear may be obtained by swabbing the vaginal canal with a cotton applicator and rolling the material onto a clean slide. The slides are immediately fixed by immersion in an alcohol-ether mixture (equal parts) for 2 to 24 hours. They are then subjected to the following procedure: (1) Stain with 0.5% pina-cyanole° in 70% methanol for 45 seconds. (2) Dilute with Wright's buffer solution, pH 6.4, for 45 seconds. (3) Wash under running tap water. (4) Decolorize with 50, 70, and 95% (1 minute in each) and absolute alcohol for 30 seconds. (5) Clear in xylene twice. (6) Mount in balsam.

As an alternative, the cresyl violet method described by Moore and Barr may be used for mucosal smears after they have been obtained in the manner described above. Then: (1) Fix in alcohol-ether for 2 to 24 hours. (2) Hydrate the slides by subsequent passage through 70 and 50% alcohol, then distilled water—5 minutes in each. (3) Stain in 1% solution of cresyl violet for 10 minutes. (4) Differentiate in 95% alcohol and dehydrate in dehydrated alcohol. (Note that it is best to accomplish this differentiation on each separate slide by slowly dropping alcohol on it, because rinsing in alcohol frequently removes all the dye.) (5) Clear in xylene. (6) Mount in balsam.

In oral mucosal smears, normal XX females show at least 25–30 cells with sex chromatin in a total count of 100 cells. There is little difficulty in inter-preting smears of the oral mucosa, and proficiency in reading them may be

---

° Pinacyanole solution may be obtained from Southeastern Biochemicals, Inc.

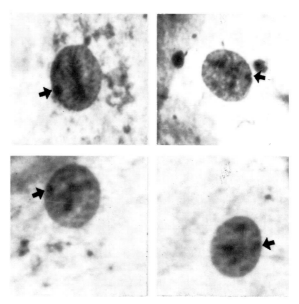

FIG. 112.—Mucosal smears showing sex chromatin. (From Greenblatt, R. B., and Martinez Manautou, J.: Am. J. Obst. & Gynec. 74:629, 1957.)

acquired with practice (Fig. 112). In those individuals where the count is less than 25–30, a mosaicism may be indicated, and leukocyte cell or tissue culture for karyotype is necessary for a complete diagnosis.

In studies on human blood smears, Davidson and Smith reported the observation of a "drumstick-like" mass projecting from the nucleus of the mature neutrophilic leukocyte of the female. Since projections of this size and shape are nearly always absent in male smears, they concluded that this "drumstick" was the female sex chromatin in the blood cells. It was their further belief, based on numerous observations, that the XY chromosomes of the male produce smaller clublike or nodular projections from the nucleus. These may, with a little experience, be distinguished easily from the "drumstick" (Fig. 113).

Blood smears.—A peripheral blood smear of even distribution should be used. When the slides are completely dry, they are fixed in absolute methyl alcohol for 1 or 2 minutes, then subjected to the following procedure: (1) Stain with 0.5% pinacyanole in 70% methanol for 30 seconds. (2) Dilute with Wright's buffer solution, pH 6.4, for 30 seconds. (3) Wash under running tap water. (4) Decolorize with 50, 70, 95%, and absolute alcohol for 30 seconds. (5) Air dry and read under oil immersion. In an alternative method, Wright's staining technic may be used.

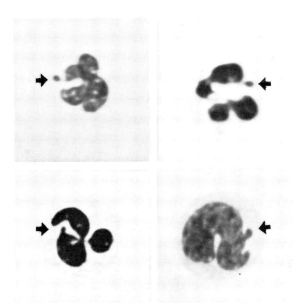

FIG. 113.—Blood smears showing typical drumsticks **(above)** in the female and nonsignificant clublike projections **(below)** in the male. (From Greenblatt, R. B., and Martinez Manautou, J.: Am. J. Obst. & Gynec. 74:629, 1957.)

The blood smears are more difficult to interpret and more time is required to study them. A total of 500 cells or less may be counted, and it is necessary to find 6 drumsticks for diagnosis of a female pattern. Some investigators believe that 1 or 2 such drumsticks in 500 cells is sufficient for a positive diagnosis. It appears, however, that the satellite body of Davidson and Smith is not identical with the heterochromatin mass and must be regarded as a sex characteristic rather than as the XX complex. This was the conclusion reported by Ashley.

One point of warning is in order. It does not follow that the genetic sex should be a deciding factor in determining the sex in which a child or individual should be reared. The sex chromatin determinations are chiefly aids to the clinician in arriving at a proper diagnosis.

Figure 114 illustrates a histologic section of skin from a female, showing the positive sex chromatin mass.

4. URINARY HORMONE ASSAYS.—In congenital adrenal hyperplasia, the excretion of urinary 17-ketosteroids is markedly increased, but of greater significance is the finding of elevated levels of urinary pregnanetriol. In male pseudohermaphroditism, urinary 17-ketosteroid excretion is normal or below normal levels. Elevated 17-hydroxycorticoids are found not only in Cushing's

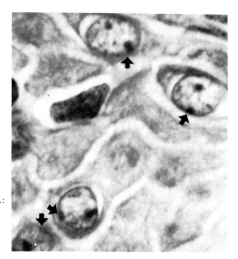

FIG. 114.—Histologic section of skin from a female showing sex chromatin bodies in nuclei. (From Greenblatt, R. B.: Am. J. Obst. & Gynec. 70:1165, 1955.)

syndrome but in the occasional patient with congenital adrenal hyperplasia and hypertension. The elevated 17-hydroxycorticoids in such instances probably represent compound S and not hydrocortisone or cortisone excretion. Markedly elevated 17-ketosteroid values are usually found in virilized patients with adrenal tumors. In these cases urinary dehydroepiandrosterone is frequently increased while pregnanetriol is quite low and may vary from 0.5 to 5 mg./24 hours. After puberty, urinary gonadotrophin excretion, as a rule greater than 52 m.u./24 hours, is found in the cases of gonadal dysgenesis, seminiferous tubule dysgenesis, and male pseudohermaphroditism with abdominal testes. If radioimmunoassays for FSH and LH are employed, values much above the normal of 3–8 mIU/ml. are usually obtained. An index of estrogen activity may be obtained by study of the vaginal mucosal smear.

5. RADIOGRAPHIC STUDIES.—In individuals with ambisexual genital development, cystograms and vaginograms not only aid in arriving at a diagnosis but contribute to the detection of anomalies of development and assist the clinician in deciding whether surgery is wise. Retrograde or intravenous pyelograms are useful in detecting anomalies, occasionally adrenal tumors, and in ascertaining the functional capacity of the genitourinary system. Study of the bone age is advantageous in showing whether bone maturation is normal, delayed, or accelerated.

6. WHEN IS EXPLORATORY LAPAROTOMY INDICATED?—The diagnosis of congenital adrenal hyperplasia should not offer too much difficulty. In the patient with ambisexual genital development and high urinary 17-ketosteroid and pregnanetriol titers, a trial of cortisone therapy has diagnostic significance if followed by a rapid decrease in 17-ketosteroid and pregnanetriol titers. Ex-

ploratory laparotomy certainly is not necessary. However, when the diagnosis is in doubt, as in male pseudohermaphroditism and in female pseudohermaphroditism that is not of adrenal origin, and when true hermaphroditism is suspected, exploratory laparotomy with proper biopsies of the gonads is indicated. When ovotestis is suspected, a small biopsy specimen taken at the periphery may reveal only ovarian tissue. The gonad should be bisected and adequately inspected.

7. KARYOTYPE.—Blood and tissue culture for chromosomal karyotyping is now available in most medical centers. An XO, XX, XY, or XO/XY, XO/XX, or many other mosaics may be obtained in gonadal dysgenesis. XY in male pseudohermaphroditism, XX in congenital adrenal hyperplasia, XXY in Klinefelter's syndrome, and XX or XX/XY in true hermaphroditism may be expected.

Management

The importance of diagnosis early in childhood and management by those skilled in the problems of intersexuality cannot be stressed too much. Indecision in selecting and assigning the sex best fitted for the hermaphroditic child will cause anguish to child and parents. Money, Hampson, and Hampson believe that gender role and sexual orientation are firmly established in childhood by the age of $2\frac{1}{2}$ years. Psychosexual orientation does not depend primarily on sex chromosomes or the gonads and does not appear to be instinctive and automatic but is a result of direction, imitation, and environment and all the associated experiences. For older hermaphroditic infants, children, and adults, Money et al. recommend that first consideration be given to the degree that a gender role has been indelibly established in the sex already assigned, and that changes of sex be scrupulously avoided except in rare and carefully appraised instances, so as to avoid hazardous psychiatric sequelae.

1. TRUE HERMAPHRODITES.—After psychiatric evaluation, a decision is made as to the sex in which the patient should proceed, and appropriate surgery is undertaken to remove the heterosexual structures. Ovotestes are best removed, and when both gonads are sacrificed, immediate substitutional therapy should be instituted.

2. GONADAL DYSGENESIS.—Females with gonadal dysgenesis and negative sex chromatin are usually quite feminine in their attitudes and aptitudes. They may receive with advantage substitutional estrogen and progesterone therapy. Frequently breasts develop adequately, and some growth in height may occur in those whose epiphyseal closure is incomplete. Menses may be induced with regularity.

In gonadal dysgenesis, a few cases are on record in which one gonad was dysgenetic, the other a testis. The dysgenetic gonads serve no useful purpose and their removal should be left to the discretion of the gynecologist. The infantile uterus in these cases need not be removed, since with cyclic estrogen and progesterone therapy menses may be induced.

3. SEMINIFEROUS TUBULE DYSGENESIS.—Males with seminiferous tubule dysgenesis and positive sex chromatin patterns may receive androgens and have improvement in well-being. If gynecomastia is present, surgical removal is advisable.

4. MALE PSEUDOHERMAPHRODITES.—The sex of a pseudohermaphrodite cannot and should not be decided from the external appearance of the genitalia. Infants who, at birth, present evidence of ambisexual development should not be immediately labeled male or female or given a permanent Christian name until studies are performed to clarify the sexual status. The appearance of the external genital pattern too frequently proves a snare for the unwary.

If male pseudohermaphroditism is diagnosed early in childhood, a trial of chorionic gonadotrophins may be instituted in the hope of inducing testicular descent. Those who respond may be managed with a view to salvaging them according to their gonadal sex. Those who do not respond and those seen at a later age who show feminine inclinations or are being reared as females should be treated at the appropriate time by surgical and hormonal methods in order to transform them in the female direction.

Experience has taught that male pseudohermaphrodites as a rule fare better as females than as males. With few exceptions, the surgeon or urologist would do well to discourage reconstructive procedures designed mainly to conform to the gonadal sex. A case that illustrates the folly of attempting to convert a feminized male pseudohermaphrodite into a functional male is that of an 18-year-old boy who now begs to be "unsexed" and transformed into a female (Fig. 115). This patient was brought up as a girl until age 6, and as a boy thereafter. At $15\frac{1}{2}$ years, a urologist decided to "reshape" him because laparotomy revealed abdominal testes. The physician disregarded the presence of gynecomastia, the effeminate nature of the patient, the beardlessness, and the high-pitched voice. The breasts were removed, and six operations were performed in an attempt to bring the testes down and correct the hypospadias. The effort proved purposeless, for the patient is now completely inadequate as a male. He lacks masculine drive and interests, he is sterile, and he is psychologically and emotionally feminine. In retrospect, it is not difficult to see that reconstructive surgery toward maleness should not have been undertaken. The patient should have been allowed to progress toward femaleness. The abdominal testes might have been removed and estrogens administered to accentuate development in the female direction. A vaginal canal could have been created and the small phallus removed. Experience has shown that such

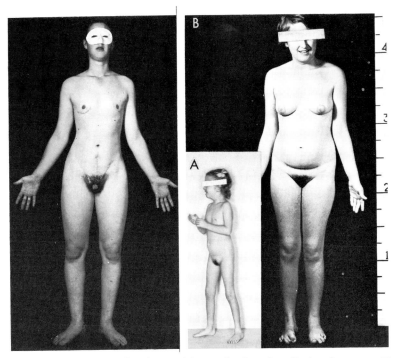

Fig. 115 (left).—Feminized male pseudohermaphrodite after ill-advised surgery. (From Greenblatt, R. B.: Am. J. Obst. & Gynec. 70:1165, 1955.)

Fig. 116 (right).—Female pseudohermaphrodite **A,** before and **B,** after 6 years of continuous cortisone therapy. (Courtesy of Dr. Robert B. Greenblatt.)

effeminate intersexuals rarely become adequate males, regardless of how well the surgery is performed or the amount of androgen administered.

When should gonads be removed? It is the conviction of many investigators that the abdominal testes should be removed from male pseudohermaphrodites being brought up as females. Of 17 tubular adenomas collected by Stalker and Hendry, 11 occurred in pseudohermaphrodites. Furthermore, Morris found seven malignant tumors in 82 patients with the syndrome of testicular feminization.

5. FEMALE PSEUDOHERMAPHRODITISM.—Since the advent of cortisone, no female pseudohermaphrodite need go on to virilization. If seen early in childhood or before marked psychic and somatic masculinization has occurred, these patients do well on cortisone-like steroids and develop as normal females. In some instances the urogenital sinus has to be transformed surgically into a functional vaginal canal, and when the clitoris is quite large, excision is advisable. On cortisone, epiphyseal maturation is considerably slowed, growth

in stature takes place, breasts develop, and ovulatory menses set in. In a few instances, conception has taken place.

Figure 116, A, shows a child with congenital adrenal hyperplasia seen at age 5 with a bone age of $8\frac{1}{2}$ years. Figure 116, B, shows the same child after 6 years of continuous cortisone therapy. The child has been feminized extraordinarily well and somewhat prematurely. Bone age advanced at a normal pace during the period. Plastic surgery had been recently performed to complete the genital transformation in the female direction by excising the clitoris, enlarging the vaginal canal, and using the skin of the clitoris to form labia minora.

Of greater concern in the management of female pseudohermaphroditism resulting from congenital adrenal hyperplasia is the neglected child or the young woman seen later in life who is completely virilized, physically and emotionally. How should she be managed? I have successfully transformed two such adult females into males. Both individuals were extremely virilized, and one in particular made a noteworthy adjustment as a reconstructed male.

Normal Menstruation

The Normal Menstrual Cycle

DEFINITIONS.—*Menstruation* is the periodic expulsion of blood from the uterus associated with necrosis of the uterine endometrium. The onset of menstruation is called the *menarche*. Many girls begin to menstruate at the age of 11 or earlier and others do not start until they are 16 or older, but the mean age is between 13 and 14 years. It is not known why some girls begin to menstruate early and others late. However, the most important factors are heredity, constitution, and environment. Early onset of menstruation is often associated with early development of secondary sex characteristics and, not infrequently, shorter stature than in those who have a late onset.

Bleeding from the uterus generally recurs at about monthly intervals throughout the sexual life of a woman and stops at the *menopause*, which usually occurs between the forty-sixth and the fiftieth year. Menstruation is nearly always absent during pregnancy and, of course, does not occur in women whose uterine or ovarian activity has been abolished by operation or irradiation. The serum FSH and LH levels present in the normal ovulatory menstrual cycle is schematically presented in Figure 117 depicting the FSH and LH surge responsible for ovulation.

FREQUENCY OF MENSTRUATION.—It has long been believed that most women menstruate regularly every 28 days, but this is a myth. Few women have a perfectly regular rhythm, regardless of the number of days that elapse between menses. A long time ago Fraenkel said that the only regular thing about menstruation is its irregularity. It is true that most women menstruate every 26–30 days, but there are many who bleed every 21–26 days and a large number whose intervals are more than 30 days. These intervals may change many times during the sexual life of a woman. Causative factors of such changes may be pregnancy, change of climate, change of occupation, and altered state of health. At the beginning of the menstrual life, the cycles are usually irregular, but after a few months or a year a pattern develops. In young girls amenorrhea frequently takes place with change of climate or on going away to school, camp, or nurses' training school. Such amenorrhea is nearly always temporary.

Bartelmez showed that abrupt fluctuations in successive menstrual cycles

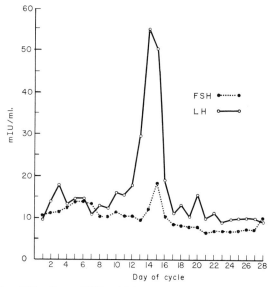

Fig. 117.—Serum FSH and LH in a normal menstrual cycle.

may occur even in "regular" women, and errors are apt to result from the application of statistical modes and means to particular cycles. Mathematically, all cycles with similar external features such as length may differ fundamentally even to the extent of one being ovulatory and the other anovulatory.

The fluctuations in the time relations during the cycle appear to be due to variations in the ebb and flow of the controlling hormonal tides. A short cycle is usually due to a short postmenstrual (quiescent) phase. Occasionally the postovulatory phase is short (7 to 10 days), yielding an inadequate luteal phase. Prolongation of the postovulatory phase occurs only with a persistent corpus luteum or perhaps a very early pregnancy that did not take root.

DURATION AND AMOUNT OF FLOW.—There is great variation in the number of menstrual days, but in most instances the flow lasts 3 to 5 days. A menstrual period that lasts more than 8 days is abnormal. The amount of blood varies enormously, the range extending from 10 to 200 ml., but the mean loss is about 35 ml.

SYMPTOMS ASSOCIATED WITH MENSTRUATION.—It is widely believed that numerous changes take place during the menstrual cycle, especially in the temperature, pulse, blood pressure, blood chemistry, blood count, and hemoglobin values, but, as Fluhmann has shown, there is considerable confusion about such changes. The cyclic preparation for menstruation does have a profound effect on the body, as evidenced by the large number of women who have premenstrual tension (see p. 285). Some illnesses are periodically aggravated by the menses. Most women, however, have little difficulty with menstruation except for the inconvenience of using vulvar pads or other means of collecting the blood that comes from the uterus. Incidentally, I have seen no harm from the use of vaginal tampons either in young girls or in married women. Occasionally, a tampon will be forgotten or lost in the vagina. A foul odor results, and this leads the woman to her physician. Removal of the foul-smelling tampon followed by a few daily douches is all that is necessary. Furthermore, girls and women who do not flow excessively may continue their usual activities just as if they were not menstruating. These include bathing, golf, swimming, and other sports. However, young girls should be cautious about indulging in competitive sports during menstruation because of the emotional strain induced by the competition.

CAUSE OF MENSTRUATION.—In spite of all the effort expended in the study of menstruation, we do not know the cause of this phenomenon, although we do possess means of controlling it. From Biblical times until the present, there has been a belief that the menstrual flow is a cleansing process. The demonstration of a menotoxin (denied by some) helps to support this idea, but there is no scientific proof of the necessity or the presence of such a purifying process. All we do know is that menstruation is a degenerative process that culminates in changes in the endometrium brought about by hormonal activity.

There is no unity of opinion concerning the method whereby the hormones involved in the process of menstruation bring about the menstrual flow. Some investigators believe that menstruation is a negative phenomenon due to the withdrawal of some hormone that is active during the building-up stage of the endometrium. Others maintain that the bleeding is a positive phenomenon brought about by the action of a specific substance on the endometrium.

The *withdrawal theory* of menstruation is based upon a number of facts, chiefly that menstrual bleeding occurs when the corpus luteum regresses and that bleeding from the endometrium follows removal of a functioning corpus luteum. Since the corpus luteum produces both estrogen and progesterone, there are two withdrawal theories, namely, the *estrogen-deprivation theory* and the *progesterone-deprivation theory*. E. Allen first propounded the estrogen-deprivation theory. In support of it is the fact that bleeding that is identical with the menstrual flow can be induced by removing both ovaries, neither of which contains a corpus luteum. Likewise, in anovular menstruation, the cyclic bleeding is clinically identical with ovular menstruation, and yet there is no progesterone present at any time in the cycle. The bleeding is assumed to be due to the withdrawal of estrogen. Furthermore, the bleeding that follows removal of ovaries that contain no corpus luteum can be prevented by administering estrogen. In women as well as monkeys, uterine bleeding can be induced by giving estrogens for a variable period of time and then suddenly stopping the medication. Bleeding will occur a few days after the last dose of estrogen.

There are a number of objections to the estrogen-deprivation theory. Fluhmann listed four, as follows: (1) Prolonged daily injections of estrogenic substances into human castrates or spayed monkeys are accompanied by uterine bleeding that occurs during the period of administration of the hormone. (2) The use of large doses of estrogens in the late postovulatory phase fails to prevent the onset of normal menstruation. (3) Menstruation normally may occur in the presence of large amounts of estrogenic hormones in the blood. (4) A rise and fall in the estrogen content of the blood may occur during long periods of amenorrhea.

Opponents of the estrogen-deprivation theory proved that it was possible to produce cyclic bleeding from a secretory endometrium by giving a series of estrogen injections followed by a series of progesterone injections. Likewise, it is well known that the onset of menstrual bleeding follows degeneration of the corpus luteum and therefore is associated with cessation of progesterone production. Another argument in favor of the progesterone-deprivation theory is the bleeding that can be induced by removing or destroying the corpus luteum. The injection of about 50 mg. of progesterone in amenorrheic women with adequate endogenous estrogens will often cause uterine bleeding in 2 to 4 days.

Anovular Menstruation

Until recent years, there was some controversy concerning the definition of menstruation. Some foreign pathologists maintained that the term menstruation could only be used when uterine bleeding took place from disintegration of a progravid endometrium. In order for such an endometrium to be present, ovulation with the formation of a corpus luteum must have taken place. However, American investigators, of whom the first was Corner, proved that menstruation can and does take place from a follicular or proliferative type of endometrium. The persistence of such an endometrial pattern is generally considered to be proof of the absence of ovulation and corpus luteum formation. Hence there can be menstruation without ovulation. The two types of menstruation, namely ovular and anovular, are usually indistinguishable as to regularity, duration of flow, color of blood, and other characteristics. Whereas the histologic difference between ovular and nonovular menstruation is an academic one, the clinical difference is of serious import, because women who regularly fail to ovulate cannot become pregnant. Nearly always when the term menstruation is used, it signifies ovular menstruation. When menstruation without ovulation is discussed, usually the two words "anovular menstruation" are used. Incidentally, only ovular menstruation is associated with premenstrual tension or dysmenorrhea, except when organic pathology accounts for the dysmenorrhea. These symptoms are often useful in distinguishing between ovular and anovular menses.

It is quite likely that in young girls menstruation for at least the first year or more is anovulatory. Otherwise it would be difficult to explain why girls who marry at an early age, as in India and elsewhere, do not conceive until they have been married a few years, despite the fact that they do not use contraceptives. Biopsy studies support the presence of anovulatory menstruation in young girls. Also, at the end of the reproductive career, in the premenopausal period, menstruation is often anovulatory. Of course, there are many exceptions, because very young girls do become pregnant and a relatively large number of women past 44 become pregnant, some even after the clinical menopause.

There is a simple method of determining whether or not a woman has ovulated. Since the endometrium reflects what occurs in the ovary, study of the endometrium will disclose whether an ovum was expelled in any particular menstrual cycle. For this purpose, a curettage is unnecessary. All that is needed is to secure two or three small strips of endometrium, which are readily obtained with a tiny curet or, better still, with a hollow suction curet such as those devised by Novak and by Randall for this purpose (Figs. 118 and 119).

Suction biopsy of the endometrium is an important aid in detecting ovulation and carcinoma of the endometrium. It is a simple procedure which is accurate and inexpensive and can be performed under local anesthesia or with no anesthetic at all. It eliminates hospitalization and curettage in many cases. The results of suction biopsy of the endometrium for the detection of

FIG. 118 (above).—Novak suction curet for biopsy of endometrium. (Manufactured by J. Sklar Manufacturing Co., Long Island City, N.Y.)

FIG. 119 (below).—Randall suction curet for biopsy of endometrium. Pieces of endometrium are readily obtained without use of suction. (Manufactured by V. Mueller & Co., Chicago.)

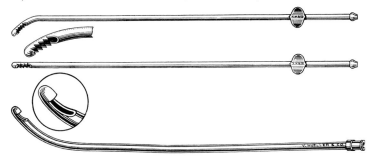

endometrial carcinoma are far better than Papanicolaou smears made from the cervical canal and the vaginal pool. A Randall or Novak curet is used and material is aspirated from all surfaces of the uterus, going around in a circumferential direction. Novak used the electric motor suction, which is more likely to yield satisfactory tissue for biopsy than is suction by syringes. Suction is made by an ordinary electric suction machine found in all operating rooms, and the curettings are drawn into a bottle. However, sufficient material may be obtained by using syringes if aspiration is used several times.

TECHNIC OF ENDOMETRIAL BIOPSY.—With the patient in the lithotomy position, a careful bimanual examination is made. The cervix is exposed with a speculum. An antiseptic is applied to the cervix, which is grasped with a single-toothed volsellum. A sterile uterine probe may be inserted to determine the length and direction of the uterine cavity; this is not essential. Then the sterile suction curet is gently introduced past the internal os up into the body of the uterus. The curet is pulled down gently but firmly along the anterior uterine wall until it reaches the internal os. Then it is pushed back into the uterine cavity and turned to one side or the other and again withdrawn gently but firmly against the uterine wall and removed from the uterus. The cutting edge of the curet is then inserted in a small bottle of formalin or other fixing fluid, and shaken, whereby pieces of endometrium will drop into the fixing fluid. The Novak and Randall curets are suction curets, but they may be used without suction, in the manner just described. The pieces of endometrium that are removed are studied microscopically after histologic sectioning and staining.

The appropriate time to obtain endometrium to detect ovulation is between the twenty-second and the twenty-fourth day of the menstrual cycle, because on these days, if an ovum was expelled, the endometrium should be in the luteal or progravid phase. Some gynecologists consider it better to obtain pieces of endometrium during the first 12 hours of the menstrual flow. There are two reasons for this opinion. First, the possibility of disturbing an early pregnancy, should it be present, is avoided. Second, if ovulation and the menstrual bleeding are for some reason considerably delayed, the endometrium will present a follicular or proliferative phase even after 25 days, and the conclusion will be drawn that the patient did not ovulate, whereas she may actually ovulate a few days after the biopsy specimen is taken. However, Brewer and Jones believe that endometrial biopsy specimens obtained the first day of menstruation do not give an accurate picture of previous endometrial responses to stimulation. The endometrial tissues are ischemic, partially necrosed, or, in some areas, necrotic and functionally may be partially or completely inactive. Often the tissues in some areas reflect antecedent stimulation and activity and in others show greatly diminished or no signs of stimulation and activity. These striking changes have been noted as soon as

1 hour after the onset of menstruation. Bartelmez found them before the onset. Accurate interpretation of functional activity is possible only by study of the endometrium during the actively functioning period of the life of the corpus luteum and endometrium. Therefore specimens for biopsy must be taken from 4 to 6 days before menstruation. Difficulty caused by variations in the time of ovulation and the length of the cycle may be solved by determination of the approximate time of ovulation by temperature shifts, vaginal smears, hormonal studies, and other methods.

If the endometrial tissue is taken a few days before the menstrual flow and it is not in the progravid phase, this is proof that no corpus luteum was present and hence an ovum was not extruded. It must be remembered that discovery of anovulatory menstruation is not an indication that the patient always has anovulatory menstruation. She may ovulate at certain times and not at others. (The word biopsy refers to the microscopic examination of a piece of tissue and not to the procedure used for obtaining the tissue. A regular curet, a suction curet, a punch instrument, or an electric wire may be used to secure tissue for biopsy.)

(For a discussion of ovulation see p. 141.)

Deliberate Delay of Menses

The voluntary delay of a normal menstrual period may be desirable for several reasons—a honeymoon, athletic event, or surgery. If a basic amount of estrogen, such as 0.1 mg. of Ethinyl estradiol (EE), is given along with a progestogen sufficient to substitute for the regressing corpus luteum, then the integrity of the endometrium will be maintained. This medication may be given as late as the twenty-second to twenty-fourth day of the cycle and continued for 10, 20, 30 days or longer. Estrogen per se in doses up to 0.5 mg. of EE per day will not suffice—but 0.1 mg. of EE with as little as 5 mg. of Norlutate, 10 mg. of Norlutin, or 30 mg. of Provera or 30 mg. of Duphaston will prove adequate. The more potent birth control pills such as Ovral 0.5 mg. (Wyeth), Ovulen 1 mg. (Searle), or Ortho-Novum 10 mg. (Ortho) may be employed from day 20 to day 40 with excellent results. To be more certain of delaying the menses, $1\frac{1}{2}$ tablets daily will provide greater assurance of success.

Menstrual Irregularities

Dysmenorrhea

MOST WOMEN are not particularly uncomfortable at the time of menstruation, but many have mild disagreeable symptoms just before and during the menses. There may be slight abdominal cramps, mild backache, pain in the legs, headache, fullness and pain in the breasts, mild depression, constipation, diarrhea, increased perspiration, and increased frequency of urination. However, some women have severe pain just before and/or during the flow. Such pain is designated *dysmenorrhea*. When no genital abnormality can be detected to account for the severe pain, the condition is called *primary dysmenorrhea*.

The pain of *primary dysmenorrhea* is characteristically intermittent, severe, cramplike, and colicky. Hence the dysmenorrhea is spoken of as spasmodic. Because the pains are usually colicky and there is frequently retroflexion of the uterus, the pain was and still is believed by many to be caused by an obstruction in the cervix. However, obstruction is rarely, if ever, a cause of primary dysmenorrhea. On the other hand, in *secondary dysmenorrhea* there may be obstruction as, for example, after amputation or excessive cauterization of the cervix and from scars caused by forcible dilatation of the cervix or from a large sessile polyp in the cervical canal.

The exact cause of spasmodic dysmenorrhea is not known. Rubber balloons placed in the uterine cavity have revealed that in some women who have dysmenorrhea, there are strong uterine contractions coincident with the pain (Moir). On the other hand, a similar technic together with endometrial biopsies and assays of blood and urine have failed to demonstrate any consistent phenomena that are peculiar to patients with primary dysmenorrhea.

TREATMENT.—A complete history should be obtained to determine the kind of work performed by the patient, the amount of exercise she indulges in, how many hours she sleeps, and how regular her bowel movements are. In addition, a careful physical examination is important; it should include not only a bimanual examination in a married woman and a rectal examination in a virgin but also a thorough study of the patient's posture. The blood should be studied for anemia. Any deficiencies in diet and blood must be corrected.

Since the psyche plays an important role in dysmenorrhea, the physician should delve into this and try to discover whether the patient has any fears, serious worries, or domestic difficulties. In nearly all instances of dysmenorrhea, suggestion and common sense must be used along with drugs and other remedies.

Whenever a cause for the pain is found, it should be removed. As a general rule, simple remedies should be tried first. These should include suggesting that the patient occupy herself during the menstrual period so as to keep her mind off the pain and not expect the pain. Patients may bathe just as often during the menstrual flow as at other times. Often a hot bath gives relief. However, women whose flow is profuse should not take hot tub baths during menstruation.

During an attack of severe pain, the patient should keep off her feet if possible and should apply a hot water bag or an electric pad to the lower part of the abdomen or back. In addition, acetylsalicylic acid may be prescribed. Edrisal, a tablet that contains amphetamine sulfate, aspirin, and phenacetin, often gives relief. Two tablets are taken and repeated every 3 hours if necessary. Edrisal also is prepared with codeine; dosage is about the same—1 or 2 tablets, repeated every 3 hours if needed.

Hormones are used extensively to relieve dysmenorrhea. The sequential contraceptive pill, Oracon (Mead Johnson) is eminently suitable for this purpose. This is sufficient to inhibit ovulation and induce withdrawal periods with regularity and without pain. Also curative is administration of a combined estrogen-progestin preparation such as Ovulen (Searle; 1 mg. of ethynodiol diacetate and 0.1 mg. mestranol) or Norinyl (Syntex; 2 mg. of norethindrone and 0.1 mg. mestranol) or Ortho-Novum (Ortho; 1 mg. of norethindrone and 0.1 mg. mestranol). If this medication is not well tolerated because of severe nausea, the retroprogesterone Duphaston (Philips-Roxanne; 10–25 mg. daily from day 5 to day 25 each month) often gives excellent results.

Stilbestrol is a much less expensive hormone than a progestin and relieves many women of dysmenorrhea. The usual procedure is for the patient to take 2 1-mg. tablets every night for 25 nights, beginning the first night of the menstrual flow. This is to prevent the pain that would occur at the time of the next menstrual flow. The rationale is that the hormone usually suppresses ovulation but not menstruation. It is a common observation that, with rare exceptions, only women who ovulate have dysmenorrhea and that women who do not ovulate do not have painful menstruation. The patient is asked to repeat this treatment for two and sometimes three menstrual periods, then skip a month. This treatment by no means gives permanent relief, and, although it relieves the pain in a large proportion of patients, it often upsets the menstrual cycle or is followed by a profuse flow. This may be avoided if a progestogen such as 5 mg. of Provera (Upjohn) is added to this regimen during the last 5 days of treatment.

If endocrine therapy fails to relieve dysmenorrhea, a stem pessary inserted in the cervical canal for 2 or 3 months occasionally may help to relieve painful menstruation for a year or more.

Numerous operative procedures have been resorted to in an effort to overcome dysmenorrhea, the oldest and the one still most popular being dilatation of the cervix with or without curettage. Although relief is often obtained, it is usually temporary.

There is an operation that cures many patients with primary dysmenorrhea. However, it should be reserved for those with extremely severe pain in whom every other remedy has been tried, because it involves abdominal surgery. The operation to which I refer is pelvic sympathectomy.

In most cases of severe dysmenorrhea, the oral contraceptives give relief by inhibiting ovulation. Hence dilatation with curettage, stem pessaries, and pelvic sympathectomies are now rarely employed.

Amenorrhea*

As is well known, menstruation may be either ovulatory or anovulatory. Ovulatory menstruation is the end point of a balanced series of physiologic events involving a dynamic relationship of the hypophysis, ovary, and endometrium. The thyroid and adrenal glands, as well as the general nutritional and emotional state of the individual, exert a profound influence on menstrual function. Amenorrhea is not a disease but a symptom and as such may imply serious endocrine imbalance or a pathologic lesion. This is particularly true in cases of primary and secondary amenorrhea. All amenorrheas due to endocrine disorders are due to some change in the hormonal milieu, be it hypohormonal, hyperhormonal, or hormonal dysfunction. Nonendocrine amenorrhea is seen following too vigorous curettage or postabortal infection (Asherman syndrome) and in those rare instances of end-organ failure in which the endometrium is not responsive to endogenous or exogenous hormones. Whenever possible in the patient with primary amenorrhea, the nuclear chromosomal sex pattern should be established, and, if feasible, a chromosome analysis and karyotype carried out.

The adult female who has never menstruated has *primary amenorrhea.* Amenorrhea is *secondary* when a woman of childbearing age menstruated more or less regularly in the past and now has shown no signs of catamenia for 1 or more years. *Oligomenorrhea* refers to the occurrence of menses irregularly at varying intervals ranging from a few months to a year. Amenorrhea is said to be *physiologic* when associated with pregnancy, the postpartum period, lactation, and the menopause.

°This discussion is based on a report by R. B. Greenblatt, J. Internat. Fed. Gynec. & Obst. 1:94, 1963.

TABLE 10.—CLASSIFICATION OF AMENORRHEA

1. Hypothalamic—pseudocyesis, anorexia nervosa, stress
2. Hypophyseal
   a) Hyperhormonal—acromegaly, Cushing's disease
   b) Hormonal dysfunction—Chiari-Frommel and Argonz-del Castillo syndromes
   c) Hypohormonal—Simmonds' disease, Sheehan's disease, and hypogonadotrophic hypo-ovarianism
3. Ovarian
   a) Hyperhormonal—incretory tumor (granulosa cell and arrhenoblastoma) and functional cysts (follicular and luteal)
   b) Hormonal dysfunction—polycystic ovary syndrome of Stein-Leventhal and small polycystic ovary syndrome
   c) Hypohormonal—delayed pubescence, gonadal dysgenesis (Turner's syndrome), premature menopause, primary ovarian failure, dysgerminoma
4. Adrenal
   a) Hyperhormonal—Cushing's syndrome, adrenogenital syndrome, congenital adrenal hyperplasia
   b) Hypohormonal—Addison's disease (rarely complicated by amenorrhea)
5. Thyroidal
   a) Hyperhormonal—thyrotoxicosis
   b) Hypohormonal—myxedema, borderline hypothyroidism
6. Anomalies of sexual development
   a) Syndrome of feminizing testes
   b) Male pseudohermaphroditism
   c) Asymmetrical gonadal differentiation
   d) Incomplete Müllerian duct development

Table 10 presents a classification of amenorrhea.

1. *Hypothalamic.* Stress, anxieties, and fears may block or derange the hypothalamic-pituitary axis, and amenorrhea may be its only manifestation. The amenorrhea associated with pseudocyesis or even fear of pregnancy, the inability to adapt to changes in environment whether climatic or social, and disturbing emotional episodes may be included in this group. During World War II a statistical study of the menstrual patterns of women in London during the blitz revealed amenorrhea in a high percentage of them. A prime example of the endocrine disorder is that which follows the psychophysical disturbance of anorexia nervosa.

Psychogenic or hypothalamic amenorrhea is often the underlying factor in secondary amenorrhea. Reifenstein believes that, with emotional trauma, there is a block to the normal release of neurohormones or impulses from the hypothalamus to the anterior pituitary gland for production and/or release of luteinizing hormone (LH). He found that small doses of estrogens taken for several months ultimately stimulated the release of LH and the return of regular cyclic menses in many instances. The induction of uterine withdrawal bleeding in these patients often has a salutary effect on their psyche, for pseudomenstruation may remove the psychogenic block.

In pseudocyesis, the hypothalamic-pituitary derangement differs from most so-called psychogenic or hypothalamic amenorrheas. Here there may be a persistence of a corpus luteum, and the patient excretes pregnanediol during the amenorrhea (Lloyd). It appears that in such cases a continuous release of Prolactin or luteotrophin (LTH) maintains the corpus luteum (thus resembling the amenorrhea of pseudopregnancy).

2. *Hypophyseal.* Amenorrhea is encountered in those hyperhormonal conditions that result from increased pituitary activity, as in acromegaly and in Cushing's disease. The Chiari-Frommel syndrome, on the other hand, may be classified as one of hormonal dysfunction, for although there is evidence of increased prolactin activity, there is a compensatory lack of gonadotrophic secretion.

Hypohormonal amenorrhea resulting from pituitary failure is seen with chromophobe adenoma, craniopharyngioma, and destructive tumors of the pituitary and parapituitary region, as well as lesions associated with calcification of the pituitary or its stalk. The panhypopituitarism of Simmonds' disease is readily recognizable by the regressive changes in secondary sex characteristics, particularly loss of sexual hair and signs of loss of multi-target organ function, i.e., thyroid, adrenals, and ovaries. Sheehan's disease in some instances is indistinguishable clinically from Simmonds' disease. The diagnosis, however, is reserved for those women who have suffered from postpartum hemorrhage and shock. The degree of pituitary insufficiency that follows depends on the severity of the anoxia and damage to the gland. In most cases the amenorrhea persists, but, in the milder forms of the disease, recovery has been known to occur (Israel and Conston). In hypogonadotrophic hypo-ovarianism, there is a selective failure by the hypophysis to produce or secrete gonadotrophins. The result is that the ovary, though normal, suffers from lack of stimulation, hence the amenorrhea. Absence of gonadotrophins on plasma or urinary assay suggests the diagnosis.

3. *Ovarian.* The amenorrhea resulting from hyperhormonal conditions of the ovary may be divided into organic (incretory tumors) and functional (persistent follicular, luteal, or corpus luteum cysts) type.

Secondary amenorrhea is one of the sequelae of most of the androgen-producing tumors of the ovary such as arrhenoblastoma, Leydig and hilar cell tumors, and of adrenal rest tumors of the ovary. Surgical extirpation of the tumor usually is followed by resumption of normal cyclic menstruation. In women with an estrogen-producing tumor such as a granulosa cell tumor, the menstrual cycle, as a rule, becomes deranged and periods of amenorrhea followed by prolonged bleeding may occur. Amenorrhea of a few weeks duration may be associated with various types of functional cysts of the ovary—follicular, luteal, and persistent corpus luteum cysts. Spontaneous regression ultimately occurs, and cyclic menses may then resume.

The polycystic ovary syndrome of Stein-Leventhal is one of hormonal dysfunction. Chereau in 1854 first described the sclerocystic ovary with its pearly capsule. In the latter part of the 19th Century, Pozzi is said to have been among the first to perform wedge resection of the ovaries. In 1935, Stein and Leventhal described the syndrome that bears their names, i.e., amenorrhea, hirsutism, infertility, and bilaterally enlarged polycystic ovaries, and the treatment of this disorder.

In many instances there is an enzymatic defect in the polycystic ovaries that hinders the proper and orderly synthesis of ovarian steroids. There is a parallel to this disorder in the enzymatic error of steroidogenesis found in congenital adrenal hyperplasia.

Mahesh and Greenblatt demonstrated by incubation of tissue slices from Stein-Leventhal polycystic ovaries that such ovaries, at least in vitro, are capable of producing excessive amounts of androgenic precursors. Wedge resection of the ovaries is frequently followed by cyclic ovulatory menses, not that the enzymatic defect is corrected, but because more gonadotrophins become available per unit of ovarian mass. Beneficial results of such a procedure last from a few months to many years.

The thickness of the ovarian capsule has been thought to prevent ovulation. That this is erroneous is suggested by the following observations. (1) The removal of one ovary alone is sufficient to allow the ovulatory process to proceed from the untouched contralateral ovary. (2) At laparotomy, a fresh corpus luteum has been occasionally observed in one of the typically enlarged pale ovaries despite the characteristic thick capsule. Histologic study of sections frequently fails to reveal any old corpora lutea or albicantes as evidence of previous ovulations. (3) The administration of human pituitary follicle-stimulating hormone (HP-FSH) followed by human chorionic gonadotrophin (HCG) results in ovulation and corpus luteum formation in patients with the classic Stein-Leventhal syndrome. (4) Clomiphene citrate (MRL-41), an analogue of the nonsteroid estrogen Tace, has gonadotrophin-releasing properties and when given orally has proved particularly effective in inducing ovulation in patients with the Stein-Leventhal syndrome.

Many patients with amenorrhea and infertility with and without hirsutism are found, at laparotomy, to have small polycystic ovaries. Wedge resection is only occasionally followed by cyclic ovulatory menses. The pathophysiology of this disorder is not understood.

Many variants of gonadal dysgenesis have been recognized since Turner's description of ovarian agenesis associated with small stature, webbing of the neck, cubitus valgus, low hair line, and sexual infantilism. Gonadal dysgenesis may occur in females of small stature but without webbing of the neck or low hair line. Rudimentary gonadal streaks are present in these cases instead of ovaries (see p. 251). It may occur in girls of normal height but with sexual infantilism. Primary amenorrhea is the common denominator in all of these cases. On the other hand, primary hypo-ovarianism, the counterpart of males with primary eunuchoidism and small testes, is frequently considered but rarely proved. Most of the eunuchoid-appearing females are found at laparotomy to have gonadal dysgenesis rather than simply small, nonfunctioning ovaries. Nevertheless, primary ovarian failure does exist and is occasionally encountered. High plasma or urinary gonadotrophins point to primary ovarian failure, whereas absence of gonadotrophins points to hypogonadotrophic hypo-ovarianism.

Delayed pubescence may rightly be considered an hypohormonal condition. It may be the result of failure of the hypothalamus to stimulate release of pituitary gonadotrophins or of temporary refractoriness of the target organ to respond to gonadotrophins.

Premature senescence of the ovary resulting in secondary amenorrhea and often accompanied by hot flushes and signs of autonomic nervous system imbalance is occasionally encountered in women after several years of apparently normal menstruation. The atrophy of the vaginal mucosa as indicated by the study of vaginal cytology suggests failure of estrogen production by the ovaries. The high urinary or plasma gonadotrophin titers help to sustain the diagnosis of premature menopause. Patients encountered with this syndrome have been aged 19 and upward.

Neuter-appearing young girls with primary amenorrhea have been encountered with nonsteroid-producing tumors such as dysgerminomas. Such young women often are thin, with poorly developed secondary sexual characteristics. The tumor may be unilateral but, not infrequently, is bilateral. Amenorrhea may also occur in women with cystic and malignant teratomas.

4. *Adrenal.* Hyperhormonal adrenal disorders include Cushing's syndrome and the adrenogenital syndrome. The former is a purely metabolic disorder of increased and constant hydrocortisone secretion and consequent hypergluconeogenesis. As a rule, amenorrhea is a prominent symptom in Cushing's syndrome, but, in cases caused by a small adenoma, the symptomatology may prove confusing, and amenorrhea may not be present early in the disease. In the adrenogenital syndrome, the combination of virilization and amenorrhea is striking, although amenorrhea is not a constant finding.

Under adrenal dysfunction may be placed congenital adrenal hyperplasia. There are two varieties, in one of which masculinization sets in early in life. Such patients are born with an enlarged clitoris, a urogenital sinus, or a normal vaginal introitus, and pubic hair appears at age 4–6. Epiphyseal maturation advances rapidly. Female secondary sex characteristics do not appear at puberty or later, nor does menstruation ever occur. In the other type the clitoris is enlarged, but pubic hair may not appear until 8 or 9 years of age or later. Menarche may set in and menses continue for a variable number of years. Secondary amenorrhea invariably follows.

Adrenal dysfunction is a diagnosis that belongs to the gray zone of medicine. Many believe that certain cases of amenorrhea, infertility, hirsutism, and enlarged polycystic ovaries are not primarily ovarian but adrenal in origin. The administration of glucocorticoids is more likely to be followed by ovulatory menstruation in this group. Suppression of adrenal gonadal steroid activity with corticoids removes some inhibiting influences on the pituitary, permitting the release of more gonadotrophins.

Differentiation between congenital adrenal hyperplasia and adrenal dysfunction is readily made because in the former the very high levels of urinary 17-ketosteroids and pregnanetriol or pregnanetriolone are readily suppressed on administration of dexamethasone or other glucocorticoids.

Addison's disease, the only true hypohormonal condition of the adrenal, is only in exceptional cases complicated by cessation of menstruation. At times there is coincident premature menopause or an autoimmune basis affecting both the adrenal and the ovary.

5. *Thyroidal.* Adequate thyroid function may or may not be essential to normal pituitary-ovarian function. Disturbances in ovarian activity, often manifested by disturbed menstrual function as either menorrhagia or infrequent and scanty menses, are observed in both hypo- and hyperthyroidism. Thyroid medication for menstrual abnormalities has so successfully ameliorated the disorder in so many instances that many physicians employ thyroid hormone empirically in all such cases. It is quite probable that only the hypothyroid and subclinical hypothyroid patients respond. A trial of thyroid extract in doses of 30–90 mg. daily for 1 or 2 months may be in order in suspected cases not substantiated by laboratory tests. If the desired result is not obtained, thyroid medication should be discontinued. Excessive and prolonged medication leads to iatrogenic hypothyroidism when therapy is terminated.

TREATMENT.—Treatment consists of the use of oral progestogens for 5 days each month in those with adequate endogenous estrogens and a sequential form of therapy such as provided by Oracon or Norquen, or by simply giving Premarin 1.25 mg. for 21 days, with the addition of a progestin such as Duphaston or Provera during the last 5 days of this regimen.

If amenorrhea cannot be overcome by time, proper hygiene, diet, hormones, and perhaps psychotherapy, the last treatment that can be applied is roentgen ray therapy to the pituitary gland alone, the ovaries alone, or to both. After such x-ray therapy, about 70% of amenorrheic patients will menstruate regularly, and about 25–30% will become pregnant within a year.

Arnold studied the effects of irradiation of the hypothalamic area of adult monkeys and found marked degeneration of the paraventricular and supraoptic nuclei of the hypothalamus. Since these nuclei exert a considerable influence on the function of the pituitary body and since the latter is relatively radioresistant, Arnold suggests that any therapeutic benefits of irradiation to the hypophyseal region may be due to the effects of x-rays on the hypothalamus. Rakoff concluded that irradiation to the ovaries rather than to the pituitary is primarily responsible for the effects of radiation therapy.

There has been considerable opposition to the use of x-rays for treatment of amenorrhea and sterility. This has come chiefly from geneticists, who have proved in several types of lower animals that the fourth and subsequent generations of offspring show enormous increase in the incidence of deformities and monstrosities.

Menorrhagia

Menorrhagia, or excessive menstrual bleeding, may be organic or functional in origin. The organic type may be due to pelvic inflammation, submucous leiomyomas, adenomyomas, intrauterine polyps, tuberculous endometritis, carcinoma, or other conditions involving the ovaries or uterus.

Functional bleeding is nearly always of endocrine origin. The exact source is unknown, but the ovaries, especially the follicle apparatus, play an important role. Hypothyroidism is frequently associated with this condition. Constitutional disability and general illnesses may also lead to menorrhagia. In many cases of functional bleeding, the endometrium presents the histologic picture of hyperplasia, but any type of endometrium may be found.

Bleeding between the periods, or *metrorrhagia*, is strongly suggestive of carcinoma, which must always be ruled out. Other causes of intermenstrual bleeding are retained products of conception, extrauterine pregnancy, and polyps, and following the use of gonadal steroids such as estrogens or while on the birth-control pill.

Irregular bleeding just before or during the menopause should always arouse a suspicion of malignancy. In nearly all cases it is imperative to perform a curettage to rule out cancer, even though in most instances the irregular bleeding is due to the change of life. Such a curettage must be done thoroughly, because a minute cancer may be present. In cases of carcinoma of the endometrium, just as in instances of uterine polyps and submucous leiomyomas, hysterography may reveal the pathologic condition (see Chapter 18).

If bleeding begins after a woman has stopped menstruating for a year or more, a careful bimanual examination must be made at once. Such bleeding usually indicates a malignancy or use of estrogens. If the cervix is the site of the malignancy, the diagnosis is readily made, if not by palpation and inspection then certainly through vaginal and cervical smears and biopsy of the cervix. If the cervix is normal, a curettage of the cervix and uterus separately should be performed. This may reveal a cancer of the body of the uterus. If, in a woman who bleeds some years after the menopause, an examination reveals a slightly enlarged uterus and a one-sided mass, especially if curettage reveals hyperplasia of the endometrium, a granulosa cell tumor of the ovary may be suspected.

TREATMENT.—Before any treatment of abnormal bleeding is begun, the presence or absence of carcinoma must be determined. When a cause for profuse menstrual bleeding is discovered, it should be removed if possible. This may mean removal of a submucous leiomyoma, a polyp, inflammatory adnexal masses, or even the entire uterus.

In young girls every effort should be made to avoid an operative procedure, even curettage, unless it is essential. In most girls the menses regulate themselves spontaneously after a number of months or years; but young girls must be helped while waiting for this to occur or serious symptoms may result from anemia.

Hormones may be used to check excessive menstrual bleeding. The best results in management of functional uterine bleeding are usually obtained when the following therapy is used.

Estrogens.—Uterine bleeding may be brought on by a sudden lowering of estrogen levels (estrogen-deprivation bleeding). Breakthrough bleeding will result from constant and prolonged estrogen stimulation. In either instance sufficiently large doses of estrogens will raise the estrogen levels and so usually arrest the bleeding. Parenteral administration of estrogen, followed by descending oral doses, may be used to good advantage. More rapid hemostasis may be obtained by the intravenous use of conjugated estrogens (Premarin, Intravenous). The dosage is 20 mg., given intravenously every 4 to 8 hours until bleeding is arrested. Then oral therapy with conjugated estrogens (Premarin) or the equivalent in doses of 3.75 mg. per day, gradually reduced to 1.25 mg. per day, is given for 3 weeks. Then a course of progesterone, such as 5 mg. of norethindrone acetate (Norlutate, Parke-Davis) or its equivalent, is administered for 5 days. Withdrawal bleeding will follow in several days that will simulate a menstrual period.

Estrogen therapy is particularly useful in the management of functional uterine bleeding that occurs at the menarche and at the menopause. A complication of high-dosage estrogen therapy is nausea. The commonest errors that are made with estrogen therapy are the use of inadequate dosages and the abrupt cessation of therapy when bleeding is arrested. Estrogen dosage should be tapered off gradually.

Progesterones.—Fortunately, many of the former disadvantages of progesterone therapy may now be avoided because of the availability of two groups of progestational agents.

1. A single intramuscular dose of 250 mg. of 17-α-hydroxyprogesterone caproate (Delalutin) will frequently arrest bleeding within 24–48 hours.

Withdrawal bleeding will be postponed for 7 to 19 days. The administration of this long-acting progesterone in this manner affords the patient a real breathing spell before withdrawal bleeding occurs. The addition of a long-acting estrogen (Delestrogen) enhances the effectiveness of Delalutin, arresting bleeding in 6 to 24 hours.

2. The 19-nortestosterone derivatives, especially in combination with an estrogen such as Ortho-Novum (Ortho), or Norlestrin (Parke-Davis), or Ovral (Wyeth), or Ovulen or Demulen (Searle), are particularly useful in arresting a bout of dysfunctional uterine bleeding. Three tablets are given daily until the acute bleeding is arrested or greatly diminished and then 2 tablets per day are continued for as long a period as desired, usually until the hemoglobin level is restored to normal. Withdrawal bleeding may thus be postponed for 10, 30, 90 days or longer, as suits the patient and her physician.

Iron alone or combined with liver should be prescribed for all women who bleed excessively.

ENDOMETRIOSIS.—The only real cure for endometriosis at present is surgery and sometimes pregnancy. There is no need to resort to operative procedures when the endometriosis is not extensive or painful unless a patient is sterile and desires children.

One of the best temporizing measures in the management of endometriosis is the prolonged administration of norethindrone or norethindrone acetate in 15- to 30-mg. doses (occasionally break-through bleeding threatens and the dosage must be gradually increased to 40–50 mg. per day) for periods up to 9 months. This has resulted in postponement of menses and marked reduction not only in pelvic discomfort but also in the size of cystic ovarian masses. Nodules in the culdesac and indurated uterosacral ligaments in many instances soften or disappear. The longer the therapy, the better the results. Kistner, who first suggested the use of Enovid for periods of 9 months or so (pseudopregnancy), employs increasing doses of the combined estrogen-progestogen birth control pills such as Enovid or Ovulen (Searle).

Freedom from pain may be lost when therapy is discontinued. A second course of prolonged therapy may be undertaken. Satisfactory results have been obtained in about half of the patients so treated.

Mittelschmerz (Mid-Menstrual Pain)

Some women experience mild or even relatively sharp pain in one or the other of the iliac fossas every month about midway between menstrual bleedings. This pain is believed to be due to rupture of an ovarian follicle and may be associated with a slight bloody discharge from the uterus. The condition is called mittelschmerz, or periodic intermenstrual pain, and has clinical significance because it sometimes leads to the mistaken diagnosis of acute appendicitis and ruptured ectopic pregnancy. Many unnecessary operations have been performed because of it. The diagnosis can usually be made from the history and the physical findings, and no treatment is necessary except to put the patient to bed and give her relief from pain. One way to prevent mittelschmerz is to suppress ovulation, as in dysmenorrhea (p. 275).

Hypomenorrhea

Hypomenorrhea, or scanty flow, is fairly common. It has no significance and actually requires no treatment. For those concerned, the administration of the sequential birth control pill usually affords them a more normal withdrawal period.

Polymenorrhea

Some women menstruate every 3 weeks or oftener. Although this is a nuisance, no harm results from it as long as the amount of blood lost is not excessive. If much blood is lost during each menstrual period, oral contraceptives should be prescribed or a curettage may be performed.

Oligomenorrhea

Oligomenorrhea, or menses every 3 or 4 months, should be regarded as a mild form of amenorrhea. No treatment is necessary for purposes of health. If the condition is associated with sterility, it should be treated as is amenorrhea.

Premenstrual Tension and Premenstrual Distress

A great number of apparently normal women undergo considerable suffering from a variety of causes during the week or so preceding the menstrual flow. With the onset of menstruation, this premenstrual distress disappears. The distress occurring may be due to one or several of the following causes: headache, nausea, bloating of the abdomen, fullness and pain in the breasts, emotional disturbances, edema of the vulva, and frank edema of other tissues of the body. Although the disagreeable character of premenstrual distress is, in many women, sufficiently mild to be tolerated, in others it induces considerable misery. Often patients suffer severe psychic alterations, such as depression, suicidal tendencies, or extreme irritability. This condition has been termed *premenstrual tension*, supposedly a distinct clinical entity. However, Freed and Greenhill noted all gradations in severity of symptoms during the premenstrual period, and it has been difficult to draw a sharp line between premenstrual distress and premenstrual tension. Owing to the similarity of symptoms, we concluded that premenstrual tension is an extreme degree of premenstrual distress rather than a separate syndrome.

Whatever the etiology, Freed and Greenhill have postulated a single mechanism for the development of the variety of changes that occur. Premenstrual distress is, according to this hypothesis, the result of sodium ion retention by the different tissues of the body under the influence of the ovarian steroids. This retention of sodium ion is associated with an increase in extracellular fluid in the tissues which may be microscopic in amount or may develop into gross edema. Under this theory, the neurologic symptoms result from edema of the nervous system, probably the brain, the nausea and bloating of the abdomen result from edema of the gut, and the other symptoms arise from the specific organs affected.

Actual proof of this working hypothesis is lacking, although many physiologic reactions can be presented in support of such conclusions. It is well known, for instance, that sex hormones are steroids that have a definite effect on water balance. Estrogens, androgens, and other hormones are capable of causing sodium ion retention. Zuckerman and his associates demonstrated that estrogens increase the water content of the extragenital tissues of the body as well as of the sex organs. Premenstrual edema is a clear example of water retention caused by ovarian activity. In this connection, many workers have noted the resemblance of the sex steroids to those of the adrenal cortex, a major function of which is to help preserve electrolyte and water balance.

On the basis of this hypothesis that premenstrual distress results from tissue edema, Freed and Greenhill institute therapy whereby the excess sodium and associated fluid are lessened. For this purpose ammonium chloride, a salt frequently used for removal of edema fluid in cardiac and renal disturbances, is administered orally.

TREATMENT.—Patients with premenstrual tension are advised to refrain from adding table salt to their food during the last two weeks of the menstrual cycle. During this time they are given 0.6 Gm. of ammonium chloride 3 times daily. A large number of women have been treated with this simple remedy, and nearly all of them have been relieved of premenstrual distress. Ammonium chloride may harm women with cardiac, renal, or hepatic disease and therefore should not be prescribed for such women.

For enormous abdominal distention, which begins about five days before the onset of the menses, G. Jones believes the cause to be triggered by the progestational phase of the cycle. Hence it should be prevented by anything which will prevent ovulation. She prescribes Norlutin from day 5 through 25 for each of two cycles. This treatment completely relieves the abdominal distention.

Another simple and effective agent is testosterone propionate. The patient may be given 25 mg. hypodermically on the tenth and the third day before the expected menstruation, or, better still, she can take a 10-mg. tablet of methyltestosterone or a 5-mg. sublingual or buccal tablet daily for 10 days before the expected onset of menstrual flow (Freed). For rapid relief at the height of premenstrual tension, the injection of a mercurial diuretic is often effective. Any of the newer diuretics given for 8–10 days prior to onset of menses has also proved effective.

Mastopathy, mastoplasia, or cystic disease of the breasts.—Excessive estrogen in the blood may produce painful breasts with or without cystic disease. Both the pain and the size of the nodules in the breasts may be reduced by testosterone therapy. Often the prompt relief is dramatic, but, of course, the treatment must be continued for several months and repeated from time to time. In patients who have mastopathia throughout the menstrual cycle, a 5-mg. sublingual or buccal tablet should be taken daily for a month. However, if the breasts are painful for only 7 to 10 days before the beginning of the menstrual flow, a 5-mg. sublingual or buccal tablet daily for the 10 days before the beginning of menstruation will often help to relieve the pain.

The Climacteric and Menopause

THE TERM *climacteric* is generally used as a synonym for the word menopause, although the two terms are not synonymous. The word *menopause* simply means the physiologic cessation of the menstrual flow, whereas the term climacteric refers to a period in the life of every woman that is a consequence of ovarian senescence. It lasts from then onward to the last of life. This period has been called the critical age because in many instances distressing symptoms appear. Many changes occur during the climacteric, including cessation of the menses; hence the menopause is only one of its phenomenon. The laity refers to the climacteric as *change of life.*

The climacteric rarely comes on suddenly, except when castration is performed on a young woman by means of surgery or radiation. Nearly always, there are premonitory signs and symptoms before the menopause actually takes place. Hence there are premenopausal, menopausal, and postmenopausal periods, only the last of which is sharply defined. The basis for the climacteric changes is an alteration in the endocrine system. The organs chiefly involved in this process are the hypothalamus, pituitary, and gonads. Other systems, particularly the nervous and circulatory, are also affected. Accompanying the climacteric is a train of emotional manifestations, either as a result of the climacteric or aggravated by it. The onset of the climacteric varies considerably and is difficult to define. This is readily understandable when one realizes that many changes take place in women long before they cease menstruating or have vasomotor disturbances such as hot flushes. Chief among the premenopausal alterations are a change in disposition, emotional upsets, deposition of fat, and gain of weight. Generally speaking, the majority of women experience the climacteric between their forty-sixth and fiftieth years. Women who begin to menstruate early in life usually have a long menstrual career and a late climacteric. However, this is far from a constant rule.

ENDOCRINE SYSTEM.—Definite changes take place in the pituitary, gonads, and probably other glands. There is an increase in the amount of follicle-stimulating and luteinizing pituitary hormones in the circulating blood owing to withdrawal of the inhibiting effect of the ovaries. For many years, the pituitary gland was considered the master gland. Now, we feel that the pituitary is subservient to a higher authority—the hypothalamus. The hypothalamus plays an important role in the symptomatology of the climacteric as it does in the control of many other functions. The hypothalamus has many centers; for instance, one controls thirst and water metabolism. A lesion of the supraventricular or supraoptic nuclei will induce unquenchable thirst, i.e., diabetes insipidus. A lesion of the anterior hypothalamus may result in sexual infantilism, whereas one of the posterior portion may be associated with sexual precocity. The hypothalamus is intimately tied to energy control—therein reside centers for appetite, temperature, and sleep. The fat boy in the *Pickwick Papers* was either eating or sleeping; he probably had an hypothalamic lesion.

Thyroid disturbances are often simulated during the menopause, resembling hyperthyroidism or, less frequently, hypothyroidism. The commonest symptoms of hyperthyroidism in the climacteric are tachycardia, palpitation, tremor, loss of weight in some cases, disturbances of the digestive tract (especially diarrhea), vasomotor disturbances (particularly hot flushes), menstrual hemorrhages, and nervousness. The symptoms of hypothyroidism are those of myxedema and include flabbiness, hoarse voice, thick skin, constant feeling of coldness, falling of the hair, mental sluggishness, headache, constipation, and cutaneous eruptions.

NERVOUS SYSTEM.—The symptoms during the menopause that are of nervous origin are headache (although sometimes it is due to hypertension), dizziness, insomnia, drowsiness, neuralgia, numbness in the legs, pruritus, and various sensory disturbances. There are a large number and variety of emotional upsets during the climacteric, varying from slight changes in disposition to actual psychosis.

CIRCULATORY SYSTEM.—The disturbances that may occur in this system are vasomotor, such as hot flushes, perspiration, sensation of choking or suffocation, tachycardia, dyspnea, and cardiac arrhythmia. Generally, the term "hot flashes" refers to the hot, tingling sensations that often involve the whole body. The term "hot flushes," which is used more often, refers chiefly to involvement of the head, neck, and upper thorax.

METABOLIC SYSTEM.—Evidence has been increasing that there is a direct relationship between diminished production of estrogens and the pathogenesis of atherosclerosis. Onset of the climacteric and diminution of estrogen production coincide with the rapid and progressive increase in the incidence of atherosclerosis. The Framingham study emphasized that coronary disease is 20 times more common among males than females during the years 30–39 and increases in frequency as the end of the reproductive period approaches.

There is overwhelming clinical and experimental evidence that there is a relationship between the levels and patterns of circulating lipids and the pathogenesis of atherosclerosis. The role of cholesterol, especially in relation to serum phospholipids, is gaining wide acceptance. Therefore, both the alterations in serum lipid patterns seen with changes in the individual's hormone status (whether brought about endogenously or exogenously) and the concomitant changes in atherosclerotic diseases appear to be parts of the same process.

Few women on estrogen therapy complain of low back pain, discomfort, or crippling associated with osteoporosis. It has been thought that the basic defect is hypofunction of the osteoblasts that are under estrogen control. Gonadal failure and the rapid decline in endogenous estrogen supply interfere with osteoblastic activity (Albright). Calcium replacement therapy alone accomplishes but little. However, a concept that has gained currency recently is that estrogens dampen the effect of the parathyroids on calcium mobilization from bone, slowing down the rate of unopposed bone resorption. On estrogen therapy, excessive mobilization of calcium is arrested and further vertebral compression fractures averted, although x-ray findings, as a rule, fail to show any definite improvement in bone remineralization (Fig. 120).

Stranjord and Lanzl developed an ingenious machine for the accurate determination of bone density. Their instrument makes it possible to measure the density of the phalanges by transmission of the gamma radiation of I^{125}. The bone density of postmenopausal patients (after bilateral oophorectomy) on exogenous estrogen therapy (stilbestrol 0.5 mg. every other day) was found to be much greater than that of postmenopausal patients without estrogen medication. This initial sampling demonstrated that estrogen replacement definitely increases bone density in castrated women. It is my custom to treat the postmenopausal or the osteoporotic woman with 1.25 mg. of Premarin

FIG. 120.—Note osteoporosis and collapsed vertebrae in a 49-year-old patient with primary amenorrhea. After many years of estrogen therapy, there was no mineralization but remarkable clinical improvement. (Courtesy of Dr. Robert B. Greenblatt.)

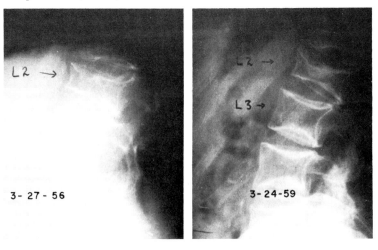

continuously for 20 to 40 days, followed by 5 days of a progestogen (2.5 mg. of Norlutate or 5 mg. of Provera or 10 mg. of Duphaston or Gynorest), increased exercise, added calcium intake orally, and a high-protein diet.

ARTIFICIAL MENOPAUSE.—The menopause may be brought about artificially and quickly by surgical removal of the ovaries or by the elimination of ovarian function by intrauterine radium or roentgen rays. Removal of the uterus alone, with retention of the ovaries, may hasten the appearance of climacteric symptoms, possibly because the blood supply to the ovaries may be compromised by the surgical interference. There is some question as to whether or not the uterus has an internal secretion that is essential in preventing the symptoms of the climacteric.

Symptoms

The symptoms of the menopause, i.e., hot flushes or flashes, sweats, etc., are believed by many to be due to a hyperpituitarism because of the marked increase in urinary gonadotrophins (Fig. 121). But high urinary gonadotrophins are also present in eunuchoidism and in primary ovarian failure. The young woman with gonadal dysgenesis and sexual infantilism has high urinary gonadotrophins and severe hypoestrogenism, yet does not have hot flushes. However, should she receive estrogen therapy for many years, in all probability she will develop hot flushes when hormonal treatment is abruptly terminated. The hypothalamus has been described as the master ganglion of the autonomic nervous system. We must think of the menopause as the

FIG. 121.—Urinary FSH titers fell while the patient was on estrogen therapy (12 mg. TACE q.i.d.). When, after 26 days, the treatment was discontinued, the vaginal cytology remained estrogenic but the urinary gonadotrophin titers gradually rose to pretreatment levels by the eightieth day. However, in spite of the rise in FSH titers, the hot flushes were held in abeyance. (From Greenblatt, R. B.: Geriatrics 7:263, 1952.)

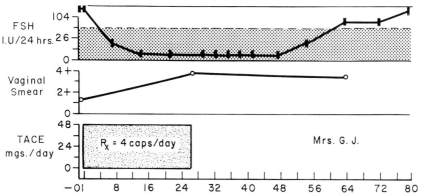

estrogen-deprivation state that occurs after years of hypothalamic conditioning. With decrease or interference in estrogenic production, the hypothalamus responds with heated displeasure. The appearance of hot flushes, sweats, globus hystericus, spasms, and a variety of symptoms are precipitated by the autonomic nervous system imbalance (see Table 11).

Another group of symptoms commonly attributed to the menopause are not primarily due to the climacteric but are inherent in the individual. The climacteric uncloaks many of the neurotic and psychogenic symptoms that many women have managed to successfully suppress. However, under the stress of the change of life, anxiety, apprehension, depression, insomnia, nervousness, headaches, frigidity for some, and increased sex drive for others, come to the surface. Nervousness and depression may have been present all the while but now blossom forth. I am reminded of Shakespeare's Lady MacBeth, whose ambition bordered on the psychopathic. She was determined to see her husband crowned King of Scotland. In the process Duncan, Banquo, and then the wife and children of McDuff were liquidated through her scheming. Then, in her middle years when the security of the throne was hers, she was heard to sigh, "Out, damned spot! Out, I say! . . . Here's the smell of blood still: all the perfume of Arabia will not sweeten this little hand." Insomnia became her relentless enemy. Shakespeare depicts the unforgettable scene:

> *Macb.* How does your patient, doctor?
> *Doct.* Not so sick, my lord,
> As she is troubled with thick-coming fancies
> That keep her from her rest.
> *Macb.* Cure her of that.
> Canst thou not minister to a mind diseas'd,
> Pluck from the memory a rooted sorrow,
> Raze out the written troubles of the brain,
> And with some sweet oblivious antidote
> Cleanse the stuff'd bosom of that perilous stuff
> Which weighs upon the heart?
> *Doct.* Therein the patient
> Must minister to himself.

And I fear we have too many physicians who maintain the Shakespearean attitude that, "Therein the patient must cure himself." The woman in the menopause with severe insomnia, depression, crying spells, apprehension, now worsened and complicated by hot flushes and sweats, is expected to help herself. To merely shrug and insinuate that the menopause is physiologic, that women must suffer through it, is not the understanding nor the compassion expected of the physician. It is within our province to temper the psychosexual upheaval of this trying period. Estrogens along with some homespun psychology, with or without tranquilizers or antidepressants, may lessen the distressful symptoms. Estrogen vaginal suppositories are helpful for cystitis.

TABLE 11.—Symptoms of the Climacteric Classified by Causes

Autonomic N.S.	Psychogenic	Metabolic
hot flushes	apprehension	demineralization
formication	depression	myalgia
globus hystericus	insomnia	skin atrophy
perspiration	nervousness	atrophic vaginitis
spasms	← headaches →	incontinence
palpitations	← increase in sexual → responsiveness	arthritism
G.I. disorders	← decrease in sexual → responsiveness	change in lipid metabolism

(Modified from Greenblatt, R. B.: The Menopause and Its Management, in Dorfman, R. I., and Neves e Castro, M. [eds.]: *Pituitary-Ovarian Endocrinology* [San Francisco: Holden-Day, Inc., 1963].)

Another group of disturbances primarily due to a metabolic disorder are brought on by the estrogen-deficient state, i.e., osteoporosis, certain myalgias, skin atrophy, vaginal atrophy, urinary incontinence, some arthritides, and reversal of the α and β lipoprotein ratio. Demineralization of bone is not merely an aging process. The young girl who has primary ovarian failure or from whom the ovaries have been removed will, in many instances, develop varying degrees of osteoporosis by the age of 35. Some patients with urinary incontinence and nocturnal frequency have noted marked improvement while on replacement hormonal therapy. Women suffering from some forms of osteoarthritis find the condition worsened at the time of the menopause, and many of them do much better on replacement therapy than on corticoids. Senile or atrophic vaginitis does not respond to douches and soothing creams. Estrogens, locally or orally, cause maturation of the vaginal mucosa, induce a return of the normal flora, and vitiate irritating discharge and pruritus.

Kraurosis vulvae, frequently seen in the menopause, is associated with an estrogen deficiency. There are, however, other factors that precipitate its appearance, because only a small proportion of women develop the condition. Many such patients have, in the past, been treated by vulvectomy because of the fear of cancer. Surgery can be avoided if the patient is adequately treated with estrogen replacement therapy orally and with hydrocortisone-like ointments locally. Local areas of leukoplakia may develop in women who continuously traumatize the vulvar area by scratching. Leukoplakia may be a precancerous condition and should be treated by surgery.

Mention was made of precipitating factors in kraurosis vulvae. In a series of 25 patients, 24 were found to have absence of free hydrochloric acid on gastric analysis. Women in older age groups will frequently have absence of free-hydrochloric acid, but the incidence of 24 out of 25 is far greater than one would expect in such a group. Though I do not know what the precipitating factors are, I do know that corticoids increase hydrochloric acid secretion by the gastric mucosa. Appropriate hormonal therapy has succeeded not only in assuaging the discomfort and mitigating the woes of the women with kraurosis vulvae but also has militated against the development of vulvar cancer.

Robert Wilson of New York and his book, *Feminine Forever*, advocated that every menopausal woman be treated and the *feminine index* be the guide to therapy. He placed much store on the feminine index which, in my opinion, may prove misleading. Many women with menopausal symptoms have moderately mature vaginal smears. Furthermore, after termination of many months of estrogen therapy, a mature vaginal smear may persist for 6 months, 1 year, or longer. One cannot always judge the need of therapy by vaginal cytology. It is my considered opinion that we should treat the patient, not the laboratory, not the smear. Then again, there are many women endowed with ovaries that continue to secrete small but adequate amounts of estrogens for 10–15 years after cessation of menses. Such women are not necessarily candidates for estrogen replacement therapy.

Management

The management of the climacteric or the menopause is a controversial one; there is room for disagreement. The more conservative physician believes the menopause is physiologic and hence warns us to keep hands off; the middle-of-the-roader feels that one need but treat the immediate symptoms for as short a period as possible; whereas I am a little to the left of center and urge that the hormonally deficient menopausal patient receive adequate replacement therapy. It is well that we disagree, for the practice of medicine would be monotonous, indeed, if all adopted the post-Galen posture toward diagnosis and treatment. The question is still being asked, "Is the menopause a disease or just an epoch?" and each physician must decide this for himself. I feel that the woman in the autumn of her life deserves an Indian summer rather than a winter of discontent.

Estrogens may be administered for 21 days each month in a dosage sufficient to minimize untoward effects of hormone deprivation and yet small enough to avoid uterine bleeding. The smallest dose adequate to keep the vaginal mucosa in an estrous state is usually, but not always, an adequate one. If break-through or withdrawal bleeding occurs, it is advisable to add small doses of an androgen to the regimen of therapy. For instance, 2.5 to 5.0 mg. of methyltestosterone may be added to a daily dose of 0.625, 1.25, or 2.5 mg. of conjugated equine estrogens (Fig. 122). However, if this complication persists, it is best to induce controlled withdrawal periods. This can be accomplished by administration of a progestational agent, in combination with an

AE	1	2	3	4	
JUNE	X				COMPLETE RELIEF. EXCESSIVE WITHDRAWAL BLEEDING.
JULY					
AUG.		X			COMPLETE RELIEF. ALMOST NORMAL PERIOD.
SEPT.			X		RECURRENCE OF SYMPTOMS, NO RELIEF.
OCT.				X	HOT FLASHES WORSE THAN EVER BEFORE.
NOV.		X			COMPLETE RELIEF. NORMAL WITHDRAWAL PERIOD.
DEC.		X			NO RELIEF, RECURRENCE OF SYMPTOMS.
JAN.				X	NO RELIEF. HOT FLASHES SEVERE (20–30 PER DAY).
FEB.	X				COMPLETE RELIEF. EXCESSIVE WITHDRAWAL BLEEDING.

Patient preferred AE-2 because withdrawal bleeding was controlled and was much less than with AE-1. Both preparations gave equally good results as far as amelioration of hot flashes was concerned.

FIG. 122.—Mrs. H. G. O., w. f. 44. Menopause. Hot flashes—severe (previously controlled with estrogens, but had severe bout of uterine bleeding following estrogen therapy). This was part of a double blind study in which an estrogen (*No. 1*), an estrogen-androgen combination (*No. 2*), an androgen (*No. 3*) and a placebo (*No. 4*) were employed in the management of severe symptoms in a menopausal patient. (From Greenblatt *et al.*, J. Clin. Endocrinol. 10:1547, 1950.)

estrogen for 21 days each month or during the last 5 to 10 days of a 20-day to 30-day course of an estrogen. Furthermore, the regular shedding of the endometrium at regular intervals will generally prevent the development of adenomatous hyperplasia of the endometrium. Treatment is greatly simplified for women who have undergone hysterectomy, and the percentage of such women is high. When orally administered medication is ineffective or un-dependable, or treatment by injections is erratic, implantation of 1 or 2 (25 mg.) pellets of estradiol and 1 (75 mg.) pellet of testosterone, at intervals of 6 to 8 months, has proved a method of therapy satisfactory to patient and physician alike.

The common belief is that all estrogens taken continuously tend to cause bleeding from the uterus. Hence estrogens are prescribed cyclically. A simple way is for the patient to take the estrogen every night for the first 21 days of the month, then stop until the first night of the next month. However, several gynecologists maintain that small doses of estrogens given continuously for many years do not lead to uterine bleeding.

Davis instituted long-term substitution of estrogens in postmenopausal women more than a quarter of a century ago. Following the administration of stilbestrol, he found a definite tendency to lowering of serum cholesterol and to elevation of phospholipids, while the level of total circulating lipids remained relatively constant. The C/P ratios were thus lowered by stilbestrol administration and appeared to be a fairly sensitive index of the estrogenic effect.

Cyclic administration of estrogens in the postmenopausal period, according to Davis, is not necessary. It has been demonstrated that small amounts of estrogens will stimulate the growth of the endometrium for a short time, following which it regresses and remains inactive despite continued therapy. He feels that cyclic therapy provokes uterine bleeding in the woman who has her uterus. Uterine bleeding in the menopausal and postmenopausal periods must always be regarded with great suspicion. It may have been induced by the cessation of estrogen therapy for a short period, or it may arise occasionally in patients while on hormone therapy. Although estrogens may be responsible for the bleeding, the possibility of early endometrial carcinoma can be ruled out only by curettage.

In conclusion, I raise a few questions. If estrogens prevent the reversal of α and β lipoproteins in the aging female, would the incidence of cardiovascular accident be reduced by replacement therapy? Would it be out of order to practice preventive medicine by anticipating the inevitable ovarian senescence to which every woman is heir by administering small doses of estrogens in cyclic fashion? For those subject to break-through bleeding, would a modified form of sequential estrogen-progestogen therapy insure shedding of the endometrium and act as a prophylaxis against endometrial cancer?

The long-term administration of exogenous estrogens to menopausal and postmenopausal women has a fourfold objective: (1) to suppress the menopausal symptoms; (2) to retard the physical atrophic changes; (3) to retard the development of atherosclerosis and its sequelae; and (4) to retard osteoporosis and other skeletal changes.

The difficulties of the menopause—the imbalance of the autonomic nervous system, the psychogenic disorders, and the metabolic disturbances—continue, from mild to severe form, until the end of life. It is unrealistic to withhold measures that may make the transition smoother or prevent disabling pathologic processes.

Atrophic (Senile) Vaginitis

By THE TERM atrophic vaginitis is meant a nonspecific inflammation of the vagina that occurs as a result of an estrogen-deficient state. The adhesive form is frequently seen in childhood, the atrophic form in the postmenopausal woman. It also is observed in young women who have been castrated by surgery or radiation therapy. For this reason the name atrophic vaginitis is preferable to senile vaginitis.

Normally, after the menopause, atrophy of the pelvic organs takes place, marked in some, less so in others. This involves the vagina, which becomes shorter and narrower. At the introitus there is considerable constriction after a few years. The mucosa is decidedly thinned out and easily traumatized. When inflammation takes place in this atrophic vaginal mucosa, senile or postmenopausal vaginitis follows. The exciting factor may be repeated minor trauma or a secondary infection. Because of the absence of epithelial glycogen and its by-product, lactic acid, pathogenic bacteria readily invade the vaginal canal in the absence of the normal flora and an acid pH. The protective lactic acid bacillus or the Döderlein bacillus, the organism normally present, disappears. Ulcerations and erosions may appear in the vaginal mucosa. The denuded areas usually fuse to close off the vagina in numerous places. If the filmy adhesions are broken down early in their formation, bleeding results, which may lead to the suspicion of carcinoma.

The symptoms of atrophic vaginitis are generally a vaginal discharge that produces a burning sensation in the vagina and on the labia, burning on urination, often pruritus vulvae, and pelvic discomfort. The discharge is usually watery and whitish, but may be blood tinged. Sometimes there is excoriation of the skin on the vulva, anal region, and inner parts of the thighs.

Diagnosis is easy. The patient has a castrate type of vaginal smear. Infection in the absence of trichomoniasis or moniliasis should suggest the diagnosis, particularly in the postmenopausal period or after castration. Vaginal examination reveals punctate superficial bleeding areas and thin adhesions between the walls of the vagina. In most instances these adhesions can be broken down easily. The vagina is much narrower than normal, the introitus is tight, and the trauma incident to digital examination usually causes bleeding. Frequently, the cervix cannot be felt. Sometimes, even one finger in the vagina causes discomfort because of tightness.

Treatment consists of the administration of estrogen, as advocated by Davis. The basis of this treatment is restoration of the atrophic vaginal mucosa to that of a normal premenopausal condition. Estrogen accomplishes this, but unfortunately the change is not permanent.

Estrogens administered orally or locally are helpful. A synthetic estrogen may be prescribed in about the dose used for hot flushes, perspiration, and the like. If there is no improvement in 2 weeks, the dose should be increased. Estrogen applied locally in the vagina is very helpful; it is best given in the form of a suppository (diethylstilbestrol, Lilly). When there is considerable pruritus not controlled by oral or vaginal therapy, it may respond to an effective salve containing 1 mg. of diethylstilbestrol to each gram of ointment or to Premarin cream (Ayerst) or Dienestrol cream (Ortho). Great relief from itching can be obtained in most cases with an ointment containing hydrocortisone (Synalar, Meti-Derm, or Cortef). Usually relief is noted within 2 weeks after treatment is started. After therapy is stopped, there may be a recurrence, and more estrogen will have to be prescribed. A number of courses may be required; caution is necessary because, regardless of the route of administration, there may be some uterine bleeding and the patient should be so warned.

Elderly women who have had extensive vaginal plastic surgery usually complain of difficulty in having intercourse. A helpful procedure is to insert a diethylstilbestrol 0.1–0.5 mg. vaginal suppository every night for 1 week in every month, or to apply a vaginal cream (Dienestrol cream 0.1–0.5 mg./Gm. or Premarin cream 0.625–1 mg./Gm.). This will maintain the vaginal mucosa in a healthful condition.

Pruritus Vulvae

PRURITUS of the vulva is a symptom, not a disease entity. It may be due to a variety of causes, the commonest of which, other than kraurosis and leukoplakia (see Chapter 35), are: pregnancy, glycosuria, candidiasis, trichomonal vaginitis, gonorrhea, obesity, menopause, uncleanliness, pediculosis, senile vaginitis, eczema, incontinence of urine, fistula in ano, morphinism, neurodermatitis, and constitutional diseases such as jaundice, Hodgkin's disease, and leukemia. Itching of the vulva may vary from a mild irritation to a most distressing affliction. The pruritus is usually worse during the night, although many women troubled with pruritus vulvae suffer both day and night. The frantic desire to scratch not only aggravates the condition but sometimes leads to infections or other serious changes in the skin.

Treatment

The treatment of pruritus depends on the cause, which usually is easy to determine, and its removal generally brings relief. In some cases either the cause cannot be found or the etiologic agent cannot be removed immediately as, for example, the itching associated with pregnancy and that accompanying obesity.

In these patients symptomatic treatment must be given at least for a while. Of greatest importance is cleanliness, not only after each urination and bowel movement but at all times. In cleansing the vulva there must be no rubbing, only patting, preferably with soft toilet paper, soft cotton, or soft tissue.

One of the best suggestions to make to the patient is that she refrain from scratching no matter how great the urge. She should be told that scratching only aggravates the itching and much greater relief can be obtained by pinching the portion of the skin that itches or by making firm continuous pressure on the involved parts with the closed fist or fingers. Sometimes hot applications help, but at times heat aggravates the itching, and many women are relieved by the application of cold compresses. Lotions and salves containing phenol, menthol, and other substances are also helpful temporarily. Various preparations may have to be tried.

The following are useful prescriptions for pruritus vulvae:

(1) Menthol   0.30 Gm.
    Phenol   0.60 Gm.
    Rose water ointment   30.00 Gm.
    Directions: Apply locally

(2) Phenol   0.30 Gm.
    Prepared calamine powder   1.30 Gm.
    Zinc oxide   2.00 Gm.
    Rose water ointment   30.00 Gm.
    Directions: Apply locally

In every case of pruritus vulvae, it is essential to obtain a complete history and to make a thorough general and local examination. Regardless of the detection of an apparently local cause for the itching, the urine should always be examined for the presence of sugar. In some patients pruritus vulvae is the symptom that leads to the discovery of diabetes. Even if sugar is found in the urine, the vaginal secretion must be examined because, in a large proportion of diabetic women who have pruritus of the vulva, the cause of the itching is not the glycosuria but a candida infection. Naturally women with diabetes must be treated for their diabetes; the systemic improvement also benefits the local condition.

If the itching of the vulva is due to the presence of candida, trichomonas, gonorrhea, the menopause, senile vaginitis, or kraurosis vulvae, these conditions must be treated along the lines suggested in the special chapters devoted to them.

In obese women a concerted attempt must be made to reduce the weight and to keep the vulva and thighs as clean and dry as possible.

Pediculosis pubis occasionally causes pruritus. Treatment consists of removing the offending parasites, the Phthirus pubis, or crab louse, and the ova. The parasites themselves are usually attached firmly to the hairs, with the head buried in the hair follicle. They produce a toxin which may cause small gray or bluish macules in the pubic area or elsewhere on the skin. The ova or nits are usually attached to the shafts of the hairs.

Gamma benzene hexachloride (Kwell) lotion is very effective for destroying both pediculi and nits. Application on 2 consecutive days with thorough bathing 24 hours after the second application is usually curative.

The treatment of eczema is often difficult. If a cause can be found, it must, of course, be removed if possible. In the acute stage it is best to avoid the use of soap and water for washing the vulva, using olive oil instead. Whenever the parts become moist, they must be dried to prevent chapping. Cotton may be applied to avoid rubbing and chafing. Application of a powder such as zinc stearate is helpful because it prevents maceration and protects the eczematous surfaces from friction and moisture. Cold wet dressings of Burow's solution (1 tablespoonful of aluminum acetate solution to 8 oz. of water) or of a 1:1,000 aqueous solution of silver nitrate are frequently very helpful. In applying silver nitrate solution, rubber gloves should be worn to prevent discoloration of the fingernails. Lotions such as the following may be used:

R	Calamine	8.00 Gm.
	Zinc oxide	15.00 Gm.
	Calcium hydroxide solution	
	Rose water, of each to make	250.00 Gm.
	Directions: Apply locally twice a day	

In the chronic stage of eczema, soothing lotions or ointments should be used, and antiseptic ointment for any associated infection.

When incontinence of urine or a fistula in ano is the cause of pruritus vulvae, it must be corrected surgically. If morphinism is the causative factor, this must be treated. If a constitutional illness is responsible for vulvar itching, an attempt must be made to treat the illness. Chemotherapy or irradiation in Hodgkin's disease or leukemia may be palliative in itching produced by these diseases.

When pruritus occurs in women past the menopause, oral hormone therapy usually gives relief. This may be in the form of diethylstilbestrol or other synthetic preparations or natural estrogens, in the doses used for menopausal symptoms (see p. 235). Additional relief from the pruritus may be obtained from application to the vulva of Premarin or Dienestrol vaginal cream.

Other valuable aids where pruritus is accompanied by inflammatory changes are topical corticosteroids. Creams and lotions containing hydrocortisone and its newer derivatives such as fluocinolone acetonide (Synalar), fluandrenolone (Cordran), triamcinolone acetonide (Kenalog, Aristocort), and betamethasone valerate (Valisone) are widely used. Local injections of corticosteroid suspensions may also give relief.

Kraurosis Vulvae, Leukoplakia Vulvae, and Lichen Sclerosus et Atrophicus of the Vulva

THERE ARE several diseases that present with white vulvar patches. Kraurosis vulvae and lichen sclerosis et atrophicus represent atrophic conditions, whereas vulvar leukoplakia is hypertrophic.

The term *kraurosis*, which means shrinkage, should perhaps be applied only to the vulva that is atrophied or shrunken (Fig. 123). The atrophy and shrinkage are similar to those seen in the vagina of very old women or following radiation therapy to the pelvis for malignancy or to induce the menopause. The general belief is that kraurosis is due to absence of estrogen stimulation of the vulva. In young women kraurosis is probably due to lack of response of the vulva to estrogen, owing to some unknown cause. Areas of kraurosis often become infected.

The chief symptom of kraurosis is itching, which may be intense, especially in the presence of local infection. There may also be a burning sensation and, if there is narrowing of the introitus, dyspareunia or impossibility of coitus.

The histopathologic features of kraurosis vulvae are identical to those of lichen sclerosis et atrophicus, and some investigators feel they represent variants of the same pathologic process.

Lichen sclerosus et atrophicus represents an atrophic process that may closely resemble kraurosis vulvae in its clinical aspects and that is identical histologically. Early lesions consist of whitish papules with hyperkeratosis and follicular plugging, usually beginning on the labia majora and perineal skin. In later stages the lesions become confluent to form symmetrical whitish atrophic patches with a "cigarette-paper" consistency. Frequently there is a "figure-of-eight" configuration with involvement of vulva, perineum, and perianal skin. Accompanying the vulvar lesions, typical lesions of lichen sclerosis et atrophicus may occur elsewhere on the cutaneous surface.

Although basically a benign atrophic process, lichen sclerosis et atrophicus may develop hyperplastic changes characteristic of leukoplakia. In this circumstance, evolution into squamous cell carcinoma is a distinct possibility. A similar hyperplastic change may occur in kraurosis vulvae.

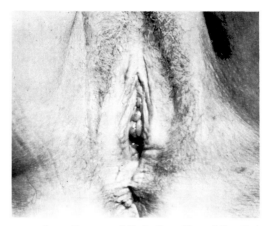

FIG. 123.—Kraurosis vulvae. (Courtesy of R. B. Greenblatt, *Office Endocrinology* [4th ed.; Springfield, Ill.: Charles C Thomas, Publisher, 1952].)

As in the case with the other vulvar dermatoses under consideration, itching is the most prominent feature and may be intractable.

Vulvar leukoplakia (Fig. 124) represents a hyperplastic process. Clinically the lesions present as rough, infiltrated gray-to-white plaques which are usually dry. Frequently involved areas include the clitoris, labia minora, and inner aspects of the labia majora. Itching is usually severe.

FIG. 124.—Leukoplakia vulvae. (Courtesy of Dr. Robert B. Greenblatt.)

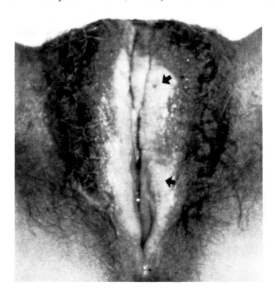

Leukoplakia is a premalignant lesion, and, if untreated, may eventuate in invasive squamous cell carcinoma.

The term leukoplakic vulvitis is frequently used in reference to these vulvar lesions, but it is not a diagnostic entity. Atrophic forms of leukoplakic vulvitis usually include kraurosis vulvae and lichen sclerosis et atrophicus, and hypertrophic forms include hyperplastic changes in these diseases and true leukoplakia.

Treatment

Therapy of these vulvar lesions will depend upon the pathologic changes. Kraurosis vulvae and lichen sclerosis et atrophicus without hyperplastic changes may be treated medically, although hyperplastic changes dictate a surgical approach. Topical preparations containing hydrocortisone or its derivatives, estrogens, and antipruritic agents such as menthol or phenol may relieve the itching and retard the pathologic process. Oral or parenteral estrogen preparations have also been used, although profuse vaginal bleeding may complicate this therapy.

Topical therapy frequently is ineffective, and in these cases many gynecologists perform vulvectomy including a margin of unaffected skin. Unfortunately, in lichen sclerosis et atrophicus the recurrence rate after vulvectomy is very high.

Leukoplakia with its malignant potential is treated surgically, and vulvectomy is the treatment of choice. Representative areas must be examined carefully in the search for invasive changes.

Diagnosis of Uterine Carcinoma by Vaginal, Cervical, and Intra-Uterine Smears

THE PROCEDURE of making vaginal smears introduced by Papanicolaou and Traut should be carried out on all women who come to an office or clinic for a routine periodic examination.

In the course of his studies Papanicolaou discovered that cancer cells can be identified in the human vaginal smear. Not only advanced cancer but the earliest lesions can be detected by vaginal smears. Therefore vaginal smears constitute a reliable means of discovering cancer in earliest forms. However, *smears must be made not only from the vagina, but also from the cervix, and, whenever possible, from inside the uterine cavity.*

All types of carcinoma of the uterus (including the exceedingly early stages of the disease) have a common characteristic, namely, they are exfoliative growths. That is, they are constantly shedding superficially placed cells. These liberated cells float singly or in groups into the secretions of the uterus, cervix, or vagina, mix with normal cells and are present in the vagina.

This exfoliative characteristic makes it possible to observe, in preparations of the vaginal, cervical, and uterine secretions, cells representing all the epithelial tissues, normal or pathologic, which line the uterus or vagina at the time of investigation. In contrast, the curettage and biopsy technics can disclose microscopically only those cells actually reached by instrumentation, which at best is a sampling procedure. Therefore these technics may not be completely thorough and are particularly ineffectual in the early stages of the disease, when the lesion is small. Moreover, preparation of vaginal, cervical, and even intra-uterine smears is so simple that the procedure can be widely applied and as often as necessary, without the restrictions of monetary and time costs imposed by curettage or biopsy.

Two criteria must be fulfilled before the vaginal, cervical, and uterine smear method of diagnosis can be successful or reliable. First, *it is not recommended as a means of ultimate diagnosis.* It should be used as a preliminary or sorting procedure and should be confirmed as a matter of routine by biopsy and tissue diagnosis. Second, evaluation of individual cells or those arranged in small groups is much more difficult and requires a greater knowledge of cytology than for the recognition of cancer in tissue preparations, where orientation of the abnormal cells to one another and to the basement membrane is of great assistance in making a diagnosis. In many respects the use of the vaginal, cervical, and uterine smear preparation for the recognition of malignant cells is analogous to the use of blood smear preparations in the diagnosis of diseases of the blood and blood-forming organs.

Preparation of Vaginal, Cervical, and Intra-Uterine Smears

The method of taking vaginal smears recommended by Papanicolaou and Traut follows:

A slightly curved glass pipet, 15 cm. (6 in.) long and 0.5 cm. in diameter, with a rounded tip and a small opening and equipped with a strong rubber bulb for suction, is used. The patient is placed on an examining table in the lithotomy position. The labia are separated, the rubber bulb is compressed and the glass pipet is introduced into the posterior fornix of the vagina. Pressure on the bulb is then released, and the suction produced serves to aspirate vaginal fluid with its cellular content into the glass tube. During aspiration the tip of the tube is moved from one side of the fornix to the other so that all parts are sampled. The pipet is then withdrawn and the vaginal material is spread on the surface of a clean microscope slide with a sudden expulsive pressure on the bulb. Further spreading with the convex side of the pipet is advisable when fluid is abundant, as when there is considerable bleeding or abundant mucus. Very thick smears are not well penetrated by the fixing fluids and cannot be stained uniformly.

The slides are plunged immediately into a solution of equal parts of 95% alcohol and ether. Drying of the smears should be carefully avoided because it results in loss of the sharp outlines of the cells and in a change in their staining reaction. Fixation does not require more than a few minutes, but smears may be kept in the alcohol-ether solution over a long period. The slides should not be kept in the fixative for more than 2 weeks because the cells slowly lose their normal staining reaction. If ether is not available, plain alcohol (95%) can be used. For shipping slides, a square bottle $1\frac{3}{4} \times 1\frac{3}{4} \times 4\frac{1}{4}$ in. may be used. Such a bottle may hold as many as seven or eight slides. An ordinary paper clip attached to each or every other slide prevents the smears from rubbing against one another. Some cytologists prefer to receive dry smears instead of wet ones.

A few precautions should be observed in obtaining material for the vaginal smear. The vaginal contents should not have been disturbed by any lubricant used for examination or treatment. Douching will, of course, dilute or completely wash away the cellular deposits for several hours, but smears should be made anyway. However, the patient should be told that the smears may have to be repeated and not to worry if this is the case. The same applies to the presence of blood in the vagina and cervix. In fact, bleeding, especially after the menopause, is an absolute indication for the making of smears.

Smears should be made in every pregnant woman at the time of her first visit unless they have been made within 6 months.

The proper staining of the slides and the recognition of cancer as well as the other types of cells require considerable knowledge and experience. Every hospital has among its personnel individuals capable of staining such slides and interpreting them because this procedure can save many lives. Important as the vaginal, cervical, and intra-uterine slides are in the discovery of early cancer of the uterus, in every case in which cancer cells seem to be present, confirmation should be obtained by biopsy and/or curettage.

Ayre advocates cervical scraping, or "surface cell biopsy," because he believes it to be far superior to vaginal smears in the detection of cervical carcinoma. He devised a special spatula by means of which surface cells from intact epithelium of the endocervix are removed (Fig. 125).

Smears may also and easily be made by rotating cotton-tipped applicators on the lateral walls of the vagina, in the posterior vaginal vault, the cervical canal, and, whenever possible, the uterine cavity, using a different applicator for each of these areas. Each applicator after use is *gently* rolled over a glass slide and not roughly smeared on the slide because this procedure will destroy many cells.

An attempt should be made to obtain cells from the endometrium, even though in many cases this is impossible because the cervical canal prevents the passage of any instrument or applicator. Where the cervical canal can be penetrated, an aspirating canula with a syringe attached is introduced into the uterine cavity. The endometrial cavity is aspirated, and the canula is withdrawn. The material that is obtained is blown onto a slide and spread with another slide. Both are immersed in 25% ethyl alcohol or other solution. Some gynecologists prefer to use the brush technic, which simply consists of inserting a very tiny brush inside the endometrial cavity, rotating it, and obtaining the material in this manner.

Table 12 shows a copy of the form used at the Michael Reese Hospital for Papanicolaou smears. The five Papanicolaou classes for cancer diagnosis are in general use but their usage, according to Wied, is discouraged by the Terminology Committees of the International College of Cytology and the American Society of Cytology. Instead, it is recommended that verbal descriptions of the diagnostic cell patterns be used, which represent an improved system of communication between cytopathologist and clinician.

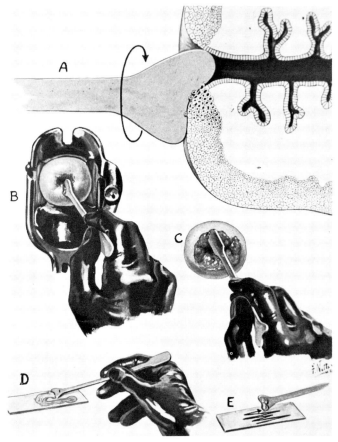

Fig. 125.—"Surface biopsy" cell method. **A,** cervical cell scraping removes surface cells from intact epithelium of ectocervix. **B,** most cervixes show red cervical os, whose marginal cells may be sampled with rotation of cervical spatula. **C,** occasional cervix with large erosion requires scraping with spade end of spatula. **D,** correct way of transferring cervical secretions from wooden spatula to glass slide, with circular motion. **E,** incorrect way of transferring cervical secretion; excessive to-and-fro action may break up organized clusters of cells in sample of secretion. (Courtesy of J. E. Ayre, *Cancer Cytology of the Uterus* [New York: Grune & Stratton, Inc., 1951] and Cyto-Diagnosis in Uterine Cancer, Ciba Clin. Symposia 3:107, 1951.)

The terminology of cells normally exfoliated from the female genital tract was changed in 1958 by the International Academy of Cytology. Essentially the following indices and values are currently used: (1) the Karyopyknotic Index which represents the relation of all mature squamous cells (regardless of cytoplasmic-staining reaction) containing a pyknotic nucleus to mature squamous cells containing a vesicular nucleus; (2) the Eosinophilic Index which

TABLE 12.—Form Used at the Michael Reese Hospital for Papanicolaou Smears

RECORD NUMBER | V | IB | MO | DAY | YR | N U |

☐ PRIVATE OUTPATIENT ☐ EMERGENCY ROOM ☐ MANDEL CLINIC

DIAGNOSIS

DEPT. 605 CODE

TOTAL CHARGE

CERVICAL OR VAGINAL SMEAR

111 ☐ NEW ☐ REPEAT
☐ RUSH

DATE AND TIME RECEIVED

DATE EXAMINED

RESIDENT OR INTERN

REQUISITION PREPARED BY

TECH.

CHART

CLINICAL DATA: GRAV. _____ PARA _____ LMP _____ PREGNANCY ☐ Yes ☐ No

CYTOLOGY NO.

POSTMENOPAUSAL ☐ Yes ☐ No   RADIATION THERAPY ☐ Yes ☐ No

HORMONAL Rx ☐ Yes ☐ No

HYSTERECTOMY ☐ Yes ☐ No TYPE

REMARKS (For lab use only)

OTHER CLINICAL DATA

M. D.

CYTOLOGIC INTERPRETATION

THE CELL PATTERN IS CONSISTENT WITH

☐ CLASS I - ABSENCE OF ATYPICAL CELLS
☐ CLASS II - ATYPICAL CYTOLOGY BUT NO EVIDENCE OF MALIGNANCY
☐ CLASSIFICATION DEFERRED INCONCLUSIVE
☐ CLASS III - CYTOLOGY SUSPICIOUS OF MALIGNANCY
☐ CLASS IV - CYTOLOGY STRONGLY SUGGESTIVE OF MALIGNANCY
☐ CLASS V - CYTOLOGY CONCLUSIVE FOR MALIGNANCY
☐ SPECIMEN NOT ENTIRELY SATISFACTORY
☐ REPEAT EXAM INDICATED ☐ CYTOLOGIC FOLLOW-UP INDICATED

☐ INFLAM PROCESS/REPAIR ☐ ADENOCARCINOMA ☐ MONILIA ENTIFIED
☐ SQUAMOUS METAPLASIA ☐ CARCINOMA (OTHER) ☐ VIRAL INCLUSIONS
☐ DYSPLASIA ☐ POST RADIATION-DYSP. ☐ ATYPICAL CELLS
☐ CARCINOMA IN SITU ☐ RADIATION EFFECT ☐ ENDOMETRIAL CELLS
☐ SQ. CELL CARCINOMA ☐ TRICHIMONAS IDENTIFIED

HORMONAL PATTERN
☐ COMPATIBLE WITH AGE & HISTORY ☐ NO HORMONAL READING POSSIBLE
☐ INCOMPATIBLE WITH AGE & HISTORY

represents the relation of all mature squamous cells with eosinophilic cytoplasm (regardless of nuclear appearance) to mature cells with cyanophilic cytoplasm; (3) the Maturation Index which represents the relation of parabasal to intermediate to superficial cells; (4) the Folded Cell Index which represents the relation of all folded mature squamous cells to flat mature squamous cells; and (5) the Crowded Cell Index which represents the relation of mature squamous cells lying in clusters of four or more cells to clusters of three or less crowded mature cells (this index is cumbersome to assess and is often similar to the Folded Cell Index); (6) the Superficial Cell Index which represents the relation of the superficial cells (mature cells with pyknotic nuclei) to all other squamous cells; (7) the Maturation Value which assigns a certain value to each cell type (superficial, 1.0; intermediate cells, 0.5; parabasal cells, 0.0). Thus, a specimen consisting only of parabasal cells would have a maturation value of zero.

The Schiller Test for Carcinoma of the Cervix

KERMAUNER AND later Rubin and Schiller proved that in carcinoma of the portio of the cervix (approximately 96% of the cancers of the cervix), there is such an early stage that it cannot be recognized with the naked eye. In this early stage there is no invasion of the underlying tissue; the only sign of malignancy is a change within the cells. It is well known that the stratified squamous epithelium of the vagina and the portio contains glycogen, provided it does not become keratinized. Most of the glycogen disappears when the squamous epithelium changes into carcinoma. Therefore the proof of the presence or absence of glycogen may serve to distinguish normal from cancerous cells. Schiller discovered a means of detecting this in the living woman in a harmless way. He found that if an aqueous solution of iodine is poured on the cervix, the normal stratified squamous epithelium of the cervix and vagina assumes a mahogany-brown stain in about 30 seconds, whereas carcinomatous areas remain unstained and therefore are whitish. Thus there is a sharp demarcation between the carcinomatous and the normal epithelium. A non-staining area is called "Schiller positive" and a stained area is "Schiller negative." (There is some glycogen in cancer cells but apparently not enough to take the iodine stain.) The iodine solution that must be used is the Gram solution. Schiller advocated Lugol's solution for his test, but he referred to the Lugol solution used for bacterial staining. This is equivalent to our Gram solution, which consists of:

Iodine	1 part
Potassium iodide	2 parts
Water	300 parts

A stronger solution is unsatisfactory. The regular tincture of iodine is useless; only a watery iodine solution should be used.

PROCEDURE.—A speculum is introduced into the vagina and all mucus and discharge are removed from the cervix and upper part of the vagina. Then 20–30 ml. of Gram's solution is poured on the cervix and upper part of the vagina from a cup or other vessel having a long, sharply pointed tip. The solution is then spread around with a cotton applicator or a cotton pledget.

After half a minute the excess of solution is gently absorbed with a pledget of dry cotton. The cervix and vagina are then examined carefully in good light. If they are mahogany brown all over, there is no carcinoma because all the epithelium contains glycogen. If, however, one or more white unstained areas are observed, there is only a suspicion of carcinoma, because not all white areas signify cancer. There are other conditions, benign ones, in which glycogen disappears from the epithelium. Glycogen is always absent in the presence of carcinoma, but not only in its presence. White areas are observed in the following conditions:

1. Trauma. Occasionally the fingers, a speculum, or other instrument may be responsible for the removal of superficial layers of epithelium that contain glycogen. Inflammation and maceration may cause the disappearance of glycogen-containing epithelium. Such traumatized areas are usually deep and sharply defined.

2. Leukoplakia. The white areas of this condition are believed by some to be forerunners of cancer, but this has not been proved.

3. Keratinization developing in a prolapse. The glycogen disappears from the squamous epithelium in various areas, which may become confluent.

4. Hyperkeratosis of the squamous epithelium of the cervix, such as occurs in syphilis. This, however, is rare.

5. Erosions of the cervix.

6. Some nabothian follicle cysts that are superficially situated in the cervix.

Since all white areas are not carcinoma, the only way to determine whether or not cancer is present is to remove all white areas and have them examined microscopically. Because the carcinoma is limited to the surface cells and there is no invasion of the underlying tissue, all that is necessary is to scrape off the white area with a sharp curet or scalpel or to lift it off with a curet. Most carcinomas of the cervix begin at the junction between the squamous and the columnar epithelium, hence they usually begin at the external os, where they may easily be detected.

The Schiller iodine test is inexpensive and easy to perform. The staining vanishes after a few minutes and there are no ill effects. It can be carried out readily as routine by every physician in his office.

It must be emphasized that this test is to be used only when the cervix appears normal to the naked eye, that is, when the squamous epithelium is intact. When an obvious carcinoma is present, with ulceration and destruction of tissue, not only is this test unnecessary but it will fail to reveal the characteristic white areas. The purpose of the test is to detect the earliest stages of carcinoma of the cervix, and these occur in intact epithelium. Hence the test may be used not only for suspicious cases but for all women. The Gram solution must be replenished frequently because it must be fresh.

Parenthetically it may be added that, whereas it is only necessary to scrape off unstained areas for microscopic study, in every case in which there is a visible ulceration or indurated area that is to be removed for histologic study, it is essential to remove a good-sized piece of tissue containing not only the suspicious area but also a portion of the surrounding healthy tissue.

The Schiller test will not often reveal an early carcinoma. However, even if only one cancer is detected among a few hundred women, detection by the test will probably mean the saving of that one woman's life. As Schiller pointed out, a preinvasive layer of cancer may remain for months or years without invading the underlying tissue. This is contrary to the general opinion that carcinoma grows rapidly from the start.

Invasive Carcinoma of the Uterus

Early Diagnosis

CARCINOMA OF the cervix is the commonest genital cancer. Formerly it was taught that the earliest signs of carcinoma of the uterus were bleeding between the menstrual periods or after the menopause and a watery serous vaginal discharge. It is now known, however, that by the time these signs appear, the cancer most likely has been present for a long time. Our task, therefore, is to detect cancer before abnormal symptoms cause the patient to go to her physician.

Despite the advances in treatment of malignant tumors, the incidence of cure is not as high as it can and should be. This is almost entirely due to the fact that too few women are seen in the early stages of carcinoma. If most cancers of the uterus could be detected in stage 1, the cure rate would be much higher. The best results of all are obtained in patients with stage 0, that is, carcinoma in situ; practically all women with this stage can be cured with proper therapy. Therefore one of our chief problems is to try to diagnose cancer early. This means, first, that all women must be examined at least twice a year, whether or not they have abnormal symptoms, and, second, that physicians must possess the necessary knowledge to detect early carcinoma. Both married teen-agers and single ones should be urged to have yearly pelvic examinations.

Since most patients go to their family physician for nearly all their ailments, general practitioners should familiarize themselves with methods of searching for and identifying cancer in its incipiency.

A speculum must be used every time a bimanual examination is made. Furthermore, the cervix should be carefully scrutinized, not given just a hasty glance. Most important is the removal and histologic study of every area that is friable, nodular, or in any way suspicious. The next best way, and one which is definitely simpler, is to make smears of the vaginal and cervical secretions, as mentioned in Chapter 36. The slides should be sent to a cytologist qualified to interpret them. The vaginal, cervical, and intra-uterine slide procedure must be part of a routine check-up once a year.

At the time of the periodic check-up, not only the pelvic organs but also the breasts should be examined (see Chapter 4).

Prophylaxis

In recent years great doubt has been cast on the theory that carcinoma of the cervix is an irritation carcinoma. Schiller and others have shown that in carcinoma of the cervix the inflammatory reaction is found only around the carcinoma. Hence the inflammatory change is a reaction against the carcinoma and is secondary to the malignancy, not a forerunner of it. Some authorities believe that carcinoma of the cervix is spontaneous. In other words, heredity and constitution play the dominant roles, whereas local irritation plays a secondary part.

In order for carcinoma to arise there must almost certainly be not only a predisposing constitutional factor but a local factor which is not definitely known. Therefore it is essential that the cervix be maintained in as normal a condition as possible. This means that during labor, trauma to the cervix should be avoided, all lacerations should be repaired promptly and properly, and all women, especially those who have had a number of children, should have periodic visual as well as tactile examinations of the cervix. Smear tests should be carried out in all women. Abnormal conditions of the cervix, particularly vascular and granular areas, should be treated with electric cautery, or conization in order to perhaps avoid carcinoma.

Detection of Early Invasive Carcinoma of Cervix

The large proportion of all uterine cancers occurs in the portio, or that portion of the cervix that protrudes into the vagina and is covered externally by stratified squamous epithelium. The area chiefly involved in carcinoma is the external os, the junction between the squamous epithelium and the intracervical columnar epithelium. To detect early invasive carcinoma, it is important to inspect the cervix carefully. To accomplish this properly, the physician must have adequate exposure and proper illumination, and he must carefully study the cervix. It is impossible with the naked eye to recognize preinvasive carcinoma, the type for which vaginal smears, the Schiller test, and the colposcope were devised. Also the cervix must be carefully palpated, especially for unusual hardness or nodules.

The thirteenth volume of the *Annual Report on the Results of the Treatment of Carcinoma of the Uterus and the Vagina*, published under the patronage of the International Federation of Gynecology and Obstetrics, presents the definitions for the different clinical stages of carcinoma of the cervix, corpus, and vagina as follows:

CERVIX

PREINVASIVE CARCINOMA OF THE CERVIX

Stage 0: Carcinoma in situ, intraepithelial carcinoma. Cases of Stage 0 should not be included in any therapeutic statistics.

INVASIVE CARCINOMA OF THE CERVIX

Stage I: Carcinoma strictly confined to the cervix (extension to the corpus should be disregarded).

Stage IA: Cases of early stromal invasion (preclinical carcinoma).

Stage IB: All other cases of Stage I.

Stage II: The carcinoma extends beyond the cervix but has not extended onto the pelvic wall. The carcinoma involves the vagina, but not the lower third.

Subgrouping of Stage II cases into IIA (no parametrial involvement) and IIB (parametrial involvement) is recommended.

Stage III: The carcinoma has extended onto the pelvic wall. On rectal examination, there is no cancer-free space between the tumor and the pelvic wall. The tumor involves the lower third of the vagina.

Stage IV: The carcinoma has extended beyond the true pelvis or has involved the mucosa of the bladder or rectum.

A bullous edema as such does not permit allotment of a case to Stage IV.

Notes to the Staging

A case should be allotted to stage IA only following microscopic diagnosis of the earliest stromal invasion performed before planned treatment. Stage IA represents that group of cases of carcinoma of the cervix which can only be diagnosed microscopically following biopsy. They have often formerly been called microcarcinoma. In the remainder of Stage I cases, a clinical diagnosis will be possible.

A patient with a growth fixed to the pelvic wall by a short and indurated, *but not nodular*, parametrium should be allotted to Stage II. It is impossible at clinical examination to decide whether a smooth and indurated parametrium is truly cancerous or only inflammatory. Therefore, the case should be placed in Stage III only if the parametrium is nodular out on the pelvic wall or the growth itself extends out on the pelvic wall.

The presence of a bullous edema or a growth bulging into the bladder or the rectum does not permit consignment of a case to Stage IV unless the invasion of the bladder is proved by biopsy. Ridges and furrows into the bladder wall should be interpreted as signs of involvement only if they remain fixed to the growth at examination, thus bearing out that the carcinoma has invaded the submucosa of the bladder.

CORPUS

Stage 0: Histologic findings suspected of malignancy but not proved.

Stage I: The carcinoma is confined to the corpus.

Stage II: The carcinoma has involved the corpus and the cervix.

Stage III: The carcinoma has extended outside the uterus but not outside the true pelvis.

Stage IV: The carcinoma has extended outside the true pelvis or has obviously involved the mucosa of the bladder or rectum.

NOTE: In rare cases, it may be difficult to decide whether the cancer actually is a carcinoma of the endocervix or a carcinoma of the corpus and endocervix. If a clear decision cannot be made at the fractional curettage, an adenocarcinoma should be allotted to carcinoma of the corpus and an epidermal carcinoma to carcinoma of the cervix.

Notes to the Staging

The presence of a bullous edema or a growth bulging into the bladder or the rectum does not permit consignment of a case to Stage IV unless the invasion of the bladder is proved by biopsy. Ridges and furrows into the bladder wall should be interpreted as signs of involvement only if they remain fixed to the growth at examination, thus bearing out that the carcinoma has invaded the submucosa of the bladder.

VAGINA
PREINVASIVE CARCINOMA OF THE VAGINA

Stage O: Carcinoma in situ, intraepithelial carcinoma.

INVASIVE CARCINOMA OF THE VAGINA

Stage I: The carcinoma is limited to the vaginal wall.

Stage II: The carcinoma has involved the subvaginal tissue but has not extended onto the pelvic wall.

Stage III: The carcinoma has extended onto the pelvic wall.

Stage IV: The carcinoma has extended beyond the true pelvis or has involved the mucosa of the bladder or rectum.

A bullous edema as such does not permit allotment of a case to Stage IV.

Notes to the Staging

The presence of a bullous edema or a growth bulging into the bladder or the rectum does not permit consignment of a case to Stage IV unless the invasion of the bladder is proved by biopsy. Ridges and furrows into the bladder wall should be interpreted as signs of involvement only if they remain fixed to the growth at examination, thus bearing out that the carcinoma has invaded the submucosa of the bladder.

Clinically detectable early cancer of the portio should not be overlooked because, if it is, this may mean a death warrant for the patient. Characteristically, an early carcinoma of the cervix is a small, red, irregular, elevated (ulceration occurs later), circumscribed growth usually situated somewhere at the external os. When touched with an instrument or cotton applicator, the area bleeds readily. Induration may be present or absent. Whenever such a lesion is observed, it should be considered cancer until proved otherwise. No time should be lost in obtaining tissue for biopsy (not "by" biopsy) (Fig. 126). This may be done in the office. There are special punch instruments devised for securing a good-sized piece of tissue for diagnosis, although actually no special instrument is necessary. To steady the cervix, a tenaculum is applied to a healthy part of the cervix and not to the area under suspicion. A piece of tissue is excised that includes not only the entire area under suspicion but also at least $\frac{1}{8}$ in. of healthy tissue all around it. The piece should be at least $\frac{1}{8}$ in. deep if cut at right angles or at least $\frac{1}{4}$ in. deep if cut wedge shaped.

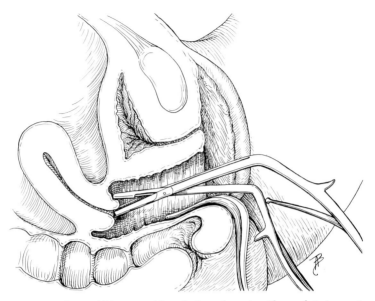

FIG. 126.—Cervical biopsy: excision of piece of cervix with punch instrument.

The tissue should be placed immediately in formalin or other fixing solution. Bleeding may be checked by cauterization or a small hemostatic pack. If more than one area is suspected or the area under consideration is widespread, a cone-shaped enucleation of the cervix should be performed. This operation is known as *conization.*

Conization is a more certain method of obtaining tissue for the diagnosis of carcinoma in situ or invasive cancer than is multiple biopsy. Biopsy can satisfactorily be done in a physician's office, but conization should preferably be an outpatient or in-patient hospital procedure.

The cervix is painted with Lugol's solution to detect any white areas (Schiller's test). The anterior lip is grasped high up with a single tenaculum. A sharp Bard-Parker knife may be used to remove the cone, but an instrument devised for this purpose, such as the Fleming, may be better (Fig. 127). Any white areas appearing after Lugol's solution is applied should be included in the cone. If there is much bleeding, a suture is placed at the upper part of the cervix on each side to ligate the descending branches of the uterine arteries. Mild oozing may be controlled with a hemostatic substance, or a high-frequency current may be applied. In most cases dilatation and curettage is advisable, but this should be done *after* conization because dilatation dislodges epithelium that is essential for a proper diagnosis.

A conization may be done during pregnancy but only if there is a high

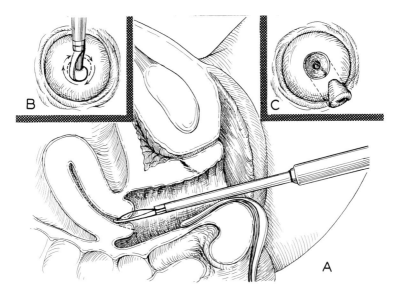

FIG. 127.—Excision of entire area of external os by conization apparatus for biopsy. **A,** proper position of apparatus. **B,** front view showing manner of excising tissue around external os. **C,** excised piece for biopsy freed from cervix. (From Greenhill, J. P.: *Surgical Gynecology* [4th ed.; Chicago: Year Book Medical Publishers, Inc., 1969].)

degree of suspicion of carcinoma. Otherwise it is wise to wait until after delivery to perform the conization. There are few complications from conization during gestation. Furthermore, following the procedure, the women can deliver living babies vaginally. The oozing area should be packed with Oxycel or Gelfoam or sutures used.

The lesion that is most often diagnosed as carcinoma of the portio is an erosion. Such a vermilion area at the external os often bleeds readily when touched, especially if it is inflamed. However, erosions are usually smooth, flat, and not indurated. They are often present in both anterior and posterior lips of the cervix or all around it, whereas early cancer is usually limited to a small area. Cancer is normally elevated and hence changes the shape of the cervix, whereas erosions do not alter its contour. When touched with an instrument, an erosion is elastic, whereas a carcinomatous area is non-yielding. Despite all these definite differences between cancer and an erosion, it is often impossible to distinguish between the conditions. A biopsy is necessary for a correct diagnosis.

The foregoing remarks deal with cancer of the portio, which may be visible to the naked eye. There are, however, some carcinomas that occur in the cervical canal and arise in the columnar epithelium. These are adenocarcinomas, in contrast to the squamous cell carcinomas of the portio. In rare cases adenocarcinoma also occurs on the portio. Carcinoma of the cervical canal cannot be detected by visual examination unless there is an extension downward onto the vaginal part of the cervix. In all other instances the diagnosis may be suspected from a bloody discharge between the menses, during coitus, or after the menopause. Frequently pyometra (pus in the uterine cavity) results from cancer inside the cervical canal because of obstruction by the cancer. The only certain way to make a diagnosis of intracervical cancer is to perform a curettage, although vaginal and cervical smears are definitely helpful and almost as reliable (see Chapter 36). Whenever a diagnostic curettage is done, both the endometrium and the endocervix must be curetted thoroughly and separately. The endocervix should be curetted first with a tiny curet and the scrapings placed in a bottle for study. The tissue obtained from curetting the uterine cavity should be placed in another bottle.

Cancer of the Body of the Uterus

Carcinoma of the body of the uterus is usually found in women who are older than those afflicted with cervical carcinoma; it is less often fatal than cervical cancer. Carcinoma of the body of the uterus occurs often in women who have never had any children, whereas most women with cervical cancer have given birth to children, many of them to large numbers of children. However, despite a common belief, many nulliparous women have cancer of the cervix. A large proportion of women with carcinoma of the body of the uterus are obese, diabetic, or hypertensive.

Carcinoma of the body of the uterus may be suspected by the presence of a watery, serous discharge and irregular bleeding. If a sound is passed into the uterine cavity, bleeding will follow because the cancerous tissue is friable (Chrobak-Clarke test). In all such patients, vaginal, cervical, and intra-uterine smears should be made and a curettage performed. In all women in whom bleeding occurs between the menstrual periods and certainly in every patient in whom uterine bleeding begins again after it has ceased at the change of life, a curettage must be performed without delay. This must be as thorough as possible because the cancerous area may be very small. Nearly always such a curettage should be performed in a hospital and not in the physician's office. In advanced cases of cancer of the body of the uterus, there is danger of perforating the uterus because of invasion of the uterine muscle by the cancer, and therefore great care must be exercised in curetting such a uterus.

In all cases of postmenopausal bleeding, the patient should be asked if she has been taking estrogens orally or hypodermically for menopausal or other symptoms. Estrogens taken injudiciously are a common cause of bleeding after the menopause.

Premarital Examination and Advice

This chapter is intended for the assistance of the ever-decreasing number of virgins.

Every physician knows of the consequences that can result from not educating children about sex matters. Much marital unhappiness and ailing among women stems from total ignorance concerning the human organs of reproduction and the mechanics, art, and psychology of sexual intercourse among human beings. Additional factors are repeated admonitions of parents to their young daughters to repress all sexual impulses and to look askance at all men who attempt to demonstrate their affection by petting.

Many states now have laws that require that shortly before marriage both partners present evidence of the absence of venereal disease. This is highly commendable. In addition, prospective brides and bridegrooms should be given instruction, not only in contraception, but also in the psychology and technic of sexual intercourse. This applies just as much to the groom as to the bride because, even though the young man has had sexual experiences for many years, he must be made aware of the fact that physical relationship with his virgin bride (if she is one) requires an entirely different technic from that which he employed with females who helped him satisfy his desires for one reason or another but seldom for love.

The ideal arrangement is for every prospective bride and groom to interview a physician, preferably the family physician whom they know well. First the girl should be seen and then the young man, and, if necessary, both together after the individual interviews. Mass instruction such as is given in some colleges is excellent, but for the practical preparation for marriage just before the latter is to take place, nothing can compare with a direct person-to-person conference in private.

Such a conference should consist of three parts, a physical examination, instruction in the art of sexual intercourse, and advice about the prevention of conception. This meeting between physician and young couples should take place at least 2 weeks before the wedding. The talk should be as informal as possible, and the physician should not write down any part of the history in the presence of the bride-to-be. He should inquire first about the girl's general health and then about her past history, especially concerning the onset of the menses and any difficulties connected with menstruation. Then he should try to find out whether the girl has any fears concerning marriage, the sex act, or childbearing. He must constantly attempt to allay any fear the girl has concerning these matters by giving rational explanations. During the conversation the physician usually obtains a good idea of whether or not the girl was brought up as a prude to repress all matters pertaining to sex or whether her parents educated her in an enlightened manner. This information will usually lead in a natural manner to a discussion of the anatomy and the physiology of the genitals. For instruction along these lines, it is necessary to produce illustrations or, better still, a model of the external and internal pelvic organs, such as is used for demonstrating the insertion of a contraceptive vaginal diaphragm. All the organs are pointed out and the function of each one is described in simple language. Then a physical examination should be made.

Physical Examination

In nearly all cases it is wise to make as complete an examination as possible, because in most instances the girl has not had a medical examination for many years. Rarely will any abnormality be found, but the patient will feel much better to learn that she is in perfect health. More important, however, is the fact that after the patient's thyroid, heart, lungs, and abdomen are examined, she will not feel as ill at ease when the genitals are examined as if the genital organs alone were examined. The breasts and nipples must also be examined; it will be a source of satisfaction to most girls to be told that they will be able to nurse their babies if they so desire.

Before examining a virgin rectally or vaginally it is best to tell her that the examination which is to be made will not hurt although it may be a trifle uncomfortable. The physician should emphasize that such an examination is necessary to be certain that all the pelvic organs are normal and to make sure that there is no physical barrier to normal sex relationships or childbearing. In most cases the bimanual examination should consist of a rectoabdominal examination and not a vaginoabdominal exploration. With a finger in the rectum it is nearly always possible to feel the cervix and the body of the uterus. Generally in virgins the uterus is small but this has no significance unless it is extremely tiny. Regardless of the size of the uterus, if the patient's menstrual history is normal, the physician need not worry about an "infantile uterus," nor should he say anything about this to the patient. Likewise no emphasis should be placed on a retroflexed uterus, because in most instances this will do no harm. If the adnexa cannot be felt on rectoabdominal examination, it is almost certain that they are normal.

In nearly all cases, before the rectal exploration, the external genitals should be inspected. Underdeveloped labia may sometimes indicate hypoplasia of the internal genitals. The clitoris should be inspected to be sure that it is not covered over completely by folds of skin or irritated by excessive secretions. The labia minora should be separated to expose the hymen and its orifice. If one finger can be inserted through the hymenal ring into the vagina, a vaginoabdominal examination should be made, but the patient should be told that the hymen is not being disrupted by this procedure.

A large number of girls use tampax or other vaginal tampons during menstruation, and, in these girls, there is rarely any trouble in inserting one finger for the examination.

Of course, a digital examination through the hymenal ring will immediately disclose whether or not the vagina or the uterus or both are absent. If the girl is not a virgin, a bimanual vaginoabdominal examination should always be done. Evidence of gonorrhea should be sought. Every prospective bride and groom must have a blood Wassermann or Kahn test.

Sexual Intercourse

A large number of prospective brides come to the office not only to discuss contraception but to seek information concerning the sex relationship. About one third of all married women experience no pleasure in the sex act. Furthermore, to a certain number of women, sexual intercourse is distinctly repulsive. In most of these instances the cause of this goes back to childhood, adolescence, or early maturity and may be due to improper education on sex matters, repulsion from having heard obscene language, unhappy love affairs, attempts at rape or having heard about rape, or some distinct psychopathologic aberration. In exceptional cases a girl may be so blasé and speak so freely about sex matters that she is cold because for her there is no glamor in the opposite sex. Some frigid women can be helped to overcome this condition. (See Chapter 14.)

One of the most critical periods in a woman's life is the time of the first sex act. Nearly all girls learn by hearsay that it is painful to have intercourse the first time. Because of this, nearly every virgin bride fears the first night after marriage. The physician can do a great deal to dispel this fear, first by explaining that the pain is usually not as great as the girl believes, but much more important is the fact that something can be done before the first act of coitus to stretch or gently enlarge the hymenal orifice so that there will be practically no pain. One simple way of stretching the hymenal opening is to teach the girl how to insert a lubricated (with soap or petrolatum), warmed douche tip or centrifuge tube into the vagina. The girl should practice inserting the douche tip or centrifuge tube a few times every night for 2 weeks before marriage. This will usually remove the sharp edge of the hymenal ring and at the same time stretch the ring. This manipulation will also accustom the vagina and levator ani muscles to a foreign body in the vagina, and this will eliminate the shock experienced by the first insertion of the penis. In some cases the girl should be given three plastic tubes, one $\frac{1}{2}$ in. in diameter, one $\frac{3}{4}$ in. in diameter and the third 1 in. in diameter. These are to be used successively to enlarge the hymenal orifice.

If one finger can be inserted in the hymen and the patient is not overly sensitive, the physician can gently but forcibly stretch the hymenal ring. He should use ample lubrication for this purpose, even more than for the ordinary vagino- or rectoabdominal examination. If, however, the physician finds that efforts not only to stretch the hymen cause pain but even the attempt to insert one finger, he should not try to make a vaginal examination. If the hymenal ring is very thick and tense, and especially if it is close to the external urethral orifice, the physician should recommend that the hymen be dilated under intravenous anesthesia. This should be done about 10–14 days before marriage to permit the introitus to heal before coitus is begun. Such a procedure is distinctly to be advised when the hymen is thick, the ring tight, and the opening too near the external urethral orifice. Frequently in such cases, if the hymen is not stretched or cut, the husband irritates the urinary meatus to such an extent that the trauma of repeated attempts to force an opening leads to urethritis and cystitis. This condition has been called "honeymoon cystitis" but in reality it is "defloration cystitis." Young brides in whom this condition develops have a most distressing honeymoon and are miserable for many weeks or months afterward. But worse than this is the fact that they have a horror of sexual intercourse even after the cystitis has cleared up, and because of this they cannot help becoming un-co-operative and sometimes frigid.

Before stretching a hymen, whether with or without an anesthetic, the physician must be certain to obtain the consent not only of the bride but also of the groom. In nearly all instances the young man will be grateful for the removal of a barrier which would present difficulties to him and pain to his bride. However, an occasional man wants to convince himself that his bride is a virgin; therefore the physician should be sure to consult the groom in every instance in which he contemplates stretching the hymenal ring.

It is not always possible to judge the distensibility of a hymen by its appearance; hence a finger should be used. Occasionally in a virgin a hymen is so soft and distensible that two fingers can be inserted readily into the vagina without producing any tear or any real discomfort. In most of these cases the hymen was ruptured by digital exploration and friction during petting or by the use of vaginal plugs during menstruation. Such girls have a marital outlet without having had sexual intercourse. Likewise, in some instances a hymen is ruptured during masturbation. Hence a physician should not conclude that a girl is not a virgin because the hymenal orifice is wide. On the other hand, some girls who have had intercourse have a hymen that looks intact; this is rare.

If a hymen is stretched forcibly but smoothly and without sudden jerks, there is usually only slight bleeding. This can be controlled by placing a piece of cotton covered with petrolatum in the introitus. The patient may go home with this cotton plug in the introitus and remove it after a few hours. If a general anesthetic is to be given, the manipulation should be carried out in the morning but the patient should be told not to have any breakfast or water that morning, before the stretching is to be done.

In practically every case in which the hymenal ring must be increased in size, it can be done by stretching with the fingers. I have never had to make any incisions for this.

After the physical barrier of pain, the hymenal ring, has been removed, a great deal will already have been accomplished in the discussion of the psychology and technic of coitus. The patient can then be told that, since there will be no pain at the first coital act, she should have no fears about co-operating to the fullest extent with her husband. Likewise, if the physician feels that the patient has repressions or fears of other kinds, he should patiently try to dispel them. Fortunately most girls nowadays do not have the false modesty that formerly often produced a shock at the time a bride first exposed herself to her husband or observed him without clothes. A large proportion of girls have seen many naked males and therefore are not at all shocked.

The fear of pregnancy can be allayed by discussing contraception. For girls whose religious tenets forbid the use of mechanical appliances, the Ogino-Knaus or rhythm method of preventing conception should be explained in detail (see Chapter 26). For others, instruction should be given concerning the use of oral contraceptives (Chapter 25) or a mechanical device (Chapter 27).

In the discussion with the prospective bride, it should be emphasized that the female can and should derive as much pleasure from coitus as the male. It usually requires time for girls to learn to enjoy the sex act, even if there is no pain connected with it. Furthermore, in most instances the female must love or at least have some affection for her partner in order to obtain the full pleasure. This is contrary to conditions in the male, because a male can have an orgasm with complete satisfaction from the very beginning of his sex career and regardless of whether or not he has any deep feeling for his partner. If this were not true, prostitution would not exist.

Since a large proportion of young girls masturbate just as do nearly all boys in their early teens, this subject should be discussed. If the girl has any fear concerning previous masturbation, she should be convinced that no harm has resulted from the habit. On the contrary, it may be a good sign because it may indicate that she will be capable of stimulation and response to her husband's caresses. If the girl admits that she still practices masturbation, the physician should find out the type indulged in. This information will be helpful to the physician because in his conversation with the young man he can tell him to be sure to stimulate the parts that produce the pleasurable sensation in his bride. Of course, the physician should not tell the young man that his bride practices autoeroticism or that she admitted that certain specific zones are erotic. The physician should simply tell the man that, because of his bride's anatomic structure, he should be sure to stimulate certain areas during the preparatory acts or at the climax or at both times. When a couple is engaged for a long time, the young man usually finds the areas that arouse his fiancée if she is capable of such stimulation, or, most likely, the couple has had sexual intercourse often before marriage.

Some girls are stimulated by other women before marriage and have certain fears concerning the effects of this. However, they also may be assured that the experience has done them no harm and that their husband can give them complete satisfaction.

The young woman should be told that sex matters ought to be discussed with her husband as frankly as are other matters. However, the usual place for such discussions is in the privacy of the bed at the proper time. If the husband arouses his wife insufficiently or not at all and especially if she knows of definite erotogenic areas, she should not hesitate to tell her husband about them or even guide his fingers or phallus to these parts. If certain types of stimulation are much more effective than others, the husband should be informed of this. In most women, the vagina but, in others, the clitoris is the most erotogenic area; hence these organs should be manipulated.

If there are times in each month when the woman's sex desire is definitely increased, this fact should also be made known to the husband so that these periods will not be permitted to go by without sex gratification.

A woman should not feel ashamed to admit that digital stimulation arouses her or even by itself can lead to an orgasm. Likewise, if she does not experience complete gratification, or any at all, by performing the coital act in the usual position, there is nothing disgraceful or abnormal about trying out other positions, such as lying on the side, entry from the rear with the woman in a modified knee-chest position, the female on top of the male, or some other position. Only by being frank with each other can a technic be developed that will give both husband and wife complete satisfaction at the same time. Fatigue usually prevents full enjoyment of sexual intercourse.

Another thing to tell a girl is that in some cases the greatest sex urge occurs during the menstrual flow and that there is no harm in indulging in coitus during the menses. To reduce or eliminate the messiness associated with menstruation, a warm douche may safely be taken before the act.

Before closing the conference with the bride, the physician should inform her that in his discussion with the groom he will repeat most of the advice he has given her, especially that which pertains to the use of the fingers when necessary, the change in posture in certain cases, the periodicity of desire in women (including its possible occurrence during the menses), and so on. Of course, the physician should specifically state that he will not divulge any secrets of the past, fears, or inhibitions.

Conference with the Groom

The approach to men is entirely different from the manner in which women are given instructions. First, a general brief history is obtained, particularly with reference to mumps in childhood and to venereal infections. Since men may also have fears and inhibitions, these should be ferreted out. Some men fear the effects of the masturbation they practiced in adolescence, but in a few words the physician can readily remove these apprehensions.

Since nearly all men have had sex experiences before they marry, instruction in the technic of coitus will not have to be as complete as it is with most women. However, the physician must point out both the psychologic and the physical differences between the former consorts of the groom and the girl he is going to marry. Many men think that they know all about sexual intercourse because of their years of experience and do not hesitate to inform the physician of this. However, nearly all of them can be told a few things that will be of help to them in their sex life with the girl they are to marry.

Some men have a fear that they have indulged in sex practices too much and therefore that they may not make good husbands. Generally this fear may also be dispelled easily. On the other hand, a rare young man has never had sexual intercourse and is afraid or ashamed that he will not know how to act. Such a young man should be given encouragement and taught the anatomy of both the male and the female. He will almost certainly have to use a finger for guidance or require aid from his wife, but he should be told that there is absolutely no disgrace in this because in some cases, even after years of marriage, such practices are carried out.

One of the most important facts to point out to a man is the difference in time required for satisfaction of the male and the female. He should specifically be told that nearly all women require a much longer period of stimulation and arousal before they reach an orgasm than do men. In fact, many men require practically no stimulation, but have an orgasm soon after insertion of the penis. Of course, there are many abnormal cases of very quick emission or premature ejaculation when the man cannot maintain an erection very long. Such men must try to train themselves to spend a great deal of time arousing their wives. They should not insert the phallus into the vagina until the wife is actually ready for the orgasm. With patience and will power, most men can do this. If they do not school themselves to do this, their wives will not be satisfied, and a bad train of events may follow. Quick emission is a frequent cause of marital maladjustment. In some cases it is responsible for frigidity in women, leukorrheal discharges, and other disagreeable signs and symptoms.

In a few married women there is a persistent discharge that results from incomplete sexual intercourse. By incomplete intercourse I mean stimulation over a short or long period of time in the sex act but absence of an orgasm. In nearly all instances, it is the fault of the husband. He either cannot or will not, or does not know how to, hold back his orgasm until his wife is ready for hers. The result is that whereas the husband is satisfied, the wife's tension is not properly released and a vaginal discharge often results. Sometimes such a vaginal discharge occurs in a woman whose husband practices coitus interruptus, or withdrawal. A similar vaginal discharge is frequently observed in girls who are engaged for a long time or who pet frequently and are thereby aroused but do not have intercourse. The remedy in the case of married women is education of the husband and in the case of unmarried girls, less ardent love-making or, preferably, coitus or marriage.

If a woman complains of pain during coitus, she will sooner or later demonstrate that she is not interested in having intercourse or that she actually dislikes it. The husband should try to remedy this condition by being most considerate during the coital act, but, if he cannot relieve the condition, the wife should consult a physician. This is better than abstaining entirely from sex relations. Otherwise, the woman will nearly always become frigid, and, if a long time is permitted to elapse, the condition may become permanent.

When a man attempts to stimulate his wife, he should realize that there are three points to bear in mind. First, the wife's mind must be aroused. This can be done by verbal expressions of love in addition to fondling of various parts of the body. Second, there are certain extragenital erotogenic areas that require stimulation, chief of these being the mouth, the breasts, and the nipples. These can be stimulated by kissing and gentle caressing. The third and most important area requires stimulation after the other parts have been aroused. This area includes the clitoris and the vagina. The latter should not be fondled until the mind has been prepared and the other erotogenic areas stimulated. Later in married life, short cuts may be taken, but not at the beginning. A great aid to increasing the satisfaction of sexual intercourse is for the male not to remove his penis immediately from the vagina but to leave it in for a few minutes after the orgasm.

Index